MIGRANT HEALTH

A PRIMARY CARE PERSPECTIVE

WONCA FAMILY MEDICINE
ABOUT THE SERIES

The WONCA Family Medicine series is a collection of books written by world-wide experts and practitioners of family medicine, in collaboration with *The World Organization of Family Doctors* (WONCA).

WONCA is a not-for-profit organization and was founded in 1972 by member organizations in 18 countries. It now has 118 Member Organizations in 131 countries and territories with membership of about 500,000 family doctors and more than 90% of the world's population.

Migrant Health
A Primary Care Perspective
Bernadette N. Kumar and Esperanza Diaz

Family Practice in the Eastern Mediterranean Region
Universal Health Coverage and Quality Primary Care
Hassan Salah and Michael Kidd

Primary Health Care Around the World
Recommendations for International Policy and Development
Chris van Weel and Amanda Howe

How To Do Primary Care Research
Felicity Goodyear-Smith and Bob Mash

Every Doctor
Healthier Doctors = Healthier Patients
Leanne Rowe and Michael Kidd

Family Medicine
The Classic Papers
Michael Kidd, Iona Heath, and Amanda Howe

International Perspectives on Primary Care Research
Felicity Goodyear-Smith and Bob Mash

The Contribution of Family Medicine to Improving Health Systems
A Guidebook from the World Organization of Family Doctors
Michael Kidd

For more information about this series please visit: https://www.crcpress.com/ WONCA-Family-Medicine/book-series/WONCA

MIGRANT HEALTH
A PRIMARY CARE PERSPECTIVE

EDITED BY

Bernadette N. Kumar

Previously Director of the Norwegian Center for Minority Health Research (NAKMI),
Now Unit for Migration and Health, Norwegian Institute of Public Health
and
Professor at the Empower School of Health, India

Esperanza Diaz

Associate Professor at the Institute for Global Public Health and
Primary Care, University of Bergen, Norway
and
Senior Researcher at the Unit for Migration and Health,
Norwegian Institute of Public Health

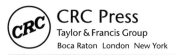

CRC Press
Taylor & Francis Group
Boca Raton London New York

CRC Press is an imprint of the
Taylor & Francis Group, an **informa** business

CRC Press
Taylor & Francis Group
6000 Broken Sound Parkway NW, Suite 300
Boca Raton, FL 33487-2742

© 2019 by Taylor & Francis Group, LLC
CRC Press is an imprint of Taylor & Francis Group, an Informa business

No claim to original U.S. Government works

Printed on acid-free paper

International Standard Book Number-13: 978-1-138-49805-1 (Hardback)
978-1-138-49804-4 (Paperback)

**Visit the Taylor & Francis Web site at
http://www.taylorandfrancis.com**

**and the CRC Press Web site at
http://www.crcpress.com**

To learning and to all patients, who teach us to be better doctors

and to

Prof. Prakash S. Shetty – teacher, guide and friend

Contents

Foreword

Western civilization will either be open for all to enter, or demolished by those excluded.

James Baldwin

It is a human property to always strive to improve quality of life, even when it implies migration to destinations far afield, when prospects for a better life are preferable to enduring troubles and suffering at home. This is in fact the driving force by which the human race has populated the earth since our origin.

The Western world is facing a surge of migration right now, as large numbers of people are leaving their home countries, fleeing from war, famine, and persecution, or just hoping to advance their economic and professional prospects. Europe is seeing the largest number of migrants since World War II.

The migrants have often endured hardships in their countries of origin. They have experienced strenuous, often hazardous journeys en route to their countries of destination, exposing them to a multitude of different health problems. On arrival they often face formidable hurdles during the vetting process, whether they apply for asylum or present other reasons for seeking residence permits. The great majority of migrants are just looking for ways and means to improve their living standard, and end up filling different niches in the local labour markets, often in low-paying jobs considered unattractive to the locals. A great number are declined residence permits and expelled immediately or are allowed to stay until conditions in their country of origin are considered safe enough for return. Many of these migrants refuse to leave and end up in increasing numbers as illegal migrants deprived of the rights of ordinary citizens. No matter the category — asylum seeker, refugee, economic migrant, expatriate, or illegal migrant — they all find themselves in a special and vulnerable situation, not least health-wise.

Even though the economy in Western countries with ageing populations depends on the influx of a great number of mainly young migrants, more often than not the newcomers are met with scepticism and rejection rather than with acceptance and understanding upon arrival on our shores. Their arrival in such great numbers has given rise to growing protectionism and right-wing populist forces accusing migrants of disrupting our culture and threatening our national identities. Bigotry and prejudice flourish, adding to the burden of suffering for the newcomers.

António Guterres, the UN Secretary General, calls on all UN member states to adopt a humane approach to migrants, encouraging world leaders to take responsibility for ending the stigma surrounding migration and dispel alarmist misinterpretation of its effects. A report entitled 'Making Migration Work for All' came ahead of negotiations on a global compact of migration adopted by the UN General Assembly in 2018.

Health services must beware of and prepare for meeting the special needs of migrants, and offer accessible, equitable, and affordable high-quality services both on their arrival and, not to forget, over time. For the ones granted permanent residence permits with the intention to stay, it will take more than a generation to familiarize themselves with their new and unfamiliar environment and to become fully integrated citizens.

This book offers guidance to health practitioners on how best to meet and treat the health needs of migrants, our fellow men, no matter what stage in the often-troubled migration process they may find themselves in.

Anna Stavdal
WONCA World President-Elect
Oslo, Norway

Preface

FROM THE EDITORS' DESK

Diversity is one of the hallmarks of twenty-first century societies. As diversity and super diversity trends tend to dominate the world over, the idea of mono-cultural or homogenous populations might well become outdated. Among the drivers of diversity, migration has in recent years undoubtedly gained attention. Migration is not a new phenomenon; however, globalization, modern transport and technology, conflicts, and climate change have facilitated waves of migration as never before with staggering numbers of over one billion migrants. Therefore, it is hardly surprising that migration has taken centre stage in influencing public opinion, which in turn, has shaped recent world events on both sides of the Atlantic.

The social sciences have dominated the research on migrants and migration patterns with a view to demographic changes, labour market mobility, nationality, political participation, and education, to name a few areas. However, health has not been on the radar of migration researchers, and neither have migrants and their health outcomes been high on the agenda for health and health care systems researchers or practitioners. Health of migrants was barely mentioned on the agenda of the first ever Global Compact on Migration held in 2018. Therefore, it is hardly surprising that 'migration and health' has often fallen between the cracks and is still evolving as an area of interest. Migration health should no longer be the domain of those with special or exotic interests, but must form an integral part of global health policies and initiatives and sustainable development goals.

European societies are increasingly more ethnically and culturally diverse. Regardless of the reasons people leave their countries of birth, migration affects the health of migrants. Addressing the health needs of migrants will require acquiring knowledge about their health, including the unique stressors and protective factors, the perceptions and attitudes both health personnel and migrants have about health, health care systems, and clinical practice. European health systems, primarily designed to cater to the needs of the majority population, are often challenged when responding to newcomers and ethnic minorities. Europe's handling of the migrant situation during the past few years has been fragmented, chaotic, and hopelessly inadequate. The variations in formal entitlements and access to health care, coupled with services that may not be 'diversity-sensitive' or 'culturally competent', could further complicate the situation for the health of migrants. Better health outcomes for all segments of the population warrant the need for adapting health care and addressing gaps.

In light of the evolving current global situation, our textbook aims to enable primary health care services, in particular general practice (including emergency room and home-based care and nursing homes), in providing adequate and appropriate treatment and managing migrants (mainly migrants), including refugees. The main target groups for this book are health professionals; students/doctors/medical pracitioners/ health personnel working directly with the migrant patient.

We have chosen to address and focus on common problems faced on a day-to-day basis through case studies and vignettes. We hope our endeavours to elaborate upon the concepts, terminology, determinants, and policies will provide our readers with the broader context of migration and health. Our intentions go beyond increasing knowledge and describing the issues of concern. We will leave our readers with a set of tools to respond to diversity. We have highlighted, where relevant, the participation and contribution of migrants to their new society, as the resilience of migrants should not be undermined. We would like to caution our readers, however, that we do not have all the answers and do not offer a set of standard solutions that will work regardless of circumstance or solve all problems.

The authors of the chapters herein reflect the expertise, competence, and skills required to put together such a book. We have been very privileged and are grateful for the opportunity to work together to put forward a book that we hope readers will find useful and enjoy reading. We would also like to thank those who read and commented on specific chapters. In particular, we would like to thank the WONCA Migration Group.

Our sincere gratitude to our publishers and editors for their confidence in us and for the foresight to embark on this important venture.

Last but not the least, we thank our families, who have been used to spending weekends and evenings on their own while we have been buried deep in our writing endeavours.

Bernadette N. Kumar and Esperanza Diaz
Oslo/Kathmandu/Bergen

Editors

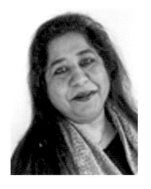

Bernadette N. Kumar, MD, PhD, is a medical graduate from India with a doctorate in epidemiology and public health from the University of Oslo, Norway, and post-doctoral research fellowship at the Institute for Psychiatry, University of Oslo. Kumar has several years of international experience working for UNICEF, WHO, WFP, World Bank, and NORAD in Asia and Africa (1989–2000). Migration and health has been the focus of her research and she is the co-editor of a textbook on migrant health in Norway. She was appointed Director of the Norwegian Center for Migration and Minority Health in 2010; and Associate Professor, Global Health at the Institute for Health and Society, University of Oslo in 2013. She has been a commissioner of the Lancet Commission on Migration and Health (2018). Currently, she works at the Norwegian Institute of Public Health, is Professor at the Empower School of Health, India and the President of the EUPHA section of Migration and Ethnic Minority Health. (Photo credit: Ram Gupta.)

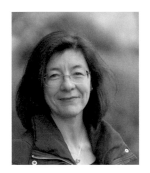

Esperanza Diaz studied medicine and became a specialist in family medicine in Madrid, Spain. In 1999, she moved to Norway, where she was certified as a Norwegian specialist in family medicine and earned her PhD at the University of Bergen. For many years she has worked as a general practitioner with a hugely diverse population. She is Associate Professor at the Institute for Global Public Health and Primary Care, University of Bergen, and is a senior researcher at the Unit for Migration and Health at the Norwegian Institute for Public Health. Diaz has several publications in the field of migrant health. She volunteers for a local non-profit organization providing care for undocumented migrants. (Photo credit: Magne Sandnes.)

Contributors

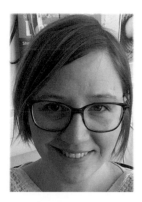

Karolien Aelbrecht is trained as a clinical psychologist and psychotherapist. Aelbrecht works as research coordinator at the Research Department of Ghent University, Belgium. She is also finishing her doctoral thesis on doctor-patient communication through the eyes of the patient: differences in medical communication according to the patient's background.

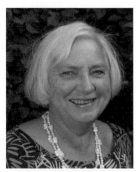

Berit Austveg, MD, received her degree from the University of Oslo, Norway. From 1976 to 1988, she led the Health Service for Migrants in Oslo. This clinic provided health care primarily for newly arrived migrant women and pioneered clinical methods in cross-cultural health work. Based on this work, Austveg authored the first Scandinavian textbook on the topic. For the past 30 years, Austveg has worked in community medicine with a focus on global sexual and reproductive health at different levels, including in and with the United Nations.

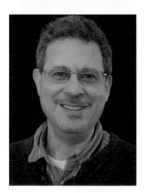

Yoav Ben-Shlomo, BSc, PhD, qualified in medicine having completed an intercalated BSc in psychology. He later earned a Wellcome Trust Fellowship in Clinical Epidemiology and completed his MSc and then PhD at London's Global University (UCL). He has been a Professor of Clinical Epidemiology at Bristol University, UK, since 2005. His major contribution has been establishing a theoretical framework around life-course epidemiology in relation to chronic diseases. Over the past decade he has worked progressively on life-course predictors of ageing. He helped set up the Indian Migration Study, looking at the impact of rural-to-urban migration in India and its impact on cardiometabolic risk, and has recently examined the impact of international migration on frailty across Europe.

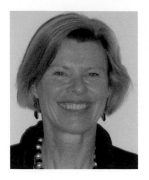

Jill Benson, PsychMed, PhD, has been a GP for over 35 years, and currently works as a medical educator for GPEx and in the clinic at Doctors' Health SA, Adelaide, as well as in mainstream general practice. For 10 years she was the Medical Director of the KWHA, an alliance of health services in three remote Aboriginal communities in the Western desert, and worked for 15 years seeing refugees at the Migrant Health Service in Adelaide. In 2012, she was awarded an Order of Australia for her work with refugees and Aboriginal people, and in mental health. She completed her PhD in 2017 on the health of refugees in Australia. She has been a member of the WONCA Working Party on Mental Health for over 10 years and is currently the Secretary.

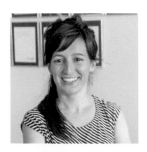

Amaia Calderón-Larrañaga, PhD, is an Assistant Professor at the Aging Research Center of Karolinska Institutet in Sweden. She holds a degree in pharmacy, a master's in public health, and a PhD from the Department of Public Health, University of Zaragoza, Spain. As a member of the EpiChron Research Group on Chronic Diseases of the Aragon Health Sciences Institute in Spain, she has published several articles on the epidemiology of multimorbidity and its impact on health systems and patients.

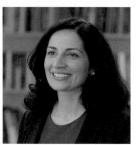

Marina Catallozzi, MD, MSCE, is an Assistant Professor of Pediatrics at the College of Physicians and Surgeons and of Population and Family Health at the Mailman School of Public Health, Columbia University, New York. Catallozzi is an adolescent medicine specialist and is board certified in both paediatrics and adolescent medicine. At Mailman, Catallozzi is the co-leader of the Sexuality, Sexual and Reproductive Health Certificate. She has an active adolescent medicine practice in Washington Heights, New York, and is dedicated to improving the health of the community.

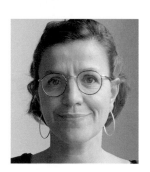

Stéphanie De Maesschalck, PhD, has worked as a family physician since 2000, currently in a primary health care centre in a superdiverse neighbourhood in Menen, Belgium. Between 2010 and 2017, she was coordinating physician for a large governmental refugee centre. She has been a Ghent University research and teaching assistant since 2001. Her PhD in 2012 focussed on 'Linguistic and cultural diversity in the consultation room: a tango between physicians and their ethnic minority patients'. She is currently Visiting Professor of 'diversity in health care' at Ghent University, Department of Public Health and Primary Care. She is a trainer for 'diversity in health (care)' for health care professionals and teams.

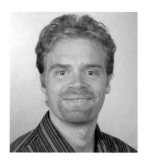

Lars T. Fadnes, MD, PhD, DTM&H, is a researcher at the University of Bergen and works clinically with family medicine. His research focuses on migration, nutrition, child health, substance use, and delivery of health care with both a global and a local perspective. He has conducted research on migrant health among children using linked National Registry data and has clinical experience with health care for migrants from his work as a general practitioner, as well as engagement for a local non-profit organization providing care for undocumented migrants.

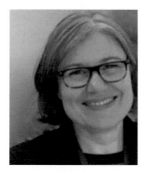

Rebecca Farrington Following study for a DTM&H in Liverpool, UK, and experiences working on four overseas projects for Médecins Sans Frontières in the 1990s, Farrington became a GP. She now works as a senior clinical lecturer in community-based medical education at the University of Manchester Medical School, as a GP with Extended Role for Greater Manchester Mental Health Foundation Trust in asylum seeker health, and as a GP in South Manchester.

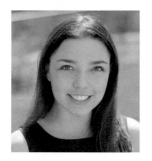

Rachel A. Fowler, MPH, received her degree in Population and Family Health from the Mailman School of Public Health, Columbia University, New York. Fowler was awarded a Sasakawa Young Leaders Fellowship Fund grant to evaluate a maternal and reproductive health programme in the Philippines. She has studied the effect of migration on internally displaced women's reproductive health in Colombia, and the effect of harmful policies on women's and girls' health and rights across the globe. She previously worked as a clinical research coordinator at Massachusetts General Hospital, Boston, Massachusetts. She grew up in the UK and Ecuador, and received a BA in neuroscience from Middlebury College, Vermont.

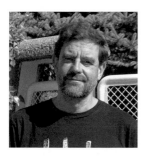

Luis Andrés Gimeno-Feliu, MD, PhD, is a family doctor in Zaragoza, Spain. He previously worked in the Democratic Republic of Congo. He holds a diploma in tropical diseases from the University Paris VI. He combines his clinical work with undergraduate teaching in general practice at the University of Zaragoza. His main areas of interest are migration and international health, social determinants of health, and multimorbidity. He is currently the National Coordinator of the Working Group on Health Inequalities and International Health within the Spanish Society of Family and Community Medicine.

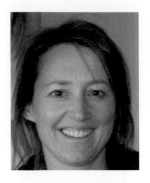

Rachel Hammonds is a Canadian post-doctoral researcher affiliated with the London School of Hygiene & Tropical Medicine and the Law and Development Research Group at the University of Antwerp Law Faculty, Belgium. Her research focuses on the intersection of development policy, health, and human rights. She has published extensively in legal and medical journals and served as a consultant to international organizations including the World Health Organization and UNAIDS. She is a New York State licensed attorney.

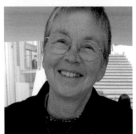

Iona Heath worked as a GP at the Caversham Group Practice in London from 1975 until 2010, caring for a mostly disadvantaged and hugely ethnically diverse population. She was President of the Royal College of General Practitioners from 2009 to 2012. She was a world executive member of the World Organization of Family Doctors from 2007 to 2012. She wrote a regular op-ed column for the *British Medical Journal* for 8 years, and has contributed essays to many other medical journals across the world. Her book *Matters of Life and Death* was published in 2007 (Radcliffe Publishing Ltd, UK) and has been translated into Italian and Spanish. Her book *Contra il Mercato della Salute* was published in Italian in 2016.

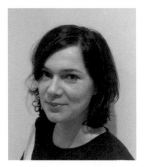

Ines Keygnaert is Assistant Professor in sexual and reproductive health at the International Centre for Reproductive Health at the Ghent University in Belgium. She is also the team leader of the 'Gender & Violence' team, focusing on violence prevention and response, sexual and reproductive health rights' violations, and gender and sexual health promotion in vulnerable populations, with specific attention to migrants. She is a founding member of the Centre for the Social Study of Migration and Refugees (CESSMIR) at Ghent University.

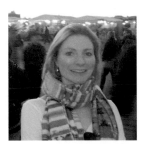

Bridget Kiely is an Irish medical doctor and has a diploma in Tropical Medicine in Lima, Peru and a master's in Public Health from University College Dublin. Kiely trained as a GP in the UK and subsequently completed a Darzi Fellowship in Clinical Leadership. In London she volunteered with clinics providing health care to vulnerable migrants. In 2015, she volunteered as part of the Ebola Emergency Response and subsequently spent 2 years in Sierra Leone, working as a clinical manager with King's Sierra Leone Partnership and as a health advisor with the Clinton Health Access Initiative. Kiely has worked with marginalized and vulnerable populations with Safetynet Primary Care in Dublin, and is now working on a PhD degree.

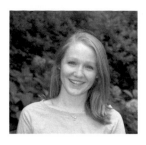 **Chelsea A. Kolff, MPH,** is the Academic Coordinator at Columbia University in the Mailman School of Public Health Heilbrunn Department of Population and Family Health (New York). Kolff previously served as a project officer and managed three federally funded grant projects focused on improving paediatric vaccination rates through the use of technology. Her interests include adolescent health and well-being, sexual and reproductive health, immunization, and education. Before graduate school, she taught high school science in Atlanta, Georgia. She received her MPH from the Columbia University Mailman School of Public Health and her AB from Princeton University in ecology and evolutionary biology (Princeton, New Jersey).

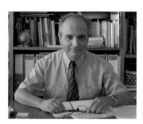 **Christos Lionis** is a Professor of General Practice and Primary Health Care at the School of Medicine, and Head of the Clinic of Social and Family Medicine at the School of Medicine, University of Crete, Greece. Lionis is also a Guest Professor of General Practice at the University of Linköping, Sweden. Since 2016, he has been the Coordinator of the Residency Training Programme of General Practice for Crete. Lionis has been awarded as Honorary Fellow for the Royal College of General Practitioners, the World Organization of National Colleges, Academies and Academic Associations of General Practitioners/Family Physicians, and for the European Society of Cardiology.

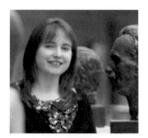 **Anne MacFarlane** is a Professor of Primary Healthcare Research at the Graduate Entry Medical School, Limerick, Ireland. She is the first social scientist to hold a Chair in Academic Primary Care in Ireland. She has specialist expertise in migrant health and participatory health research. She leads the Public and Patient Involvement Research Unit at the Graduate Entry Medical School.

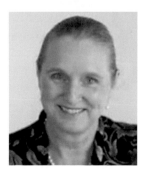 **Jeanette H. Magnus, PhD,** is a specialist in rheumatology. She earned her PhD from the University of Tromsø, Norway in 1992. She has had several positions in Norway and in New Orleans, Louisiana. Currently, she works at the University of Oslo as Senior Advisor at the Department for Leadership.

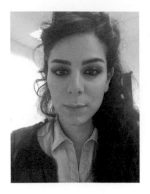

Loubaba Mamluk, PhD, MSc, earned her PhD in epidemiology at Queen's University Belfast and an MSc in human nutrition at the University of Glasgow. She is a Senior Research Associate in Epidemiology and holds a post in Population Health Sciences at the University of Bristol. Most of her work is on the effects of early life influences on long-term health outcomes. Recently, she developed and formulated the hypothesis of a multi-regional project on the mental health and well-being of Syrian refugees in the UK: 'Syrian mental Health Assessment and MIgration Study (SHAMIS)'.

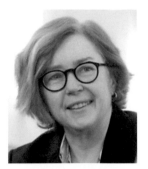

Terry McGovern, JD, serves as the Harriet and Robert H Heilbrunn Professor and Chair of the Heilbrunn Population and Family Health Department at the Columbia University Medical Center in New York. She founded the HIV Law Project in 1989 and served on the National Task Force on the Development of HIV/AIDS Drugs. She previously worked at the Ford Foundation as Senior Program Officer in the Gender, Rights and Equality Unit. McGovern has published extensively and has testified numerous times before Congress and other policy-making entities.

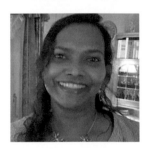

Kathy Ainul Møen, MD, was born in Sri Lanka and completed her MD degree at the University of Bergen in Norway in 2007. She has worked as a GP since 2011, and is currently working on a PhD thesis studying migrant health at the University of Bergen. She volunteers for a local non-profit organization providing care for undocumented migrants.

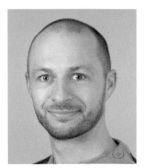

T. Rune Nielsen, PhD With a background in clinical neuro-psychology, for the last 10 years Nielsen has been involved in research on cross-cultural dementia diagnostics, including neuropsychological assessment and barriers to care, focussing on non-Western migrant populations in Western Europe as well as populations in low- and middle-income countries. As part of this research, he has participated in validation and implementation of the Rowland Universal Dementia Assessment Scale (RUDAS) in several countries.

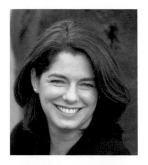

Nicole Nitti has been practicing family medicine for over 20 years and has specialized in the care of migrants and refugees for the last decade. Her interest in chronic disease prevention and management stemmed from her observing the lack of attention paid to supporting excellent control of conditions such as diabetes and hypertension in these populations. She is currently Medical Director of Access Alliance Multicultural Health and Community Services and a Primary Care Lead in the Toronto Central Local Health Integration Network, Toronto, Canada.

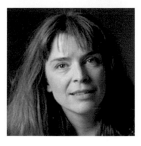

Marie Nørredam, MD, PhD, DMSc, is an Associate Professor at the University of Copenhagen, Denmark. She has contributed internationally to the field of migration and health and is the co-founder of the Danish Research Centre for Migration, Ethnicity and Health, Copenhagen, Denmark. Her research especially illuminates the need to focus on risk factors related to migration processes, as well as actual access in contrast to the rights to care of vulnerable migrant groups including asylum seekers and undocumented migrant and refugee children. She initiated the Danish Society for Immigrant Health, which works cross-disciplinary and cross-sectionally to facilitate equity in health in relation to migrants.

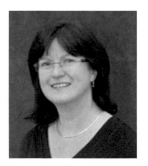

Catherine A. O'Donnell is a Deputy Director of the Institute of Health & Wellbeing and Professor of Primary Care Research and Development at the Department of General Practice and Primary Care. She is the current Chair of the Society for Academic Primary Care, where she champions the role of academic primary care and supports both clinical and non-clinical early career researchers. She is on the Advisory Board of the European Forum for Primary Care and a member of the NAPCRG International Committee. In recognition of this, Kate was recently awarded an Honorary Fellowship of the Royal College of General Practitioners.

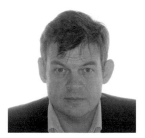

Gorik Ooms, Professor of Global Health Law and Governance at the London School of Hygiene and Tropical Medicine, is a human rights lawyer and a global health scholar.

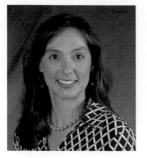

Krista M. Perreira, PhD, earned a PhD in health economics, University of California, Berkeley, 1999. She is a Professor of Social Medicine at the University of North Carolina, Chapel Hill. Her research focuses on the relationships among family, migration, and social policy, with an emphasis on gender and racial disparities. Integrating both economic and sociological models, she studies ways to improve the well-being of migrant youth. As a scholar actively engaged in community service, Perreira also serves as an advisory committee member or on the boards of directors for national task forces, local non-profit organizations, and state agencies seeking to improve the provision of services to Hispanic populations and migrants.

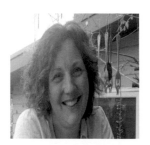

Christine Phillips, MBBS, BMedSc, MA, MPH, DipEd, MD, FRACGP, is an Associate Professor at Social Foundations of Medicine, Australian National University. Her research interests are primary health care systems, refugee health, the health of vulnerable persons and interprofessional working in health settings.

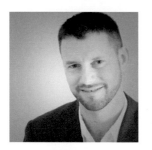

Kevin Pottie, MD, CCFP, MCISc, FCFP, is a Professor and Practicing Physician at the Departments of Family Medicine and Epidemiology and Community Medicine and Scientist at the Bruyère Research Institute, University of Ottawa, Canada. He has led GRADE equity methods and evidence-based guidelines for refugees and other migrants in Canada and EU/EEA.

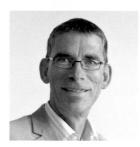

Oliver Razum, Dr Med, MSc Epidemiology (London), is Dean of the School of Public Health, Bielefeld University, Germany. He is also Full Professor and heads the Department of Epidemiology and International Public Health. His main research field is social epidemiology with a particular focus on the health of migrants, and on the role of contextual factors in the production of health inequalities. Razum has published over 220 scientific papers and numerous book chapters. Before moving into epidemiology, he worked as District Medical Officer in a rural district of Zimbabwe.

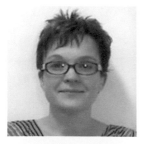

Sabi Redwood has a background in paediatric nursing and clinical leadership. In 2009, she joined the Collaborations for Leadership in Applied Health Research and Care, funded by the English National Institute for Health Research at the University of Birmingham and the University of Bristol since 2014. Redwood is Deputy Director and Ethnography Team Lead.

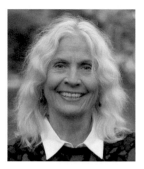

Anna Stavdal is a family doctor and university teacher in Norway. She is the President-Elect, WONCA World and the Immediate Past President, WONCA Europe.

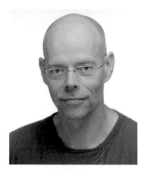

Edvin Schei is a GP and Professor of General Practice at the University of Bergen, Norway. Since he was a medical student in the 1980s, he has been critically aware of a lack of person-oriented competence in medical education, research, and clinical practice. Seeking advice from philosophy, psychotherapy, and the social sciences, Schei has sought to strengthen the humanistic aspects of medical education and practice. He has published a number of books (*Listen. Physicianship and Communication*, 2014, Fagbokforlaget, Oslo, Norway), and developed new ways of teaching professionalism.

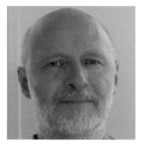

Morten Sodemann specialized in infectious and tropical diseases, started the first hospital-based Migrant Health Clinic in Europe as a Senior Consultant at Odense University Hospital and is a Professor of Global and Migrant Health at the University of Southern Denmark. He has conducted health systems research and field epidemiological studies of primary health care in Guinea-Bissau, Uganda, Cameroon, Sudan, and Tanzania. He was involved in a national training programme aimed at medical doctors to conduct health assessment of refugees and was co-producer of national clinical guidelines for health assessment of refugees in Denmark. He is engaged in training doctors and interpreters in bilingual patient communication.

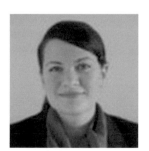

Hürrem Tezcan-Güntekin is a Professor at the Department of Epidemiology and International Public Health, School of Public Health, Bielefeld University, Bielefeld, Germany.

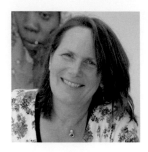

Maria van den Muijsenbergh is a GP and Professor in Health Disparities and Person-Centred Integrated Primary at Radboudumc Department of Primary and Community Care, Nijmegen, the Netherlands; and at Pharos, the Dutch centre of expertise on health disparities. Her research and teaching includes underserved groups with a focus on refugees and other vulnerable migrant groups. Until 2018, she was Chair of the WONCA Special Interest Group on Migrant Care, International Health, and Travel Medicine.

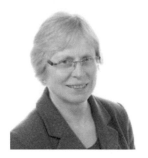

Berit Viken is a Public Health Nurse and Anthropologist in Norway. She has many years of experience in public health and health promotion with children and families. Her research is on migrant women and health services. She has been an associate professor and has taught nursing education, with further education in coaching and supervision, a master programme in health promotion and a master's degree in Social Anthropology from the University of Bergen in 1995.

Introduction

RATIONALE, PURPOSE, AND SCOPE

Globalization and diversity are part and parcel of the twenty-first century. The number of international migrants has grown at an unprecedented rate during the past 15 years, accounting now for more than 10% of the total population in Europe, North America, and Oceania (1). However, given the very nature of migration, migrants are a heterogeneous group and their health will vary accordingly. Some refugees, asylum seekers, and undocumented migrants might be considered vulnerable, while others are resilient and demonstrate the 'healthy migrant effect', with better health status on arrival than the host population.

Most countries in Europe and Western Europe attempt to provide equitable health care services to their citizens, disregarding their ethnicity, religion, country of origin, and other characteristics. Most of these health care systems are organized into primary and secondary level care. Typically, general practitioners (GPs) are the cornerstone of primary health care, representing the first point of contact of the patient with health care services. In addition to being gatekeepers for secondary care, GPs often have the responsibility for both preventive care and most of the curative care for the majority of patients.

Notwithstanding the diversity among migrants, a number of health-related differences in need (2,3), entitlements (4,5), use of services (6,7) prevalence of disease (8,9), and mortality (10,11) between migrants and their host populations has been documented. These differences can be attributed to the individual, the health professional, and at the system level. From the health professionals' point of view, a large body of literature describes challenges in providing health care across cultures, especially when the patient is a migrant with a substantially different cultural background or when the patient is unskilled in the language of the host country. These challenges apply not only to GPs (12), but to other primary health care professionals, such as nurses or pharmacy professionals (13,14), and are indeed related to the entire patient pathway as shown by studies pointing to differences in diagnostic procedures undertaken (15), number of consultations needed to be referred to secondary care (16), specificity of diagnoses provided (17), treatments given (13,18), and outcomes achieved (19) for various migrant groups across different countries. A study in Norway observed that non-Western migrants were less satisfied with primary care than native Norwegians (20). These and other differences indicate possible challenges to access and that services to certain migrant groups might not be equitable.

Undergraduate medical training and postgraduate training for GPs usually include elements of the patient-centred clinical method (21), according to which the doctor elicits information about the patient's relevant beliefs and values and takes these into account in his or her interaction with the patient. However, the patient-centred clinical method neither encourages practitioners to reflect upon the significance of their own culture and the cultural settings underlying health care nor teaches specific cultural competence approaches (22). The educational programmes for health care professionals in Europe rarely include mandatory training for tackling the challenges due to cultural difference and migration (23,24). Swedish GPs state that they avoid addressing or engaging with cultural differences in consultations (25). A recent study conducted in Norway shows that GPs lack core elements of cultural competence and specific strategies to deal with migrant patients, including refugees, as well as basic knowledge of key differences in the prevalence of diseases and use of preventive and curative health care services for some of the main migrant groups in the country (26). It is imperative that GPs and other primary health care professionals, and indeed all health care professionals, develop skills and competencies when meeting patients with diverse backgrounds in order to ensure equity in health care and better patient satisfaction (27).

Since there are no indications that migration will either abate or cease, and with the early transfer of refugees to general practice, there is an urgent need to address key issues related to migration and health, including cultural competence in pre- and post-grade curricula. A practically oriented book on migration and health targeting GPs and other primary health care providers is needed to support the development of this curriculum. We believe this book, which balances theory and practice with clinical vignettes that enrich the text throughout the book, will be widely used in both undergraduate and postgraduate training. Several themes that are targeted in this book, such as health literacy, communication, and the cultures and subcultures of systems, to name a few, will help health care providers to improve their provision of care not only to migrants, but to other vulnerable groups and society as a whole.

Before embarking on this journey with us, we would like to caution readers that the terms and definitions used in the field of migration health are a minefield and often lead to confusion. We refer to the World Congress on Migration, Ethnicity, Race and Health (MERH) 2018 Glossary and have tried to be consistent with terminology. We address all migrants in this book, not only refugees. The term *migrant* is often used in communicating to a broad audience, but the complexities of the many subgroups under this terminology are often lost. Refugees are a subset of the wider migrant term. The UN Refugee Agency (UNHCR) report uses the term *people of concern*; this includes refugees, asylum seekers, internally displaced people, and stateless people. The fact that these terms are often used interchangeably can lead to confusion, and the introductory chapters address this. Thereafter we use the term migrants and in some cases *immigrants* unless otherwise indicated.

REFERENCES

1. International Organization for Migration (IOM). *World Migration Report 2015. Migrants and Cities: New Partnerships to Manage Mobility*. Geneva, Switzerland: International Organization for Migration; 2015.
2. Gimeno-Feliu LA, Calderón-Larrañaga A, Diaz E, Poblador-Plou B, Macipe-Costa R, Prados-Torres A. The healthy migration effect in primary care. *Gac Sanit*. 2015;29(1):15–20.
3. Nørredam M. Migration and health. *Dan Med J*. 2015;61(4).
4. Rechel B, Mladovsky P, Ingleby D, Mackenbach JP, McKee M. Migration and health in an increasingly diverse Europe. *Lancet*. 2013;381(9873):1235–45.

5. Bozorgmehr K, Razum O. Effect of restricting access to health care on health expenditures among asylum-seekers and refugees: a quasi-experimental study in Germany, 1994–2013. *PLOS ONE*. 2015;10(7):e0131483.

6. Diaz E, Calderón-Larrañaga A, Prado-Torres A, Poblador-Plou B, Gimeno-Feliu L-A. How do immigrants use primary healthcare services? A register-based study in Norway. *Eur J Public Health*. 2015;25(1):72–8.

7. Berens EM, Stahl L, Yilmaz-Aslan Y, Sauzet O, Spallek J, Razum O. Participation in breast cancer screening among women of Turkish origin in Germany – a register-based study. *BMC Womens Health*. 2014;14:24.

8. Diaz E, Poblador-Pou B, Gimeno-Feliu L-A, Calderón-Larrañaga A, Kumar BN, Prados-Torres A. Multimorbidity and its patterns according to immigrant origin. A nationwide register-based study in Norway. *PLOS ONE*. 2015;10(12):e0145233.

9. Diaz E, Kumar BN, Gimeno-Feliu L-A, Calderón-Larrañaga A, Poblador-Pou B, Prados-Torres A. Multimorbidity among registered immigrants in Norway: the role of reason for migration and length of stay. *Trop Med Int Health*. 2015;20(12):1805–14.

10. Nørredam M, Olsbjerg M, Petersen JH, Bygbjerg I, Krasnik A. Mortality from infectious diseases among refugees and immigrants compared to native Danes: a historical prospective cohort study. *Trop Med Int Health*. 2012;17(2):223–30.

11. Ikram UZ, Mackenbach JP, Harding S et al. All-cause and cause-specific mortality of different migrant populations in Europe. *Eur J Epidemiol*. 2016;31(7):655–65.

12. Varvin S, Aasland OG. Legers forhold til flyktningpasienten [Physicians' relation to refugees]. *Tidsskrift Norske Legeforening*. 2009;129(15):1488–90.

13. Hakonsen H, Lees K, Toverud EL. Cultural barriers encountered by Norwegian community pharmacists in providing service to non-Western immigrant patients. *Int J Clin Pharm*. 2014;36(6):1144–51.

14. Debesay J, Harslof I, Rechel B, Vike H. Facing diversity under institutional constraints: challenging situations for community nurses when providing care to ethnic minority patients. *J Adv Nurs*. 2014;70(9):2107–16.

15. Royl G, Ploner CJ, Leithner C. Headache in the emergency room: the role of immigrant background on the frequency of serious causes and diagnostic procedures. *Neurol Sci*. 2012;33(4):793–9.

16. Lyratzopoulus G, Neal RD, Barbiere JM, Rubin GP, Abel GA. Variation in the number of general practitioner consultations before hospital referral for cancer: findings from the 2010 National Cancer Patient Experience Survey in England. *Lancet Oncol*. 2012;13(4):353–65.

17. Sandvik H, Hunskaar S, Diaz E. Immigrants' use of emergency primary health care in Norway: a registry-based observational study. *BMC Health Serv Res*. 2012;12:308.

18. Gimeno-Feliu LA, Calderón-Larrañaga A, Prados-Torres A, Revilla-López C, Diaz E. Patterns of pharmaceutical use for immigrants to Spain and Norway: a comparative study of prescription databases in two European countries. *Int J Equity Health*. 2016;15(32).

19. Tran AT, Straand J, Dalen I et al. Pharmacological primary and secondary cardiovascular prevention in a multiethnic general practice population: still room for improvements. *BMC Health Serv Res*. 2013;13(182).

20. Lien E, Nafstad P, Rosvold E. Non-Western immigrants' satisfaction with the general practitioners' services in Oslo, Norway. *Int J Equity Health*. 2008;7(1):1–7.

21. Stewart M, Brown J, Weston W, McWhinney I, McWilliam C, Freeman T. *Patient-centered Medicine. Transforming the Clinical Method. 3rd ed.* London: Radcliffe; 2013.

22. Saha S, Beach MC, Cooper LA. Patient centeredness, cultural competence and healthcare quality. *J Natl Med Assoc*. 2008;100(11):1275–85.

23. van den Muijsenbergh M, van Weel-Baumgarten E, Burns N et al. Communication in cross-cultural consultations in primary care in Europe: the case for improvement. The rationale for the RESTORE FP 7 project. *Prim Health Care Res Dev*. 2014;15(2):122–33.

24. Diaz E, Kumar BN. Health care curricula in multicultural societies. *Int J Med Educ*. 2018;9:42–4.

25. Wachtler C, Brorsson A, Troein M. Meeting and treating cultural difference in primary care: a qualitative interview study. *Fam Pract*. 2006;23(1):111–5.

26. Møen KA, Terragni L, Kumar BN, Diaz E. Cervical cancer screening among immigrant women in Norway - the health care providers' perspectives. *Scand J Prim Health Care*. 2018;36(4):415–422.

27. Govere L, Govere EM. How effective is cultural competence training of healthcare providers on improving patient satisfaction of minority groups? A systematic review of literature. *Worldviews Evid Based Nurs*. 2016;13(6):402–10.

Overarching themes

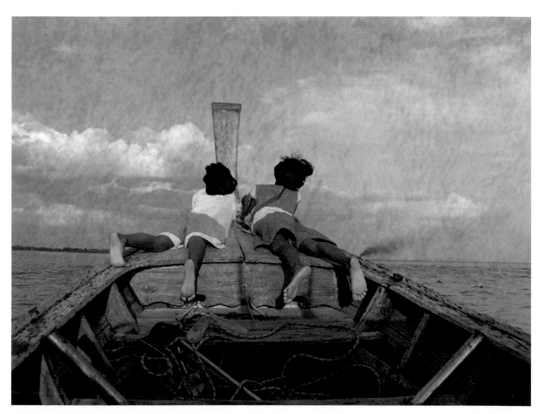

Photo credit: Sue Macartney.

CHAPTER 1

Migration and migrants: What we know about worldwide mobility and why it matters

Bernadette N. Kumar and Esperanza Diaz

LEARNING OBJECTIVES

At the end of this chapter, the reader should be able to:

- Gain a better understanding of the development of the field of migration health
- Acquire an overview of the salient features and definitions of migration, the migratory process, and the current trends in migration
- Understand the migration cycle and its implications on health
- Acquire an overview of the main policy implications, the actions taken so far, and directions for the future

Note: Chapters 1 and 2 of this book provide an overview of the subject matter and should therefore be considered as general and overarching.

INTRODUCTION

Migration, an age-old human phenomenon, encompasses a wide variety of movements and situations. These migrations have influenced the composition and structure of societies, as well as other aspects of the existence of groups and individuals, including health. Health has been, is, and will always be an integral part of the human existence. The 'Migration Period' of the Middle Ages (300–700 AD) resulted in dramatic changes in the architecture of populations in Europe. Many would argue that we are in the midst of a similar 'Migration

Period' of our times (1). Today, migration contributes significantly to global demographics as advancements in modern technology have enabled the ease, speed, distance, and numbers that can travel. The numbers of migrants and those interacting, working, and living with them are growing. While source, transit, and destination countries are constantly evolving and changing, migration has improved millions of lives, but not all migration occurs in positive circumstances. More than ever before, migration touches everyone as it intertwines with geopolitics, trade, economic, social, and security aspects affecting our daily lives.

Notwithstanding walls, fences, barbed wires, legislation, and the political climate, globalization can hardly be reversed. Current migration affects practically all nations and individuals in one way or the other. Over 250 million people reside outside their country of birth; this characterizes the sheer scale, scope, and extent of migration that undoubtedly makes the phenomenon a contemporary global issue. The 'ecological space' travelled by migrants in all phases of the migration cycle — pre-, peri-, and post-migration — will in one way or another affect health. Besides recognizing the need for better planning and management of migration and its health dimensions, it is critical for countries, health care providers, and health professionals to respond to these challenges (2). Failure to respond to the emerging realities of diverse populations in a timely and adequate manner could prove to be myopic from a political, economic, and social perspective for all concerned.

WORLDWIDE MOBILITY: STATE OF THE ART

Historical perspectives

One million years ago, *Homo sapiens* moved across and out of Africa to Eurasia and 500,000 years ago to Northern Europe. Though these early forms of migration are not well documented, much like today, they would have occurred across very long distances, albeit at a much slower pace. Fossil and climate records suggest that these population movements were most likely driven by food and environmental factors — similar to many of the underlying climate change influences today (3). Migration, whether through outright conquests or slow cultural infiltration and resettlement, shaped the grand epochs in history, e.g. the fall of the Western Roman Empire that transformed the world, and the prehistoric and historic settlements of Australia and the Americas (2).

The drivers, patterns, and dynamics of migration have persisted for centuries, though the types and forms have varied and changed considerably. There are as many reasons to migrate as there are migrants; however, the push-and-pull factors that contribute to worldwide mobility are common. Positive pull factors include better jobs, family reunification, and search for love, adventure, and new experiences. Negative push factors include famine, environmental disasters, war, religious persecution, poverty, and household financial crises. At the macro level, landmark events that govern the social, political, and geographical conditions largely determine migration. At the micro level it is the informal social networks, family, and community linkages that play an important role in both country of origin and country of settlement. Collective or personal circumstances lead to the decision to leave one's country or nation for another (2).

Forced or involuntary migration reflects aspects of humanity's inglorious history such as war and conflict, slave trade, trafficking, and ethnic cleansing (4). It could also take the form of voluntary migration (for education or employment) within one's region, country, or beyond. Regardless of the nature of migration voluntary or involuntary, every migrant has a unique and personal story. Despite the variations in motivation, the ultimate goal is the quest to improve the overall quality of life. However, migration histories do indicate that risks often taken as other values of life are given more importance than the risks. Throughout history, individuals and families have been forced or opted to migrate for a variety of reasons, often based on the hope of a better, safer, more financially secure life (3).

During the twentieth century, researchers and policy-makers, especially in Europe, paid only sporadic attention to the health of migrants. Migration health research has often fallen between the cracks, as migration researchers explore the socio-demographic aspects of migration often excluding health, whereas health researchers prioritize disease and disorders. In the twenty-first century, migration health has rapidly gained prominence and changed its course. The phases and areas of interest in the fields of migration and health have over the past decades developed rapidly and evolved, as summarized in Table 1.1. These phases and their focus have in turn influenced the evolution of migration health theories, and vice-versa.

Historically, the approach to migrant health has been either to address the immediate health and humanitarian needs of refugees and asylum seekers or conduct medical assessments of labour migrants to ensure compliance with administrative health requirements of the migration process. The growth, diversity, and extent of migration warrants more modern approaches to migrant health, and these are still evolving. On the one hand, 'endemic' diseases, either inherited (e.g. haemoglobinopathies) or a result of the gene-environmental interactions (diabetes, cancer) post migration should be given due consideration. On the other hand, considerations should include migrant communities and their descendants' travel patterns, i.e. journeys to countries of origin posing travel-related health risks and possibly involving different treatments. Thus, migrant-related programs and policies to prevent and manage these risks are increasingly gaining attention in host nations (5). Newer approaches build upon on broader global health and development strategies (6) and are directed towards sustaining and improving the health of all migrants to reduce disparities and sustain health equity. These newer approaches reflect understanding that migration is also an independent determinant of health. Migrants have largely been excluded from most studies or routinely collected data, or at least remain undescribed and uncounted as a category (7).

The main preoccupation in the last century with the health of migrants was the provision of health services, especially treatment (8). However, treating migrants when they become

TABLE 1.1   Phases in the development of interest in the health in migrants

Phases	Focus	Example
1. Exotic disease phase	Early interest in the unusual or seldom-occurring diseases of minority ethnic groups	Infections, especially STDs, Lepros
2. Biological differences	The study of biological differences with a focus on genetically inheritable diseases	Hemoglobinopathies
3. Population differences	Population patterns of disease; group comparisons with white as majority	Somatic diseases/mental health
4. Adapting health care to diversity	Adapting health care policy, research, and services to meet the needs of ethnic minority groups Challenge: Trying to ensure that the health care system as a whole is primed to meet the challenges of multicultural health care	Access to health systems Discrimination Intervention studies

Source: Johnson MRD. *Journal of Royal College Physicians London* 1984;18: 228–232. https://www.ncbi.nlm.nih.gov/pmc/articles/PMC5370889/. With permission.

ill limits protecting their health. As Michael Marmot put it, 'why treat people then send them back to the conditions that made them sick?' (24) Over the last century, multilateral agencies and nation-states have moved the migration and health agenda and policies forward to address the entire gamut of upstream and downstream interventions (9). Notable initiatives and events have led to a series of documents from international governmental organizations (IGOs) addressing migrants' health over the last 12 years, and there is a high degree of consensus about the interventions needed to protect migrants' health and are supportive of healthy migration (10–14). However, much remains to be done to attain 'health for all' including migrants (3).

Migration: Salient features, definitions, migratory process and current trends

To put it simply, the movement of populations is called migration and the people who move are migrants or, more specifically, emigrants, migrants, or settlers, depending on historical setting, circumstance, and perspective. Migrants are different from the host population and regardless of the reasons for migration they find themselves having to deal with economic struggle and hardship; they do not have the knowledge of resources and shortcuts that the existing population takes for granted and some, particularly in the early years after migration, tend to live in the shadows of society. The term 'immigrant' is usually pejorative, a label used by the settled pre-existing (or 'host') population!

Migration seldom involves a single long journey from one place to settle in another. The diversity and complexity of migration patterns include people traveling long and short distances, within and across borders, for temporary or permanent residency and often undertaking the same and different journeys multiple times (3). A clear delineation or rigid categorization of different types of migration is challenging, as the categorizing process attempts to classify a large, heterogeneous population according to limited criteria that is unsuited to capture the complex social dynamics of human mobility or the perspectives or needs of the people on the move.

Types of migration vary in regard to distance, duration, and reason. Permanent migration is for the purposes of permanent or long-term stays from rural to urban areas, more common in developing countries as industrialization takes effect and in developed countries due to a higher cost of urban living. International migration could entail both permanent and rural-to-urban migration simultaneously.

While terms such as 'voluntary' or 'forced' migration and categories such as 'refugees', 'asylum seekers', 'international', and 'internal' migrants can partially help to explain migration dynamics, they are generally administrative definitions used to classify migrants for protection, assistance, or research rather than serve as a true representation of individual circumstances. Migrant categories are not necessarily objective or neutral; distinctions frequently reflect particular assumptions, values, goals, and interests of the parties who assign these labels (3). People seeking safety from conflict may be classified as refugees, asylum seekers, or internally displaced persons, but before and during transit — especially in protracted conflicts where aid resources are insufficient — migration decisions may also relate to livelihoods and employment, similar to labour migrants. 'Distress migration', or migration due to entrenched poverty, food insecurity, and household economic shock (e.g. illness, debt), is common worldwide. Distress migration is linked to local unemployment, household financial crises, poor crop production (from climate change or soil exhaustion), and in some instances, forced evictions — for example, linked to rising real estate prices, large development projects, and land confiscation (3).

The definitions, use, and registration of migration-relevant variables differs greatly and often influences and defines policy initiatives such as national health policies and access to health care. The implications and consequences of non-uniform terminology complicate the international collection and analysis of comparable information for migrant populations (15). Interestingly, there is considerable symmetry in the terminologies for refugees, as these are often governed by covenants and guidelines. In this textbook we use existing definitions from the Glossary of MERH 2018 (the entire list can be found in [16]), but the most important ones are summarized in Box 1.1.

BOX 1.1 DEFINITIONS AND TERMINOLOGY

Migrant/Immigrant: While there is no formal legal definition of an international migrant, most experts agree that an international migrant is someone who changes his or her country of usual residence, irrespective of the reason for migration or legal status. Generally, a distinction is made between short-term, or temporary, migration, covering movements with a duration between 3 and 12 months, and long-term, or permanent, migration, referring to a change of country of residence for a duration of 1 year or more. The term is sometimes wrongly applied to the offspring of migrants born in the country of settlement. An error of the opposite kind is made when people born abroad, but with ancestry in the country of settlement, are not referred to as migrants (e.g. the Aussiedler in Germany, descendants of colonists, or possibly expelled from other countries).

Migration: The movement of people, either across an international border or within a country, including refugees, displaced persons, economic migrants, and persons moving for other purposes, including family reunification.

Asylum seeker: A person seeking asylum (i.e. leave to stay) in a foreign country on the grounds of fear of persecution or actual persecution/serious harm in their country of origin. Often erroneously used as a synonym for refugee but having a different legal status in most cases.

Irregular migrant: A person who (for example) owing to unauthorized entry, breach of a condition of entry, failure to gain asylum, or the expiry of his or her visa, lacks legal authorization to reside in the country where they are living. Synonyms in use include clandestine/undocumented migrant or migrant in an irregular situation.

Refugee: A person who, owing to a well-founded fear of persecution for reasons of race, religion, nationality, membership of a particular social group, or political opinion, is living outside the country of his nationality. In the European Union, this term is used for a person who has specifically sought and received legal asylum.

Majority population: The population, excluding ethnic minority groups. When used in race/ethnicity studies, this phrase is usually used as a synonym for white or European.

Ethnicity/ethnic group: The social group a person belongs to, and either identifies with or is identified with by others, as a result of a mix of cultural and other factors including language, diet, religion, ancestry, and physical features traditionally associated with race. All people have an ethnicity — not only minorities.

Equity: The absence of avoidable or remediable differences among groups of people, whether those groups are defined socially, economically, demographically, or geographically.

Racism (individual, institutional, direct, and indirect; also *racial discrimination)*: Belief that some races are superior to others, used to devise and justify individual and collective actions which create and sustain inequality among racial/ethnic groups. Racism is against international law. Individual racism is usually manifested in decisions and behaviours that disadvantage individuals or small groups.

Internalized racism occurs when victims of racism internalize the race-based prejudicial attitudes toward themselves and their racial or ethnic group, resulting in a loss of self-esteem and potentially in prejudicial treatment of members of their own racial or ethnic group.

Structural or *institutional racism* is race-based unfair treatment built into policies, laws, and practices. It is often rooted in intentional discrimination that occurred historically but exerts its effects even when no individual currently intends to discriminate. Racial residential segregation is an example, whereby people of particular ethnic minority groups are coerced into less desirable residential areas.

Indirect racism occurs when an apparently neutral provision, criterion, or practice would put persons of a particular racial or ethnic origin at a disadvantage.

Regardless of migration motives, economic contributions, or people's rights, amidst populist rhetoric, the amorphous labelling of people who move as 'migrants' has seemed to become a condemnatory marker for populations who have fewer resources, such as refugees, asylum seekers, and low-wage workers. The term 'expat' is in this context rather interesting — if you are a resourceful person, you can keep your culture, because you are seen as temporarily outside your true habitat. The issue of citizenship (foreigner/national citizen) as well as migrant status often comes up and is used frequently for administrative purposes. If one uses the official categories (as in the United Nations Department of Social and Economic Affairs [UNDESA] or Eurostat), the definitions are rather straightforward. Moreover, in an era of xenophobic politics, the catch all term 'migrants' obscures the net benefits of migration for destination communities and contributions to places of origin that support families and supplement development aid, which, in sum, promise greater global health (3).

Trends in international migration

By their very nature, the complex dynamics of global migration can never be fully measured, understood, and regulated. However, as the World Migration Report 2018 shows, we do have a continuously growing and improving body of data and evidence that can help us make better sense of the basic features of migration in an increasingly interconnected and interdependent world. Some of the main findings are summarized below (17):

- *Population growth*: The globalization of migration has meant a greater number of countries are affected by migratory international movements simultaneously (2). The International Migration Report 2017 shows that international migration makes an important contribution to population growth and even reverses population decline in some countries or areas. Between 2000 and 2015, migration contributed 42% of the population growth in North America and 31% in Oceania. In Europe, the size of the total population would have declined during the period 2000–2015 in the absence of migration. Not surprisingly, the number of migrants as a fraction of the population residing in high-income countries rose from 9.6% in 2000 to 14% in 2017.

- *Age*: Around three-quarters (74%) of all international migrants were of working age, or between 20 and 64 years of age, compared to 57% of the global population in 2017. Because international migrants comprise a larger proportion of working-age persons compared to the overall population, a net inflow of migrants lowers the dependency ratio — that is, the number of children and older persons compared to those of working age.
- *Gender*: While migration before the 1960s was male dominated, the current trend indicates the feminization of migration with women playing an increasingly significant role in all regions and types and making up 48.4% of all migrants in 2017. Women migrants outnumber males in all regions except Africa and Asia; in some countries of Asia, male migrants outnumber females by about three to one.
- *Destination and origin of international migrants:* If international migrants were considered as residents of a single nation, they would represent the fifth largest country in the world by population. In 2017, two-thirds of all international migrants were living in just 20 countries, and half of all international migrants were residing in just 10 countries. Migrants (foreign born) make up 10% of the population of high-income countries, whereas foreign-born people made up a large majority in Qatar (86%), United Arab Emirates (70%), and Kuwait (69%). The largest number of international migrants (49.8 million, or 19% of the global total) reside in the United States. Saudi Arabia, Germany, and the Russian Federation host the second, third, and fourth largest numbers of migrants worldwide (around 12 million each), followed by the United Kingdom (nearly 9 million). The number of Indian-born persons residing abroad numbered 17 million in 2017, ahead of the number of Mexican-born persons living outside Mexico (13 million). In 2017, Asia and Europe were the regions of origin for the largest numbers of international migrants — 106 million and 61 million, respectively. While the traditional countries of migration have been the United States, UK, Canada, and Australia, newer destinations include Ireland, Italy, Norway, and Portugal.
- *Growth*: Between 2000 and 2017, Africa experienced the largest relative increase in the number of international migrants who had originated in that region (+68%), followed by Asia (+62%), Latin America and the Caribbean (+52%), and Oceania (+51%).

This quantitative growth increases both the urgency and difficulties of government policies. Governments are further challenged by the differentiation of migration; that is, that most countries have a whole range of types of migration (i.e. labour migration, asylum seekers and refugees, family reunification, to name a few) at the same time.

Approaching migrant health: The migration cycle
Migration and health are dynamic by nature, and therefore it is very important to consider phases that can be cyclical. For health, the life-course perspective is well established and is dealt with in further detail in the following section. The migration cycle is best described in the

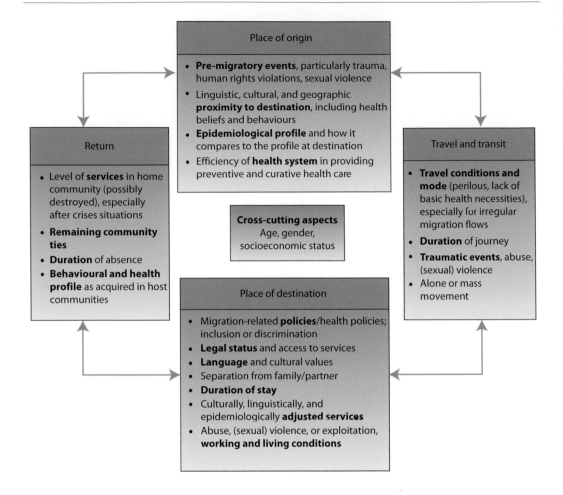

FIGURE 1.1 Phases of migration.

following phases: pre-departure (in the country of origin), transit (the journey — the interim country of destination), post-arrival (in the country of destination), and return (to country of origin) (18). These phases are summarized in Figure 1.1. While these phases are not a new concept, the time between the phases will vary depending on the wave and type of migration — the push-and-pull factors. In recent years, the transit period can take several years and become a semi-permanent situation, and return may not happen at all in the later years of life.

PUBLIC HEALTH ASPECTS OF MIGRATION: POLICY FRAMEWORKS SUPPORTING MIGRANT HEALTH

Building the right 'architecture' for global public health is a priority for all. This architecture must rest on a solid foundation. In order to build and support this foundation, it is important to understand both the determinants of health and the broader framework within which health care services operate.

Public health should not merely constitute the maintenance of a state of absence of disease but should be proactive, striving for social justice and equity with human rights at its core, and health as the main intended outcome. Collective action for sustaining good population health includes a multi-pronged drive for health development and security that includes many sectors other than health, including the political process. This gives us engagement and the power to go after the root causes of the problems. This is critical for building the foundation for good health for large populations in a long-lasting way. It also means moving from a curative to a preventive approach.

Policy development in Europe: The 22 steps

Migration health policies and priorities have evolved over time and increasingly reflect principles that support global human rights and global development goals (19,20). The advent of the Sustainable Development Goals saw confirmation from the international community that the attainment of the highest possible level of health is a basic right and that that attainment must include migrants. As migrants represent significant proportions of the global population, supporting and improving migrant health is necessary to ensure that migrants can fully contribute to the health of their communities at origin, transit, and destination. Differing processes and population flows reflect historical patterns of differences in national legislation and policies regarding nationality, citizenship, and residency. Hence, the development of policies and programs focussed on or directed towards the health of refugee and migrant populations are not always coordinated or symmetrical. Until the last decade of the twentieth century, migrant health policies, where they existed, tended to reflect issues of national importance and history.

The twenty-first century saw the forces of globalization, coupled with the dissolution of the former Soviet Union and the end of the Cold War, create profound changes in the nature, scope, and kinetics of migration. Migration flows and patterns rapidly evolved across the world, including the European Region. At the same time, issues of global public health, the role of social determinants in health outcomes, and the reduction of global health disparities assumed greater prominence in national and global health policy development. As noted earlier, sustained migration will be an increasingly important component of population growth dynamics in several high-income countries with aging populations and low birth rates. Healthy migrants have fewer health and medical needs and are more able to play active roles at their destination and supporting their families and communities. Supporting migrant health in the context of infectious disease is an important aspect of global public health safety.

In 1990, WHO and IOM held the first international conference on what was then called Migration Medicine (21). Much of the focus was access to and provision of health services for refugees and other migrants as defined in several international legal and policy instruments (see also Chapter 4). In 1999, at the Tampere EU Summit, an agreement was reached on the need for a common EU migration policy including standards for procedures related to granting refugee status, ensuring the quality of those decisions and the return of failed claimants (22). Standards for the emergency care, essential treatment, and necessary medical care of asylum seekers were developed by the Council of Europe in 2003 (23). In 2006, Resolution 1509 was adopted by the Council of Europe dealing with the Human Rights of irregular migrants defined in Article 13. However, it was not until 2007 that the road map for policy development actually took off in Europe. See Table 1.2 with the 22 Steps (24).

As seen previously, migrant health issues had become health policy priorities at national, regional, and global levels. Slowly but surely coordinated, collaborative strategies with shared

TABLE 1.2 22 Steps: Road map of soft policy instruments on migrants' health

No.	Date	Organization	Title	URL
1	2007	Portuguese EU Presidency	Conclusions of Conference on Health and Migration in the European Union	https://bit.ly/2zWgRwL
2	2007	Council of Europe	Bratislava Declaration on Health, Human Rights and Migration	https://bit.ly/2OJzht1
3	2007	Council of the European Union	Draft Council Conclusions on Health and Migration in the EU	https://bit.ly/2pKebwq
4	2008	World Health Assembly	Resolution WHA61.17 (Health of Migrants)	https://bit.ly/2RwwcLg
5	2009	International Organisation for Migration	Consultation on Migration Health: Better health for all in Europe	https://bit.ly/2y7LVZr
6	2010	WHO and IOM	First Global Consultation on Migrant Health, Madrid	https://bit.ly/2RxnwUW
7	2010	WHO Euro	Policy Briefing: How health systems can address health inequities linked to migration and ethnicity	https://bit.ly/2zCe2ls
8	2010	European Commission	Communication on Solidarity in Health: Reducing Health Inequalities in the EU	https://bit.ly/2Psxky0
9	2011	Council of Europe	Recommendations on mobility, migration and access to health care	https://bit.ly/2qJ5u8a
10	2014	WHO Euro HPH-Task Force MFCCH	Equity standards in health care	https://bit.ly/2upRq1V
11	2015–2018	WHO Euro Health Evidence Network (HEN)	Nine synthesis reports on migration and health	https://bit.ly/2RAjlYL
12	2016	United Nations	New York Declaration for Refugees and Migrants	https://bit.ly/2cUNoqS
13	2016	WHO Euro	Strategy and Action Plan on Refugee and Migrant Health	https://bit.ly/2dfcqRB
14	2016	WHO and IOM	Second Global Consultation on Migrant Health, Colombo	https://bit.ly/2kv0obL
15	2017	WHO	Framework of priorities and guiding principles on Promoting the Health of Migrants and Refugees	https://bit.ly/2Kq9yEw
16	2017	WHO & IOM	Proposed health component, Global Compact for Safe, Orderly and Regular Migration	https://bit.ly/2OliZAl
17	2017	IOM	Migration Health in the Sustainable Development Goals	https://bit.ly/2u46AJA
18	2017	World Health Assembly	Resolution 70.15 on 'Promoting the health of refugees and migrants'	https://bit.ly/2D6itXD
19	2017	WHO	Beyond the Barriers: Framing evidence on health system strengthening to improve the health of migrants experiencing poverty and social exclusion	https://bit.ly/2Dp6cwP
20	2018	IOM and Swiss Agency for Cooperation and Development (SDC)	Migration and the 2030 Agenda	https://bit.ly/2Pplo01
21	2018	United Nations	Global Compact for Safe, Orderly and Regular Migration (Final Draft)	https://bit.ly/2zuZ8yj
22	2018	United Nations	Global Compact on Refugees	https://bit.ly/2ATrj5o

responses and actions are replacing fragmented, ad hoc sporadic national migration health activities. With a growing evidence base, as seen in the increase since 2000 in research articles and reviews on migrant health (25), these developing strategies and the policy frameworks need to reflect both regular migratory movements and responses to acute large-volume refugee and humanitarian flows.

What works and what does not? The challenges with policy implementation

Despite the presence of existing and developing protocols and directives, the process of ensuring global migrant health is neither easy nor simple. Pre-existing national legislative and administrative frameworks, often based on historical patterns of regular, organized migration, can influence determinations of nationality, citizenship, right of residence, and access to or availability of services. Migration today is frequently more diverse than previous patterns, and health needs may be more complex than and/or differ from the experiences of past migratory flows. Those variations, both historical and current, have influenced national policy direction and development across Europe.

Policies directed at developing standardized and equally accessible health systems designed and supported to meet the acute-, medium- and longer-term health needs of migrants are founded in principles of equity and basic human rights. The policies support and promote health across the life course of the migrant while recognizing the impact of the various stages of migration on both individual and community health. However, the size and diversity of the migrant population may affect the achievement of some of those goals.

There is global agreement and consensus on what needs to be done to meet the health needs of migrants, as seen by the high level of consistency among the documents of the 'road map', each contribution building on the ones that have gone before. Most of these are based on extensive reviews of research evidence as well as consultations seeking the views of various stakeholders. The main recommendations of these documents are summarized briefly in Table 1.3. Recommendations 1, 2, and 3 concern 'upstream' measures; it is with regard to these that the 'road map' departs from received wisdom prior to 2007, which was almost entirely concerned with health services. Since 2007, importance has been placed on coordinated, structural, sustainable, and evidence-based measures rather than the ad hoc efforts that had traditionally characterized the field of migrant health.

Some recent documents recognize that migration does not always affect health negatively, and that migration does not make a person 'vulnerable' in the individual sense. An 'intersectional' approach (not to be confused with 'intersectoral') is recommended, focussing not only on the main effects of migrant status but also on its interactions with other variables. Recognizing the enormous diversity among migrants makes it possible to focus on the migrants who are most 'left behind' or likely to be excluded and most in need of supportive policies. Instead of recycling static notions about who is or is not vulnerable, the selection of groups should be evidence based.

The temptation to continue to deal with the low-hanging fruit of the downstream initiatives at the regional or global level is further impeded by the lack of terminologies and definitions that define and support health policies that adequately address the generational health issues associated with migrant populations. Policy-driven activities in this regard can include the collection or capture of specific migration-relevant information in national surveys, census or program level. Reflecting individual national history and migrant health experience,

TABLE 1.3 Summary of main recommendations in the 22 Steps 'road map'

1. Data and Research
   Improve data collection and research on migrants' health, including health status, health services, and background information on the migrant population and its situation in the receiving society.
2. Governance
   Strengthen the leadership of efforts to improve health protection for migrants in each country; ensure coordination between stakeholders (including Non-Governmental Organizations [NGOs] and Civil Society Organizations [CSOs]), as well as regional and international collaboration. Raise the awareness of policymakers, managers, and professional bodies concerning migrant health. Promote the involvement of migrants in all activities concerned with protection of their health.
3. Intersectoral action on Social Determinants of Health (SDH)
   Apply an intersectoral, 'whole-of-government' approach to protecting migrants' health, including health impact analyses of policies outside the health sector.
4. Access to health services
   Facilitate migrants' access to health services by improving entitlements and tackling both supply-side and demand-side access barriers (e.g. through better information for migrants about their entitlements, the health system, and how to use it, removal of practical and linguistic barriers to access, and ensuring that migrants need not fear being reported to migration authorities by health services).
5. Quality of services
   Improve the appropriateness, acceptability, and effectiveness of health services for migrants by adapting treatments and service delivery to their needs, paying particular attention to language or communication barriers and 'cultural competence' or 'diversity sensitivity'. Target preventive activities where necessary to ensure they reach, and are effective for, all migrants.
6. Attention for 'vulnerable groups'
   The term 'vulnerable' can refer either to the properties of individuals or of the situation they are in. In the 'road map', these two meanings are often not distinguished. Special attention should be paid to both types of groups, including women, children, elderly, and refugees, victims of trafficking, and undocumented migrants. In addition, attention is often recommended for certain health conditions (e.g. infectious and noncommunicable diseases or mental health problems).

national migrant health policies vary in focus and areas of interest. Some are illness or disease focussed, where concerns are directed towards the presence of conditions on or around the time of arrival. Historical public health or communicable disease control policies provide the policy basis for some national migration health programs. The migrant health experience of other nations produce policy frameworks directed towards maternal child health or psychosocial health. In some nations with large migrant or migrant-origin communities and population, cohorts' migrant health policy directions may take on an ethnic, cultural, or minority focus that is broader in scope than approaches used in other countries. The direction of the policies will from time to time be determined by the political climate. Regardless of the other determinants, if policies do not provide opportunities for migrants to become directly involved in the processes and systems that affect the lives of themselves and their families, they are unlikely to realize their potential.

SUMMARY

As the scale, scope, and complexity of international migration grows, its importance has risen to the top of the global agenda and has led to the politicization of migration. Domestic politics, bilateral and regional relationships, and national security policies of states and countries around the world are increasingly affected by international migration. Policies and regulations concerning migration are rapidly changing and have become more restrictive. Though this might reflect some signs of a growing xenophobia, it can be largely attributed to the fact that migration is generally unplanned, relatively unregulated, and poorly managed.

Despite varying needs of countries and perceptions surrounding migration, it is undoubtedly an integral part of global, social, and economic development. Migration Health has been largely neglected by both receiving and sending countries except in the case of refugees and in conflict situations. Countries have not been able to respond to the rapid pace of current migration, and acknowledging the needs and concerns of migrants to some extent entails recognition of liability and responsibility. The myth that migration ultimately succeeds has lulled authorities into complacency, whereas evidence indicates massive human wastage in terms of avoidable illness, injury neglect, and mortality.

Besides recognizing the need for better planning and management of migration and its health dimensions, it is critical that countries respond to these challenges. The response must include concrete measures suitably adapted to meet the needs of migrants. This does not imply a parallel health system for migrants, as that is both a waste of resources and unsustainable. Failure to respond to the emerging realities of poor health and disease of migrants in a timely and adequate manner could prove to be myopic from a political, economic, and social perspective by all concerned. Effective, coordinated, and integrated policies and initiatives with regard to the health of migrants will be necessary to support those initiatives.

ACKNOWLEDGEMENTS

The authors would like to thank Prof Mark RD Johnson (UK) and Prof David I Ingleby (Netherlands) for their contributions and valuable comments.

REFERENCES

1. Kumar B, Siem H, Haavardsson IK, Winkler AS. *Migrant Health Is Global Health*. Tidsskr Nor Laegeforen. 2017, doi: 10.4045/tidsskr.17.0656 2018.
2. Kumar BN. Health and migration. *Michael*. 2011;8:240–50.
3. Abubakar I, Aldridge RW, Devakumar D et al. The UCL–Lancet Commission on Migration and Health: the health of a world on the move. *Lancet*. 2018;392(10164):2606–54.
4. Kumar BN, Viken B. *Folkehelse i et migrasjonsperspektiv*. Fagbokforlaget; 2010.
5. Leder K, Tong S, Weld L et al. Illness in travelers visiting friends and relatives: a review of the GeoSentinel Surveillance Network. *Clin Infect Dis*. 2006;43:1185–93.
6. WHO Regional Office for Europe. Strategy and action plan for refugee and migrant health in the WHO European Region. 2016. http://www.euro.who.int/__data/assets/pdf_file/0004/314725/66wd08e_MigrantHealthStrategyActionPlan_160424.pdf (accessed 27 January 2018).
7. Bradby H, Humphris R, Newall D, Phillimore J. Public health aspects of migrant health: a review of the evidence on health status for refugees and asylum seekers in the European Region. Copenhagen: WHO Regional Office for Europe; 2015 (Health Evidence Network synthesis report 44).
8. Bollini P, Siem H. No real progress towards equity: health of migrants and ethnic minorities on the eve of the year 2000. *Soc Sci Med*. 1995;41(6):819–28.
9. CoE. *Recommendations on Mobility, Migration and Access to Health Care*. Strasbourg: Council of Europe; 2018. https://bit.ly/2qJ5u8a
10. EU. The EU Health Programme's Contribution to Fostering Solidarity in Health and Reducing Health Inequalities in the European Union 2003–13. Action on Health Inequalities in the European Union. Luxembourg: European Union 2014. https://bit.ly/1kW1VBo
11. Portugal R, Padilla B, Ingleby D, de Freitas C, Lebas J, Pereira Miguel J, editors. *Good Practices on Health and Migration in the EU*. Lisbon: Ministry of Health; 2007.

12. Priebe S, Sandhu S, Dias S et al. Good practice in health care for migrants: views and experiences of care professionals in 16 European countries. *BMC Public Health*. 2011;11:187.
13. Devillé W, Greacen T, Bogic M et al. Health care for immigrants in Europe: is there still consensus among country experts about principles of good practice? A Delphi study. *BMC Public Health* 2011; 11:699.
14. Mladovsky P, Rechel B, Ingleby D, McKee M. Good practices in migrant health: the European experience. *Clin Med*. 2012;12(3):248–52.
15. WHO Migrant Health Report Europe 2018. Report on the health of refugees and migrants in the WHO European Region: no public health without refugee and migrant health. ISBN 978 92 890 5384 6
16. Johnson MRD, et al. MERH2018 Glossary http://www.merhcongress.com/
17. International Organization for Migration. World Migration Report 2018. https://www.iom.int/wmr/world-migration-report-2018 (accessed 25 June 2018).
18. Zimmerman C, Kiss L, Hossain M. Migration and health: a framework for 21st century policy-making. *PLOS MED*. 2011;8:e1001034.
19. Ingleby D, Krasnik A, Lorant V, Razum O, editors. *Health Inequalities and Risk Factors among Migrants and Ethnic Minorities*. Maklu; 2012.
20. Mladovsky P, Rechel B, Ingleby D, McKee M. Responding to diversity: an exploratory study of migrant health policies in Europe. Health Policy. 2012;105(1):1–9.
21. IOM, WHO. Migration medicine. IOM/WHO Conference. Geneva, February 3–6, 1990.
22. European Parliament. Tampere European Council 15 and 16 October 1999, Presidency Conclusions. http://www.europarl.europa.eu/summits/tam_en.htm
23. Council of the EU. 2003. Council Directive 2003/9/EC of 27 January 2003. Laying down minimum standards for the reception of asylum seekers. Brussels: Council of the European Union: L 31/18. *Official Journal of the European Union*. http://eur-lex.europa.eu/LexUriServ/LexUriServ.do?uri=OJ :L:2003:031:0018:0025:En:PDF
24. Ingleby D, Nordstrom C, Magnus HJ, Dias S, Kumar BN. EU JAHEE PFA. 2018. https://jahee.iss.it/wp-7-migration-and-health/
25. Sweileh WM, Wickramage K, Pottie K, Hui C, Roberts B, Sawalha AF, Zyoud SH. Bibliometric analysis of global migration health research in peer-reviewed literature (2000–2016). *BMC Public Health*, 2018;18(1):1.
26. Johnson MRD. Ethnic minorities and health. *Journal of Royal College Physicians London* 1984;18: 228–232. https://www.ncbi.nlm.nih.gov/pmc/articles/PMC5370889/

Migration health theories: Healthy migrant effect and allostatic load. Can both be true?

Bernadette N. Kumar and Esperanza Diaz

LEARNING OBJECTIVES

At the end of this chapter, the reader should be able to:

- Understand some key concepts related to migration health such as ethnicity, race, and multicultural societies, including the relationship they have to each other
- Gain a better understanding of some of the key hypothesis related to migration health

---

INTRODUCTION

The interest in variations of risk of disease and differences in health experiences and outcomes of individuals and groups has been key to forming public health, epidemiology, and clinical practice over centuries. Historically, clinical attitudes to diversity in medical histories and conditions were attributed either to 'racial' differences or to problems related to migration (1). The racial explanation falls short, as the premise of biologically discrete races is inaccurate. Two main approaches emerged over the past three decades as a result — the socio-cultural-political approach, based on social scientist Helman (1984) (see Reference 1), and the biomedical approach, based on Cruickshank and Beevers (1989) (see Reference 1). Several attempts to bridge the gap of this rather segregationist approach have been made over the last decade by explaining diversity in biomedically measurable health conditions due to determinants and factors that include social, cultural, and political factors that can be called 'ethnic'. While these scholarly pursuits must be pursued with rigor, we cannot wait until consensus is reached regarding these approaches. This current migration period poses new challenges for health service providers, policy makers, and professionals in particular in achieving equity in health care. Therefore, it is imperative to gain a better understanding of some of the underlying concepts of: diversity, multicultural societies, race, and ethnicity, how these are interlinked, and why their application is essential to providing better health for all.

KEY CONCEPTS: RACE, ETHNICITY, DIVERSITY, AND MULTICULTURAL SOCIETIES

Given that human beings are one species, it is not surprising that we have more similarities than differences; nonetheless, humans are mentally equipped to differentiate between individuals and groups (2). Race and ethnicity are only two of many ways of trying to differentiate and group humans. Race and ethnicity are complex intertwining concepts and have been used and misused by individuals and societies to identify, classify, and categorize individuals and groups. Despite the shortcomings and harm from stereotyping and stigma, race and ethnicity have been extremely useful in demonstrating inequalities. The potential value of these concepts can only be realized by analysis of the terminology underlying these concepts and by advancing their application in modern multi-ethnic societies.

Race and ethnicity: The historical significance

Race is a concept traditionally used by biologists as a synonym for 'subspecies'. These subspecies were meant to denote isolated populations of a species that contain individuals genetically more closely related to one another than to the rest of the species. Research on race has an inglorious history. Nineteenth century scientists ranked races according to biological and social worth (2). For example, measurements of the head were to gauge intelligence, and Northern Europeans ranked at the top. This kind of research justified slavery, imperialism, and anti-migration policies. Medical practitioners too contributed to racialized science by describing diseases such as drapetomania (irrational and pathological desire of slaves to run away) or explanations that coloured children weighed less due to physical degeneration (3).

Humans are a single species, and massive efforts for over 150 years to classify races have largely failed. Crude classifications included those of Linnaeus: *Homo afer* (Negroid), *H. europaeus* (Caucasoid), *H. asiaticus* (Mongoloid), and *H. americanus* (American Indian). These arbitrary classifications were largely based on discredited theories of innate genetic differences between human populations. The paradigm of race as a marker of fundamental genetically driven biological differences between human subgroups has been deeply undermined by advances in biology showing that genetic differences between human races are small (4). It is known that 85% of all identified human genetic variation is accounted for by differences between individuals whereas only 7% is due to differences between what used to be called 'races'. Describing human variation by race should have clarified the genetic basis of disease. However, since no race has a discrete package of genetic characteristics, genetic diseases are not confined to specific racial groups. The concept of race declined at the end of World War II due to the sensitivities that the era of the Nazis brought to this concept (2).

The modern post-war concept of race evolved in the United States, with race being viewed as a social construction associated with a range of biological and social variables. The importance of social factors in the creation and perpetuation of racial categories has led to the concept broadening to include a common social and political heritage. In the past, race was identified by an observer or assigned, but now to a great degree it is self-identified. The biological concept of race was ill defined, poorly understood, and invalid. In the past few decades, race and ethnicity have been used synonymously, leading to the hybrid term race/ethnicity. Over the past two decades, the ingredients making up race have moved beyond the biological ingredients. However, despite this large overlap, differences between race and ethnicity still persist, and a clear understanding of ethnicity is key to understanding these differences.

Ethnicity: Measurement and importance

> Only when we move beyond race as a proxy and directly measure those concepts believed to be measured by race, will we make truly important advances in describing the true nature of racial variation in health.
>
> **Thomas La Veist (2)**

The need to understand social and cultural factors in health and disease and describe the health and health care of people from ethnic minorities led to the use in health studies of the term ethnicity (2). 'Ethnicity' is derived from the Greek word *ethnos*, meaning nation. Bhopaldefines ethnicity as a multifaceted quality that refers to the group to which people belong, and/or are perceived to belong, as a result of certain shared characteristics, including geographical and ancestral origins, and particularly cultural traditions and languages (5,6). The nature of ethnicity is fluid and dynamic, as the defining characteristics are not fixed or easily measured. Ethnicity focuses on a complex of factors that groups share and that lead to group identity, and in this aspect is close to the post-war sociopolitical concept of race. Ethnicity may include race, nationality, religion, and migrant status, but cannot be reduced to any one of these. Figure 2.1 illustrates that fluid and complex make-up of ethnicity.

In recent years, epidemiological and public health research has witnessed a growing interest in ethnic inequalities in health. However, the concepts of ethnicity and race raise difficult scientific and ethical issues and are controversial variables (7). The fuel of epidemiology is the analysis of differences in the pattern of ill health and disease in populations. This raises the key question, why is a disease more common in one racial or ethnic group of people than another? The answer to this question will help explain the causes of disease and bring benefit to all populations, contributing to one crucial aspect of the epidemiological strategy: demonstration of population variations in disease. The mysteries behind the myriad of ethnic differences are, however, not easily unravelled, as most ethnicity and health research is 'black-box' epidemiology. The causal mechanism behind an association remains unknown and hidden ('black'), but the inference is that the causal mechanism is within the association ('box') (8). The dangers of blindly applying this black-box approach loom large and the possibility of misinterpreting or misusing the data has been documented throughout history, unleashing harm.

Key concepts and ingredients of ethnicity and race are not well understood or defined, thereby making measurements challenging. There have been many challenges in conducting research in the field of 'health, ethnicity, and race' because of a lack of standards in defining race and ethnicity (2). To date there is no consensus on appropriate terms for use in the scientific

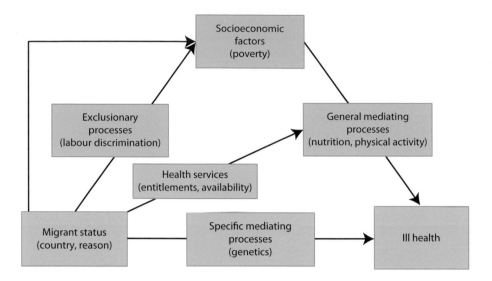

FIGURE 2.1   General model for effects of migrant status on health.

study of health by ethnicity and race, though it is clear these terms are not interchangeable and are not synonymous. We are in the midst of a paradigm shift and may also witness the evolution of a new word or phrase altogether. 'Identifiable populations' is one idea already in the literature but has not caught on (9). An emerging practice is the compound use of the terms race and ethnicity. For science, the worst-case scenario would be undermining the free exchange of ideas and generalizing research data based on differences in concepts. In other words, the term race dominates in the Americas and ethnicity in Europe.

'Racial' and ethnic categories rarely reflect genetically or socioculturally discrete or homogeneous populations. Though these categories also reflect the consequences of the structural forces within societies, and not just individual characteristics, they are rarely viewed as such. Some of the most common measures used are listed here (2,3):

- *Skin colour* is mainly genetically determined, but its measurement is subjective, imprecise, and unreliable and it is a poor proxy for either race or ethnicity.
- *Country of birth* is objective but crude. People of many ethnic or racial groups might be born in a particular country, and an ethnic group (think of the Chinese) may be scattered over many countries. Country of birth also does not enable us to distinguish between the children of migrants and native-born citizens, which can be an important source of inequalities.
- *Parents' and grandparents' national origin or country of birth* is rigid, ignores acculturation of the new generations, current lifestyle, or self-perception, and yields a large heterogeneous 'mixed' group.
- *Names* can identify people's origins; e.g. China and the Indian subcontinent.
- *Algorithms*, e.g. by using father's surname, mother's maiden name, place of birth, self-assessed ethnic identity, and stated ethnicity of grandparents, algorithms can be developed. This method requires a great deal of data and is complex for use in surveys and screenings.

It is important not to throw out the baby with the bathwater, and though it is hard to resist overplaying the colour-blind or colour-conscious paradigms, we need to learn from the past and avoid errors such as inventing ethnic groups, not comparing like with like and lumping dissimilar groups together. Administrative categories as used in census of various countries should not be blindly replicated for research purposes without considering the context. Developing population group categories is complex, as it entails capturing a range of exposures both in a life course and between generations.

However, these categories are merely 'labels' and a first step to understanding and defining a person's ethnicity or race; such labels are often shorthand for potentially important information. For example, the label 'South Asian' refers to a heterogeneous population and must only be used after careful consideration as to the purpose and context. Whilst popular terminology for ethnic minority populations (Asians, Blacks, Chinese, etc.) may suffice for everyday conversation or political exchange, it is too crude for research or practice, and when used needs accurate definition. In clinical practice it is important to understand why these labels exist; however, one needs to tread with caution lest these labels lead to stereotyping.

Some of the harmful effects of using race/ethnicity data include a one-sided focus on the problems of minorities (e.g. stressing health disadvantages at the expense of advantages), fuelling racial prejudices, and interpreting and using data in an ethnocentric way. Notwithstanding these dangers and limitations, the key role of race/ethnicity is in capturing heterogeneity within populations and thereby inequalities in health. The divide between those who want to collect data in order to help minorities ('no data, no progress'), and those who see this as potentially stigmatizing, racializing, and open to abuse has always existed and therefore caution must be exercised lest these dangers are forgotten altogether.

The discussion regarding the categories and labels is ongoing, but it boils down simply to where your ancestors came from (or where you like to think they came from) — i.e. a geographical region. We are getting bogged down in arguments about which label to use, but there is no longer much argument about what we should be measuring. We all agree that traditional racial categories are a pretty useless indicator of genetic differences that can directly influence health (though 'gene pools', defined differently, might have more heuristic value). However, what about indirect influences? Skin colour and other visible physical features are the main drivers of social exclusion. They are the best predictors of getting picked up — and shot dead — by the police. Some nonbiological features, especially hairstyle, language, accent, and clothing, can also be powerful drivers, so there is a need to unpick all the different strands of race/ethnicity. Maybe different indicators are needed for different purposes; some examples are:

- Many physiological determinants of good or bad health may be linked to gene pools.
- Social exclusion is mostly driven by visible and audible characteristics.
- Lifestyles are strongly linked to religions, but also to 'culture' (whatever that may be).

Low socioeconomic position (SEP) is linked to having poor qualifications in the first place, in combination with social exclusion.

Diversity and multicultural societies
Rapidly changing demographics and world events, natural and manmade, have paved the way for increasing diversity. Diversity as a virtue in a nation is an idea from the rise of modern

democracies in the 1790s, where it kept one faction from arrogating all power. Diversity today is not limited to the original idea, but in the modern sense includes several other dimensions such as ethnicity, gender, sexual identity, and so on. Along with globalization of economy, technology, and transportation, migration is a major driver for diversity (10). People move within their country from rural areas to urban ones, and internationally from low-income countries to high-income ones. This leads to the development of multi-ethnic and multicultural societies.

Culture, besides being a complex concept in itself, has as many definitions as those trying to define it. However, what is constant is that everyone has a culture or several cultures or subcultures. Often in this context, culture is seen as something that the 'other' possesses, disregarding one's own culture and leading to the well-known dichotomy of 'us' and 'them'. These concepts are further complicated by the coexistence of many cultures or subcultures. Multiculturalism is an ideology advocating that society should consist of, or at least allow and include, distinct cultural groups, with equal status. Multiculturalism is a term often used to describe the cultural and ethnic diversity of a nation and recognizes that this rich diversity is a positive force in furthering society's nationhood or cultural identity. Multiculturalism contrasts with the mono-culturalism often historically striven for by nation builders in their attempt to produce homogenous nation-states. As opposed to multiculturalism, mono-culturalism implies a so-called cultural unity. The term multiculturalism nowadays is often applied to distinct cultures of migrant groups in developed countries, whereas earlier indigenous peoples were often the mascots of multiculturalism (11).

Multiculturalism began as an official policy in English-speaking countries in Canada in 1971 (12). Given the contentious nature of this ideology, it is hardly surprising that multiculturalism has since then sparked off several debates. Supporters see it as a self-evident entitlement of cultural groups, as a form of civil rights grounded in equality of culture, and hope it will lead to interculturalism – beneficial cultural exchanges. Its opponents often see it as an imposition without consent. They fear it will lead to cultural ghettos, undermining national unity. In Europe especially, opponents see multiculturalism as a direct assault on the national identity, and on the nation itself, and sometimes as a conspiracy against the idea of Europe. In recent years, in several European states, notably the Netherlands and Denmark, right-of-centre governments have reversed the national policy consensus and returned to an official mono-culturalism (12). Similar reversal is the subject of debate in the United Kingdom and Germany, among others.

Several European Union countries have introduced policies for 'social cohesion', 'integration', and (sometimes) 'assimilation'. The origins of these terms are different; they are perceived differently and are not interchangeable, yet applying them synonymously leads to misunderstandings. These policies are a direct reversal of earlier multiculturalist policies and seek to assimilate migrants with a belief to restore a de facto mono-cultural society (13). Although these policies often have the stated aim of increasing national unity, they have often resulted in increased polarization and open criticism of the culture and values of specific minorities. The rejection of multicultural consensus by the mono-culturist political groups in Europe included the revival of a traditional national identity, often defined by ethnicity. Paradoxically, that excludes not only first-generation migrants, but their identifiable descendants, from full membership of a nation. New terms for minorities of migrant descent, for example, *Norwegian born of migrant descent*, have come into use with a renewed emphasis on historical culture that places stricter demands on cultural assimilation.

MIGRATION AND HEALTH

Migration denotes any movement by humans from one locality to another, often over long distances or in large groups. The reasons for migration vary greatly but require the presence of both push and pull factors, and these could be economic, political, cultural, and environmental. Migration policies usually impose barriers to free movement. Migration is often determined by landmark events that govern the social, political, and geographical conditions leading to movements of people either as individuals or masses. The migration of every ethnic group, family, and individual has its own story. Collective or personal circumstances lead to the particular decision to leave one's country or nation for another. Regardless of the motivation, the ultimate goal is the search for a better life.

Migration is now acknowledged as a determinant of health, along with other social factors. With migration, the direction of change in health is not constant, depending on the disease, population studied, and other factors. There are several theories that attempt to explain this complex relationship, but these theories have many limitations, including diversity of migrant populations, ethnocentric assumptions, and their inability to examine the underlying processes. However, a few of the most important theories are outlined here.

Concepts of migration, ethnicity, and race imply major differences in environment and culture, and some differences in biology, which inevitably lead to inequalities in health. Often the underlying cause for inequality is poverty. These concepts and their importance on health are summarized later.

Migrant status refers not just to the fact of being a migrant, but also to particular characteristics such as the type of migrant (e.g. regular, asylum seeker, or irregular) and the country of origin (or ethnicity). Adding a life-course stage perspective and a gender lens further increases and diversifies the complexity of the social determinants of health impact (13).

The exclusionary processes, such as discrimination mediating between migrant status and socioeconomic position, are the barriers that prevent migrants from realizing their full potential in the new country.

General mediating processes are the well-known links between low socioeconomic position and ill health, such as poor living conditions or nutrition. Poverty is largely responsible for these, whether one is a migrant or not. However, these mediating processes may themselves be influenced by migrant status: migrants may have enough money for decent housing, but discrimination by landlords or house agents may deny them access to it. Migrants may not be eligible for the social benefits that protect national citizens in precarious employment who lose their jobs.

Specific mediating processes are ones that do not involve socioeconomic position. For example, migrants at any level of SEP may experience direct, individual hostility – so-called 'race hate' – leading to stress and physical or mental ill-health. Both negative and positive influences on health may be linked to genes or cultural traditions. Migration policies themselves may undermine health, not only by limiting access to health services but also by increasing the difficulties experienced by migrants. Of the social determinants of health (SDH) that are most likely to affect migrants, the fundamental exclusionary processes that impede migrants' successful integration top the list.

Changes in risk/risk factors

Migration is synonymous with changes, and these can be both positive and negative and are both physical and psychosocial. For many it is a huge leap from low-middle-income countries to high-income countries, from rural to urban areas, often occurring in the course of a few hours or days. The most apparent and tangible change is often in the physical environment and includes also climate (warm to cold in general). The health status and determinants of health will differ from country to country depending on which phase of the demographic, epidemiological, and nutritional transition the migrants find themselves in. Migrants from low-income countries are likely to find themselves caught between phases of these transitions when moving from their home countries to their high-income host countries. In some ways their move accelerates these transitions, which may have already started in the home countries and are close to completion in the host countries. A key contributor is urbanization. This is a phenomenon often associated with adverse lifestyle changes, including energy-rich diets far exceeding caloric requirements coupled with physical inactivity, increased levels of smoking, and alcohol (3). In addition, adult populations of rapidly developing countries have dietary and activity patterns vastly different to those of their youth. Many of these adults also faced fetal and early childhood deficiencies related to inadequate nutrition (3).

There is increasing evidence that chronic disease (non-communicable diseases- [NCDs] — see also Chapter 12) risks begin in fetal life and continue into old age (14,15). Adult chronic disease therefore reflects cumulative differential lifetime exposures to damaging physical and social environments. The known risk factors are recognized as being amenable to alleviation throughout life, even into old age. The well-known risk factors for NCDs, such as diet, smoking, alcohol, and physical activity, will change with migration; however, the direction of change, positive or negative, will vary with gender, ethnic group, and countries of origin and destination. Ethnic differences in susceptibility to risk factors require understanding of the gene-environmental interactions. In addition, the gene-environment interactions play a role in the development of chronic disease. Examples of this are association between low growth in early infancy (low weight at 1 year) and increased risk of coronary heart disease (16), blood pressure highest in those with retarded fetal growth and greater weight gain in infancy, short stature associated with increased risk of coronary heart disease and stroke, and to some extent, diabetes (17).

The life-course perspective (refer also to Chapter 7) emphasizes that there is an accumulation of risk, either positive or negative (18). Migration will impact these risk factors depending on where in the life-course migration happens. A critical period of growth and development in the lifecycle, adolescence establishes behavioural patterns that might predict future lifestyles. The real concern about these early manifestations of chronic diseases is that once developed they tend to remain with that individual throughout life. On the other hand, this group is more likely to be responsive to changes in lifestyle if they are targeted early in life, and considering that their differences with the host population are not as great as the first generation. Physical changes are usually accompanied by psychosocial changes that might be harder to visualize and subtler in nature. These are related to a loss of cultural identity and professional status, inability to comprehend societal norms, loss of kin as well as of local milieu — all contributing to an increased stress level (6,11). However, most subtle, hard to visualize, and measure are the loss of family, friends, social network, and the difficulty of establishing new relationships in places where the societal norms/rules are different.

Migration and health theories and hypotheses

Over the past few decades, several hypotheses attempting to explain the differences in health between migrants and non-migrants and between minorities and the majority population have been launched. Some of the most important among them include the following:

- *Healthy migrant effect*: Often migrant populations tend to comprise individuals in a particularly good state of physical and mental health, perhaps reflecting a selection bias. The similarity with the 'healthy worker effect' (19), due to the exclusion of unhealthy workers from employment, has given rise to the term 'healthy migrant effect' (20). The selective migration theory is based on a selection process that determines the type of person that migrates. Often younger people migrate, and they are as a rule healthier; therefore, age bias can be one source of the healthy migrant effect. Younger people are usually healthy people willing to take risks, and are able to deal better with the hazards of migration. Younger migrants might be healthier than the non-migrant population of the area to which they migrate, and also compared to those left behind in the country of origin. The 'migrant health paradox' indicates that when migrants arrive in the country of destination, their health status is usually better than that of the hosts (21). However, the health advantage deteriorates rapidly as the length of stay in host countries increases, leading to what has been termed the 'exhausted migrant' effect (22). Post-migration cultural dislocation and stress might also adversely affect health, leading to worse health profiles among migrants. In addition, as described previously, some gene environment interactions result in higher risk for certain diseases and conditions among migrants.
- *Theories of ill health*: The intersection of health and migration is very specific because populations differ greatly, especially considering the vulnerability of migrants. Migration might adversely affect health, starting with perilous migrant journeys. Later, cultural dislocation and stress (see below) might add to the disease burden and eventually the next generation, as seen with migrant women with adverse pregnancy outcomes. The health status of some migrants deteriorates in the country of destination due to several factors (the determinants of ill-health). As is widely known, health depends on a combination of interrelated factors that are usually divided into specific groups: constitutional factors, individual lifestyles, social and community networks, living and working conditions, and general socioeconomic, cultural, and environmental conditions.
- *Negative effect*: The theory of the negative effect of migration states that a new environment adds a new set of health risks, and morbidity and mortality are increased by movement from low-risk to high-risk areas. An example could be in the case of cancer; many migrants from low-income countries will have a lower risk for certain types of cancer that are more common in high-income countries. The migration process is stressful, and adjustments in the new environment take their toll on health and contribute to high prevalence of ill health and disease, such as mental health, illustrated by high levels of depression.
- *Allostatic load*: This refers to the price the organism has to pay for its efforts to maintain stability through change. This goes to the core of migrants' need for adjusting to a new environment. Factors that can ease this process of adjustment are, for example, well-functioning coping strategies, physical activity, and adequate nutrition (23).

- *Cultural theories/acculturation*: Cultural differences impact environmental factors such as lifestyle — diet, exercise, and smoking, to name a few. The beliefs of migrants may be very different from the beliefs of health care professionals, and so there can be difficulties in understanding and barriers which inhibit health promotion and effective clinical management. The behaviour of health care professionals towards those of a different race can lead to feelings of discrimination and lack of sympathy, so that a gulf can develop. This gulf can be bridged if simple measures are adopted: training in communication, culturally sensitive health-promotion programmes, specific programmes relevant for those of defined ethnic groups, and as a basic means to increase confidence and trust, elementary skills in the migrants' native language. The acculturation theory implies taking on cultural values and practices of the host population, and there are several models for this, some of which are mentioned below (6,11):
    - *Single continuum*: This is where migrants accept the host culture with time and the host accepts them, thereby maintaining a mono-cultural society with migrants moving towards assimilation (with dominance of ties with new host culture).
    - *Two-culture model*: Here migrants accept the new culture or reject the new culture; marginalization — they do not adopt the new culture but do not retain the old culture either; separation/segregation — dominance of own culture that leads to isolation.
    - *Multidimensional model*: Integration — keeping one's own culture plus acquiring ties to the new is the first phase of this model, but this is a process of acculturation that will ultimately lead to a mixture of the two cultures, depending on the arena, such as assimilation at work but separation with regard to food habits.

Research on acculturation and health shows that given the diverse patterns of adaptation, different exposures/behaviours that shift morbidity and mortality acculturation are not only context specific but also ethnic group specific. Acculturation can be a risk factor as well as a protective factor. One study from the United States on obesity among Latinas found 75% of less acculturated Latinas thought it worse to be a smoker than to be obese, but 75% of the more acculturated thought the opposite (24). Another illustration among Turkish children in Germany showed that lower acculturation was associated with lower prevalence of asthma, atopic dermatitis, and allergy (25). The complexities of these issues lead researchers to suggest that the use of these measures of acculturation should be abandoned or they will inadvertently fuel weak explanations of health disparities by focusing only on culture. It is therefore important to focus on structural constraints that are as important to examine as the societal contexts that promote or inhibit health.

- *Differences in SEP or material circumstances*: This has been a highly debated and discussed theory. In 1990, Navarro (31) claimed that ethnic inequalities were predominately dominated by socioeconomic inequalities, whereas Smaje (9) argued that SEP might play a role along with cultural and genetic elements, and Wild and McKeigue (26) claimed that SEP played a minimal or no role in ethnic inequalities (1). It has been proposed that differences in the health of migrants and ethnic minorities are just a proxy for the SEP differences, as migrants and ethnic minorities often represent the lower socioeconomic strata. This explanation is fraught with several methodological challenges. The indicators of SEP available in most studies do not adequately account for ethnic differences in SEP, and secondly, any attempt therefore to adjust for or address these indicators has serious problems. While controlling for socioeconomic factors might suggest that they do not contribute to ethnic inequalities, the process for standardizing SEP when making comparisons across groups is not straightforward. Limitations include traditional class groupings (not internally homogenous), unemployment (not per se, but length of employment is the key issue), and most indicators do not give a lifetime risk estimate. Interactive effects and advantages and disadvantages throughout life must be considered, as in the case of migrants where socioeconomic disadvantage accumulates — also called the weathering hypothesis by Geronimous (1). Another phenomenon is the downward social mobility of migrants post migration — those with a higher social class in their home countries find themselves suddenly classified into a lower class (i.e. a Syrian doctor working in a restaurant), and this poses a great challenge in classification. As described previously in the discussion on acculturation theories, it is not unusual that migrants or ethnic minorities live in areas that are deprived, with worse environmental conditions or poorer services that impact health. This effect, called the 'area effect', adds to individual socioeconomic disadvantage.

- *Genetic or biological differences*: Neither cultural practices nor biology are static. It is also important to consider that biological differences are often a consequence of both genetic and environmental determinants over time. Ethnic identity changes over time and is dependent on the social context, and other elements contribute to cultural practices. Genetic or biological differences in risk impact disease outcomes, and in particular this might be intergenerational, with the risk being transmitted from mother to child. Some health issues like sickle cell anaemia can be linked to genetic factors.

- *Racism and discrimination*: A growing body of robust evidence shows that racism, stigma, prejudice, and discrimination are bad for health (27). Racial discrimination occurs on three levels: (i) interpersonal (interactions between individuals), (ii) systemic (production, control and access to labour, material, and symbolic resources within a society), and (iii) internalized (i.e. the incorporation of racist attitudes, beliefs, or ideologies into one's worldview) (28). Laboratory and community-based studies show the harmful health effects of all forms of discrimination, including both acute and chronic stressors, across a range of physical and mental health outcomes such as depression, psychological distress, anxiety, and well-being (28,29). As a result of racism and discrimination, poorer access to health care influences health-seeking behaviour and often results in poorer health. This access to health care may be measured by studying utilization patterns or clinical outcomes like morbidity and mortality. Migrants' access to health care may be affected by several factors relating to formal and informal barriers. Informal barriers include economic and legal restrictions. Formal barriers include language and psychological and sociocultural factors.

- *Transmission of disease*: Are migrants carriers of disease? Although there are historical examples of the introduction of disease into new settings through human mobility (e.g. the spread of infection from European colonial settlers), the risk of transmission from migrating populations to host populations is generally low. Studies on tuberculosis, for example, suggest that the risk of transmission is elevated within migrant households and migrant communities, but not in host populations (27). Nonetheless, several high income countries (HICs) screen migrants for tuberculosis as part of pre-migration visa application checks. Migrant populations may come from countries with a high burden of disease or as a result of socioeconomic disadvantage, comorbidity and malnutrition, poor health access and low immunization coverage (27). It is not uncommon for disease outbreaks to correspond to the drivers or circumstances of migration, especially in situations of conflict which dismantle already weak public health systems. Economically disadvantaged migrants often live in overcrowded conditions, suffer from poor nutrition, which can lower their immunity, and have poor access to clean water and sanitation, inhibiting personal hygiene (27). Illness and infections may also be acquired or spread via transit routes and transport means. For example, air travel can facilitate rapid geographic spread of infections. However, even risk of air travel-related outbreaks is low to modest if the destination setting has strong surveillance and inclusive public health services, which are also crucial to prevent pandemics — whether associated with population movement or not (27). Epidemiological patterns and related risks are readily addressed by assessing the infectious disease burden among populations and using data to design targeted interventions to contain outbreaks, prevent new infections through immunization, and promote early presentation and treatment through well-conducted awareness activities. Because of the prejudice and unfounded fear that can be generated by misuse of surveillance data, caution is required when releasing potentially stigmatizing disease prevalence figures for public consumption.

- *Statistical artefact*: This theory is the least likely of all explanations, that the differences observed are only the result of bias due to errors in methodology.

CONCLUSION

While the discussion regarding categories and labels is still ongoing, it all boils down simply to ancestry. While we are not caught up in arguments about which label to use, race or ethnicity, any longer the challenge remains in picking the right indicator for the right purpose, as no single measure or indicator can be used universally.

Migration provides a naturally occurring experiment, which may establish the etiological importance of factors acting at different points in the life course (11). Studies of migration are a powerful means of generating and testing hypotheses despite problems of bias and the difficulties of making comparable measurements due to indicators of socioeconomic position that might be appropriate for migrants/ethnic minorities. When migrants and their offspring are compared with other groups, changing socioeconomic circumstances within and between generations in different migrant and ethnic groups can be linked to changing health patterns (11). This perspective can explore the health of adults as related to factors that they have been exposed to across their life course. We must consider this life-course approach also in light of sociopolitical economies — global forces over a period of time. An advantage of studying both migrants and their offspring is that changes in lifestyle after migration might be easier to capture and contrast. If the risk of cardiovascular disease (CVS) increases among migrants from low-risk to high-risk areas, it is highly probable that factors are acting later on life. However, if the risk of the country of origin is retained then it is likely that genetic factors exert a greater influence. According to Forsdahl, migrants exposed to relative deprivation in childhood encountering abundance in adult life face an even greater risk of coronary heart disease than the host population (14), as might be expected in the case of a large majority of first-generation migrants born in developing countries.

A more nuanced approach to the factors underlying ethnic and migrant differences is required rather than simply attributing them to socioeconomic, cultural/behavioural, or racial/genetic. Migration impacts the health of a population in several ways: first by contributing to the sociodemographic changes, as migrants include a broad category of individuals and therefore will affect the age-sex structure or the socioeconomic characteristics. Second, more specifically related to health issues, migration contributes to increase or decrease in place-specific rates of illness and mortality. Ethnicity and migration are interacting concepts which may act as determinants for migrants' health and access to health care. Socioeconomic differences are key but are not the only determinants of ethnic and migrant health inequalities. We have by no means found all the theories, hypotheses, or explanations; there are still unidentified components that increase the risk of poor health for migrants over and above SEP disadvantage. Therefore, in trying to understand these issues we often use the 'silo approach', separating each explanation. In contrast Balarajans' term multiple jeopardy includes these explanations together: lower SEP, area effect, racism and discrimination, lower jobs, less education, living in crowded areas, poorer access to health care. Last but not least, discrimination is not only unfair and illegal, but is a threat to health at all stages of the migration process (1). The ability of individuals to mitigate the impacts of discrimination varies, reflecting several factors, including early childhood, formative adulthood experiences, and the migration process itself as well as the cumulative burden of stressors such as job insecurity, lack of social contacts, and environmental stressors (30). This highlights the importance of taking a life-course approach to understanding the health impacts of racial discrimination.

In our migration times, some politicians try to curry electoral favour by migrant-blaming. Stigmatizing rhetoric has meant that the rights of migrants are under attack by the same structures and processes that are supposed to protect them. That is, views, words, and actions by those in power instigate discrimination and restrict access to education, work, justice, and health (27). In a previous Lancet Commission on Global Governance, which addressed the political origins of health inequity, the authors outline the major influences and governance deficits which affect health and the power disparities that govern health inequity (27). The report highlights how the goals of the health sector, which are inclusive towards better health for all, commonly come into policy conflict with the interests of influential global actors who prioritize national security, safeguarding of sovereignty, and economic goals. Migrants often suffer even deeper exclusion, despite their participation as workers, parents, consumers, and investors in the economy; nonetheless, they are frequently left out of decision-making democratic processes. With these profound governance gaps, voices are few and far between to combat the current highly charged political rhetoric that demonizes migrants and which will lead to ever-deepening health disparities.

ACKNOWLEDGEMENTS

The authors would like to thank Prof David I Ingleby (Netherlands) for his contributions and valuable comments, and Prof RS Bhopal for the inspiration and his extensive work on this subject.

REFERENCES

1. Macbeth H, Shetty PS. *Health and Ethnicity*. London: Taylor & Francis Group; 2001. Chapter 1. Pgs 1-5.
2. Bhopal RS. *Migration, Ethnicity, Race and Health in Multicultural Societies*. Oxford University Press; 2014.

3. Kumar BN, Viken B. *Folkehelse i et migrasjonsperspektiv*. Fagbokforlaget; 2010.
4. Bhopal R. Is research into ethnicity and health racist, unsound, or important science? *Br Med J*. 1997;314:1751–9.
5. Chaturvedi N. Ethnicity as an epidemiological determinant: crudely racist or crucially important? *Int J Epidemiol*. 2001;30(5):92.
6. Bhopal R. Glossary of terms relating to ethnicity and race: for reflection and debate. *J Epidemiol Commun Health*. 2004;58(6):441–5.
7. Whitehead M. Life and death across the millennium. In: Drever FaW M, editor. *Health Inequalities*. London: The Stationery Office; 1997.
8. Skrabanek P. The emptiness of the black box. *Epidemiology*. 1994;5(5):553–5.
9. Smaje C. *Health and Ethnicity: A Review of the Literature*. London: King's Fund Institute; 1994.
10. Kumar B, Siem H, Haavardsson IK, Winkler AS. *Migrant Health is Global Health*. Tidsskr Nor Laegeforen. 2017, doi: 10.4045/tidsskr.17.0656
11. Kumar BN. *Ethnic Differences in Obesity and Related Risk Factors for Cardiovascular Diseases among Immigrants in Oslo*. Norway: Unipub; 2006.
12. WHO Migrant Health Report Europe 2018. Report on the health of refugees and migrants in the WHO European Region: no public health without refugee and migrant health.
13. Ingleby D, Nordstrom C, Magnus HJ, Dias S, Kumar BN. EU JAHEE PFA. 2018. https://jahee.iss.it/wp-7-migration-and-health/
14. Forsdahl A. Are poor living conditions in childhood and adolescence an important risk factor for arteriosclerotic heart disease? *Br J Prev Soc Med*. 1977;31(2):91–5.
15. Barker DJ. Fetal origins of cardiovascular disease. *Ann Med*. 1999;31(Suppl 1):3–6.
16. Eriksson J, Forsen T, Tuomilehto J, Osmond C, Barker D. Size at birth, childhood growth and obesity in adult life. *Int J Obes Relat Metab Disord*. 2001;25(5):735–40.
17. Rich-Edwards JW, Colditz GA, Stampfer MJ et al. Birthweight and the risk for type 2 diabetes mellitus in adult women. *Ann Intern Med*. 1999;130(4 Pt 1):278–84.
18. Kuh D, Ben-Shlomo Y. *A Life Course Approach to Chronic Disease Epidemiology*. 2nd ed. New York: Oxford University Press; 2004.
19. Li CY, Sung FC. A review of the healthy worker effect in occupational epidemiology. *Occup Med (Lond)*. 1999;49(4):225–9.
20. Newbold KB. Self-rated health within the Canadian immigrant population: risk and the healthy immigrant effect. *Soc Sci Med*. 2005;60(6):1359–70.
21. Chen J, Wilkins R. *The Health of Canada's Immigrants in 94–95*. Health Reports Canada Statistics; 1996.
22. Bollini P, Siem H. No real progress towards equity: health of migrants and ethnic minorities on the eve of the year 2000. *Soc Sci Med*. 1995;41(6):819–28.
23. McEwen BS. Stress, adaptation, and disease: allostasis and allostatic load. *Ann N Y Acad Sci*. 1998;840(1):33–44.
24. Abraído-Lanza AF. Do healthy behaviors decline with greater acculturation? Implications for the Latino mortality paradox. *Soc Sci Med*. 2005;61(6):1243–55.
25. Grüber C. Is early BCG vaccination associated with less atopic disease? An epidemiological study in German preschool children with different ethnic backgrounds. *Pediatr Allergy Immunol*. 2002;13(3):177–81.
26. Wild S, McKeigue P. Cross sectional analysis of mortality by country of birth in England and Wales, 1970–92. *BMJ*. 1997;314(7082):705–10.
27. Abubakar I, Aldridge RW, Devakumar D et al. The UCL–Lancet Commission on Migration and Health: the health of a world on the move. *Lancet*. 2018;392(10164):2606–54.
28. Paradies Y, Ben J, Denson N et al. Racism as a determinant of health: a systematic review and meta-analysis. *PLOS ONE*. 2015;10:e0138511.
29. Khan M, Ilcisin M, Saxton K. Multifactorial discrimination as a fundamental cause of mental health inequities. *Int J Equity Health*. 2017;16:43.
30. Williams DR, Mohammed SA. *J Behav Med* 2009;32:20.
31. Navarro V. Race or class versus race and class: Mortality differentials in the United States. *Lancet* 1990;336(8725):1238–1240.

CHAPTER 3

Culture, language and the clinic: Three stories, two keys

Iona Heath and Edvin Schei

LEARNING OBJECTIVES

This chapter should be able to:

- Help clinicians broaden their range and solve more problems
- Offer strategies and skills
- Inspire practice

We hope this will help the reader to become a better professional helper, and to appreciate the privilege of being able to ease the suffering, pain, and disease of an ethnically mixed, culturally heterogeneous, and constantly evolving patient population.

THE TWO KEYS

When invited to write this chapter, we asked ourselves, 'What makes patients from a migrant population fundamentally different from other patients?' Our answer is that the difficulties presented by ethnicity, language barriers, cultural ignorance, and incongruent expectations are differences in degree and frequency but constructed from the same materials as the challenges posed by any other group of patients. We believe that if clinicians are enabled to work in ways that are properly patient-centred, they may, with experience, acquire curiosity, relationship skills, and a conception of medicine's ethos, which will allow them to devise ways to be of some help even in the most complex of circumstances, when all seems hopelessly difficult, muddled, and confusing. At the risk of oversimplifying, we suggest that two keys are all that clinicians need to open up therapeutic spaces and possibilities. The doors to such possibilities are, paradoxically, often hidden or obstructed by doctors' genuine attempts to help — especially by conscientious adherence to the conventional, diagnosis-fixated, algorithmic approach to treatment that is taught at medical school and dominant in hospital medicine.

The first magic key is to realize that emotion is crucially important in clinical work, on more than one level. Emotional reactions to traumatic life events manifest themselves through powerful physiological mechanisms that can cause or intensify bodily symptoms, which in turn may trigger second-order feelings of fear and worry with their concomitant physiological arousal, and so on, in a self-reinforcing spiral that often ends in the doctor's office (1). On a different level, emotional rapport determines whether people, including physicians and patients, come to trust others and engage in the kinds of dialogue and collaboration that lead to change (2). The second key is to be persistently curious about how 'the world' is seen and understood by the patient and relatives, acknowledging that every single person on earth has a unique view of reality, with its own logic (3).

Both keys require listening skills that can be quite difficult to learn, depending on the clinician's background. They need to be practiced over time, as part of a clinician's personal, professional learning. Both keys will make it easier to act in pertinently open-minded ways and seek out the kind of information and insight that may allow helpful ideas and strategies to emerge in both doctor and patient. We must underline that there is a third essential key to good doctoring in complicated landscapes: a solid grasp of biomedicine. But despite what medical education seems to imply, this key rarely works without the other two, which is a cause of much suffering and bewilderment in patients, as well as frustration and feelings of inadequacy in knowledgeable clinicians.

In this chapter, we use several versions of a chest pain consultation within which the biomedical concerns remain constant, while the personal characteristics vary. We start with a version in which the patient belongs to the majority, non-migrant population.

An Example: Chest Pain without Heart Disease

CLINICAL VIGNETTE

A 28-year-old man, Bodvar Berg, enters a general practice consulting room in Norway, complaining of chest pain. He is pale, clearly frightened, and clutches his left chest with both hands, telling the nurse that he is afraid it might be something wrong with his heart. The nurse in the reception discovers that an electronic discharge letter from the local hospital has arrived today. The patient had been admitted two days ago with chest pain and had undergone all the appropriate tests for heart disease, with negative results.

SCENARIO A: DR HANSEN MEETS A NON-MIGRANT PATIENT

Dr Helene Hansen orders another ECG before seeing the patient. When he enters, she greets him kindly and starts asking about his symptoms, when and how it started, the intensity, duration, and location of the chest pain, whether it is related to physical exertion, and so on. When questioned about the family history, Bodvar tells her that his father died of a heart attack at the age of 50. Dr Hansen does a thorough clinical examination. She summarizes for Bodvar: all the findings are completely normal. She shows him the discharge letter from the hospital, smiling warmly: 'As you can see, there are absolutely no signs of heart disease. I suggest you take a few days of sick leave and then return to work. There's nothing to worry about!'

Bodvar makes no sign that he is ready to leave. He again clutches his chest and asks in an insistent tone of voice: 'But doctor, surely there must be something wrong when I am in so much pain?!'

Doctor and patient argue back and forth for a while, until Bodvar reluctantly rises, accepts a 2-day sick leave, and leaves the office with a sullen expression on his face.

We will shortly present scenario B, in which this patient meets a doctor who uses the two keys to explore his lifeworld. But before we get there, we want to point out some of the mechanisms that make otherwise excellent physicians ineffective when faced with difficult situations like the one in the example. A kernel of the problem stems from medical education and science itself – it is absorbed with the biological and diagnostic facets of healing to such an extent that many doctors end up unaware of the fundamental need to understand and influence people and relationships. In the example, Dr Hansen follows an established algorithm for coronary disease detection, seemingly unaware that the final effect of all her effort and expertise on the patient's health depends entirely on the patient's trust and cooperation, which both hinge on how the patient thinks and feels about his problem and the help offered. Or, if she knows this, she seems unable to use professional behaviour to achieve the mutual trust needed to be medically effective.

Another explanation for Dr Hansen's and other doctors' tendency to avoid working with emotion and patients' subjective experiences is that it may be emotionally threatening on a subconscious level (4). Explicit guidance of clinicians' emotional development has been largely absent from medical education, where open display of emotion tends to be seen as a sign of weakness or being unprofessional (5,6). Yet medical novices are frequently confronted with emotionally laden experiences, including death, suffering, constant competition, inadequacy, and the fear of failure and shame (7–9). Psychological defence mechanisms to emotional overload include disengagement and emotional distancing from other people's suffering, which are disturbingly prevalent among medical students and young doctors (10). Such defence mechanisms clearly establish barriers to the development of rapport, trust, and a therapeutic alliance between helper and patient – which happen to be just the therapeutic tools that doctors most need (11). The censorship on emotion in medical education is compounded by the learning mechanisms of socialization and professional identity formation, whereby behaviours and values that are prevalent in role models and 'the system', such as a tendency to treat emotional and lifeworld aspects of patients' experiences as medically irrelevant, are adopted by newcomers (12).

This professional acculturation usually happens tacitly (13,14). Hence, it may be difficult to change problematic aspects of professional behaviour unless one actively seeks feedback and guidance, in collegial groups for instance (15).

SCENARIO B: DR JENSEN MEETS THE SAME NON-MIGRANT PATIENT

We now present a second version of our example. This time, Bodvar meets a Norwegian doctor who realizes that the biomedical approach has been fully explored at the hospital, that information about heart disease has not helped him, that a new ECG or physical exam will contribute nothing, and that she needs to address his anxiety and his understanding of the causes of chest pain. Her best strategy for helping Bodvar adjust his emotions and cognitions is to behave in ways known to foster trust and generate shared understanding (3). To achieve this, the second doctor consciously aims to show Mr Berg that she respects and understands his emotions, such as pain and fear, and that she is keenly interested in understanding not only what his signs and symptoms are, but also how he interprets them, and what he does not understand and might possibly gain by sharing in her biomedical knowledge, once enough trust has been established.

Dr Joanna Jensen reads the discharge letter and sees that the hospital's diagnostic clarification has not been helpful to the patient, since he has come again today. The clear evidence that Bodvar has the healthy heart expected at his age makes it necessary to look in other directions for a way of providing help. Clearly one goal will be to help him modify his belief that the chest pain has a cardiac origin.

Dr Jensen asks Bodvar to explain why he has come to see her today and what he would like her to help him with. As he describes the symptoms, she focusses all her attention on him, listening respectfully and communicating empathy with his distress both nonverbally and with explicit statements such as 'that must have been frightening'. When he pauses and looks at her, she asks: 'What do you think might cause this pain in your chest?' He replies that he does not really know, but he thinks it must be the heart, since it's in the left side. 'And my dad died from a heart attack when he was only 50 years old. Earlier today I called my mother, she cried on the phone and insisted I should see the doctor again'. Dr Jensen thanks him for this information and tells him that fortunately chest pain often has other causes, especially in younger people. Pain can sometimes emerge if people are living under strain. Has there been any strain in Bodvar's life recently?

She learns that he is a computer engineer who has been trying to save his business from bankruptcy. He's tremendously overworked and for the last 18 months he has mostly slept on a couch in the office, eaten fast food from a nearby petrol station, and has hardly seen friends or taken a break.

As Bodvar shares his story with the listening doctor, his face regains normal colour, he seems to forget his pain. He stops and looks at her. 'To me it seems obvious that a life like yours would be very difficult for anybody!' she says. 'It certainly would make my body ache, I'm sure', she adds with a smile. 'So you think it is only that, and not the heart?' he replies, looking at her now in a non-defensive, inquisitive manner. 'Yes I do, and I think you are very fortunate to have been so thoroughly examined at the hospital, so that maybe you can let go of your fear now. I guess the loss of your dad was awful, that may add to the pain, that's how humans work, you know. And who knows, perhaps you have been working so much in order to keep your thoughts busy with less painful stuff?' Bodvar nods his head thoughtfully and grasps her hand. 'Thank you so much, doctor'.

BARRIERS AND MORE BARRIERS

Within every conversation between people, there are barriers to shared understanding, many of which have nothing to do with culture or language differences. Some stem from differences in personal experience, the use and command of words and expressions, and social context. In any relationship, the other person can never be fully knowable. Things constantly get 'lost in translation'.

Within the clinical consultation, in conversations between professionals and people who are or believe themselves to be sick, such barriers become more intrusive. Awareness of what a story or a complaint means has to be carefully constructed while consciously negotiating as many of the barriers as possible, balancing hypotheses, doubt, curiosity, and careful checking of one's developing understanding (16). Differences between the experiences of patient and clinician may prevent the latter from grasping the existential and lifeworld implications of the patient's predicament (3). These problems are likely to be exacerbated by the technical language of medicine, by the patient's relative ignorance of biomedical facts and thought processes, and by the power differential between professionals and patients (17) as well as by the effects that sickness and worry have on mental and social functioning. As if this were not enough, health care professionals are required to face at least two things: we have unavoidable responsibilities not only to the patient but also to the state and to the professional standards of medicine.

Robb and Greenhalgh point out that 'almost all actual conversations … are a mix of communicative and strategic action', expressing the distinction made by the philosopher Jürgen Habermas (18,19). Communicative action is sincere, open, and directed towards achieving understanding and consensus, whereas strategic action is oriented to success (an ulterior motive) rather than to understanding. It seems clear that strategic action predominated in Bodvar's consultation with Dr Hansen, with both patient and doctor trying to manipulate the other, whereas communicative action and the will to understand clearly prevailed in the consultation with Dr Jensen.

When health care professionals attempt to provide care to migrants, another whole tier of barriers is superimposed on this complex infrastructure. There may not be a single word of shared language. And even with the help of language education, or interpretation or advocacy services, the scope for misunderstanding remains huge, even for the well-educated executive migrant. For those fleeing extreme poverty and refugees fleeing violence, persecution, imprisonment, and torture, the gap between their lifeworld and that of the professional can seem unbridgeable: the realities of life become unspeakable by the patient and unimaginable by the doctor. Also, religious and political values and practices may be very different, or in active conflict. What is the clinician to do, then? How can he or she bridge the gap, cross the barriers, and achieve a workable understanding of the patient's plight and potential?

Medical education teaches the complex taxonomy of medical diagnosis as the route to, and the justification of, subsequent treatment, and in so doing, encourages reductionist generalization and the classification of individuals into categories who hold something in common. This something is usually but not always a diagnostic category. The danger is that the ability to classify tends to prioritize one aspect of an individual existence above all other possibilities. Even with the best of intentions, generalizations can too easily stray beyond biomedical diagnosis into the arenas of race, culture, and religion, tipping into bias discrimination and prejudice — additional barriers that too often become insuperable. As literary critic Christopher Ricks points out in his discussion of the anti-Semitism in the work of the poet TS Eliot (20), the word 'discrimination' is a two-edged sword with its dual meanings of fine judgment and prejudice insufficiently separated so that one bleeds into the other all too readily.

Clinicians need to find ways to bridge these gaps and become working partners and healers for people with whom they seem to have nothing in common, and where the usual tools of biomedicine are useless, or counterproductive. One answer is the access we all have to a basic source of understanding, and of healing power, which are the fundamental conditions of human existence — the vulnerability, mortality, dependence, and existential loneliness shared by all humans, however different their lives might be (21). To the extent that the clinician acknowledges these dimensions in her own experience, she will find common ground with others who suffer. From this place, where the health care worker allows her own personhood, and experiences of longing and uncertainty, to be tools for professional understanding and connection, ways of supporting the other can emerge. In ancient mythology, the healer was always wounded (22).

SCENARIO C: DR JENSEN MEETS A MIGRANT WORKER

In the next iteration of our chest pain consultation, the patient is a migrant craftsman. We shall see how this adds layers to his suffering, while also offering more clues to the physician looking for connections between lifeworld and symptoms.

A 28-year-old man of East European origin, Wladimir Smolensk, comes to a consultation in Norwegian general practice with our previous Norwegian GP, Dr Jensen, complaining of chest pain. He speaks a mixture of Norwegian and English and, apart from the hesitancy of his language, his presentation is as Bodvar's was.

Dr Joanna Jensen, the exemplary physician of this chapter, begins as she did for Bodvar Berg. She asks Wladimir to explain why he has come to see her today, and what he would like her to help him with, and when he replies she again takes care to signal, verbally and nonverbally, that she is listening and is affected by what she hears. Then she asks: 'I have my thoughts about the cause of your pain, but I would very much like to hear what you have been thinking.' 'It must be my heart, since it's here on the left side'. He clutches his chest again, frowning. 'And my dad died 6 months ago from a heart attack at the age of 55. I was here then; I had this big job and couldn't get home until it was too late'. Tears fill his eyes. 'I called my mother this morning; she cried on the phone and made me promise to see a doctor again'. Jensen thanks him for this information. She then tells him that chest pain often has non-cardiac causes and can develop if people live under strain. Has there been any strain in Wladimir's life recently, in addition to the terrible shock of his father's death?

She learns that Wladimir has worked for 3 years as a painter in Norway, and now runs his own business with four employees. He works 12–14 hours a day, including weekends, and has a very unhealthy life style. Lately, an important client has refused to pay for a big paint job, and he has become increasingly worried about his financial responsibilities. Back home in Poland, his wife is depressed and constantly complaining on the phone – she is pregnant and has to take care of their two little children as well as his aging mother, who seems to be getting increasingly confused.

As he talks, Wladimir's face regains normal colour, he seems to forget his pain. He looks at the doctor, waiting for a response. 'Maybe you can hear that a life like yours would be very difficult for anybody? It certainly would make my body ache, I'm sure', she says with a smile. 'So you think it could be that, and not the heart?' he replies, with an open expression in his face. 'Yes I do, and I think you are very fortunate to have been so thoroughly examined at the hospital, and I hope you can let go of your fear. I think your body is reacting to the stress of responsibility you've been under for so long. And the death of your dad before you could return home was awful – that may add to the pain, that's how human bodies work, you know. They can mimic symptoms affecting those who are very close to them. The good thing you can get out of this pain is a reminder that you need to make changes in your life, maybe?' In view of his hesitancy in both Norwegian and English, Dr Jensen is careful to check her own understanding of his particular life situation by summarizing what she has heard and his understanding of her explanations by asking him to repeat what he has understood from her. She arranges a follow-up appointment, saying that she would like to check how he is getting on in a few weeks' time.

Dr Jensen offers a little more to Wladimir than she did to Bodvar because she has read and understood the economist Amartya Sen's insistence that 'equal consideration for all may demand very unequal treatment in favour of the disadvantaged' (23). Wladmir seems enabled to leave the consultation much less worried and distressed than he appeared when it started.

Sometimes, asking 'what do *you* think' may cause misunderstandings, more so in certain cultures depending on the level of trust created. This can sometimes be avoided by meta-communicating, in words and nonverbally, that the doctor knows, and is in authority, yet wants to know how the patient interprets the situation and the symptoms.

Scenario D: Dr Jensen meets an asylum seeker

Again a 28-year-old man comes to a consultation in Norwegian general practice, complaining of chest pain. His name is Mohamed Al Ahmed. He speaks no English, but he has brought along his 14-year-old brother Abdullah to translate. The clinical story is the same as before but as Abdullah translates, Dr Jensen is careful to place her right hand on her own chest, at the site of the reported pain, and winces to express pain so that Mohamed is able to see that she has understood his symptom. When she goes on to ask Mohamed and Abdullah to explain about their life situation, she learns that they are refugees from Syria and that their mother and two sisters older than Abdullah but younger than Mohamed were killed during bombing of the Damascus suburb in which they lived. After this terrible tragedy, they fled Syria with their father, but he suffered a heart attack and died during their exhausting trek across Eastern Europe. Abdullah has clear difficulty recounting this story without breaking down, but he manages. While listening, Dr Jensen again puts her hand to the left side of her chest, but this time uses her face to express sadness and concern. At the end of the story, she thanks Abdullah for telling her this story and acknowledges how difficult it must have been to tell. As with our two previous patients, Dr Jensen carefully and slowly explains her understanding of Mohammed's chest pain, checks that Abdullah has understood and that this understanding has reached Mohamed. She asks about their immediate life circumstances now. They are staying with an older cousin and his family, but they are very overcrowded and feel that they are a burden to these relatives. She asks whether they are in contact with refugee support services. Very aware of how vulnerable the two brothers are, she arranges a follow-up appointment for the next week and arranges for a professional interpreter to be present, while making it clear that Abdullah is still welcome to come with Mohamed if that would be helpful to either of them. It is clear that Mohamed is dependent on Abdullah's language skills, but at the same time feels very responsible for his younger brother. Nonetheless, both of them seem calmer at the end of the consultation and much less overtly worried about Mohamed's chest pain, which is not mentioned again.

Dr Jensen is fully aware that the use of children as interpreters is now prohibited under Norwegian law. However, she deems a presentation of chest pain to be an emergency and knows that she must make sure that it is safe to delay a consultation until a professional interpreter is available. She is also aware of research showing that children and young people can be bewildered and upset by the conventional practice of treating an interpreter as a neutral disembodied voice, and so she is careful to involve Abdullah in what becomes a three-way consultation (24). Although ostensibly Abdullah is interpreting for his brother, it is clear that both brothers have been severely traumatized, are suffering ongoing and unresolved feelings of grief, and have clear health care needs. Little can be accomplished in a single consultation, but the first steps towards a trusting therapeutic relationship between patients and doctor can and have been achieved. Trust has been built on the doctor's explicit interest in the lifeworld and experience of the two brothers and on her insistence that the communicative will trump the strategic within the consultation. (At the same time, it is important to recognize that if Mohamed had presented with symptoms more suggestive of a medical emergency, as perhaps happened in the hospital visit 2 days before, the system priorities of biomedicine would have become relatively much more important.)

Dr Jensen wants to build trust between all three parties to the consultation and she is committed to that trust being voluntary. Robb and Greenhalgh describe it as follows (19):

> Three different types of trust are evident in these different relationships — voluntary trust (based on either kinship-like bonds and continuity of the interpersonal relationship over time or on confidence in the institution and professional role that the individual represents), coercive trust (where one person effectively has no choice but to trust the other, as when a health problem requires expert knowledge that the patient does not have and cannot get) and hegemonic trust (where a person's propensity to trust, and awareness of alternatives, is shaped and constrained by the system so that people trust without knowing there is an alternative).

Dr Jensen is aware that voluntary trust has by far the greatest therapeutic potential and is actively encouraged by continuity of care, which is another reason why she has been so careful to arrange a follow-up appointment in the very near future. She is well aware that both Mohamed and Abdullah will need help from different agencies, but she recognizes that she has an important ongoing role to play that will depend on their trust in her.

INTERPRETATION IN PRIMARY CARE

Interpreted consultations are essential to the health care of many migrant populations, but they are fraught with difficulty. As Robb and Greenhalgh demonstrate, the triadic nature of such consultations creates six distinct trust relationships (patient-interpreter, patient-clinician, interpreter-patient, interpreter-clinician, clinician-patient, and clinician-interpreter) and the failure to establish trust in any one of these can severely undermine any possibility of a therapeutic relationship between patient and clinician (25). For too long, policymakers, academics, and many clinicians have conceptualized interpretation within consultations as a simple technical exercise, and as a result have simply assumed that a formal professional interpreter is always better than an informal interpreter from the patient's own family or community. This ignores the importance of the patient's lifeworld to their medical problem and prioritizes the accuracy of translation over the understanding of the patient's particular context, which consistently prioritizes strategic action above communicative action (19). One other result of this simple technical approach has been to neglect a particular problem which is well known to front-line clinicians working particularly with refugee populations. The patient and the interpreter may share a common language but may be irretrievably divided by issues of religion, politics, persecution, and prejudice. In such situations, while an informal interpreter who has already earned a position of trust in relation to the patient might be preferred, it is imperative to raise the overall quality of interpreters for health care services and to provide them with adequate educational and emotional support.

CURIOSITY AND THE STORY OF MIGRATION

Stories of displacement and migration are as old as human history. Yet people who have never experienced the trauma of loss of place still remain profoundly ignorant of the nature and reality of such an experience and are sometimes reluctant to show interest or seek understanding. Health care professionals are by no means immune to such attitudes. And yet these stories have much to tell us about human nature, and about suffering, courage, survival, and endurance, about love and loss. The lessons learned from people with unimaginable life experiences will enhance our understanding of the yearnings that humans share, such as attachment and meaning, as well as hone our curiosity and intensify our respect for that which falls outside our ability to understand. Such experiences, if we invest in them, will enrich our lives and enlarge our repertoire of healing skills. Yet finding the time and summoning the commitment and the curiosity to really listen in the highly pressured context of contemporary primary care remains immensely difficult.

Each of us is born into a specific place in the world: into a family, a culture, a nation. We grow up developing attitudes and skills appropriate to that particular context. Those who are displaced by economic necessity, educational or professional aspiration, political or ethnic persecution, violence or war, lose not only place and home but also every dimension of the surrounding context, and once displaced, they may long for what has been lost but can never fully regain, even if eventually they find themselves able to return to the by now almost mythical 'home'.

Loss of place devalues all the skills specific to it. Lost skills are lost identity, which further exacerbates the bewilderment that usually results from life-changing displacement. The writer Timothy O'Grady describes the profound loss of skill experienced by an economic migrant from rural Ireland to inner-city England (26):

What I could do.

I could mend nets. Thatch a roof. Build stairs. Make a basket from reeds. Splint the leg of a cow. Cut turf. Go three rounds with Joe in the ring Da put up in the barn. I could dance sets. Read the sky. Make a barrel for mackerel. Mend roads. Make a boat. Stuff a saddle. Put a wheel on a cart. Strike a deal. Make a field. Work the swarth turner, the float and the thresher. I could read the sea. Shoot straight. Make a shoe. Shear sheep. Remember poems. Set potatoes. Plough and harrow. Read the wind. Tend bees. Bind wyndes. Make a coffin. Take a drink. I could frighten you with stories. I knew the song to sing to a cow when milking. I could play twenty-seven tunes on my accordion.

...

What I couldn't do.

Eat a meal lacking potatoes. Trust banks. Wear a watch. Ask a woman to go for a walk. Work with drains or with objects smaller than a nail. Drive a motor car. Eat tomatoes. Remember the routes of buses. Wear a collar in comfort. Win at cards. Acknowledge the Queen. Abide loud voices. Perform the manners of greeting and leaving. Save money. Take pleasure in work carried out in a factory. Drink coffee. Look into a wound. Follow cricket. Understand the speech of a man from west Kerry. Wear shoes or boots made from rubber. Speak with men wearing collars. Stay afloat in water. Understand their jokes. Face the dentist. Kill a Sunday. Stop remembering.

A gifted storyteller is rendered almost deaf and dumb in the hostile environment of an alien language. New communicative skills may take years to master or may never be achieved, isolating people within the migrant community. Most children adapt and learn much more quickly, and this can create divisions and tensions within families as parents become disempowered in relation to their children.

THE PRIVILEGE AND JOY OF PROVIDING CARE TO MIGRANT POPULATIONS

The anthropologist Clifford Geertz insists that 'The reach of our minds, the range of signs we can manage somehow to interpret, is what defines the intellectual, emotional and moral space within which we live' (27).

We live only one life, within which we can seek to enlarge this intellectual, emotional, and moral space. As privileged providers of health care to people whose understanding and experience of life is completely different from our own, we have the opportunity to learn from lives that would never impinge on our own in any other circumstances, and so extend both our understanding of what it is to be human, and the reach of our minds.

REFERENCES

1. Dube SR, Felitti VJ, Dong MX, Giles WH, Anda RF. The impact of adverse childhood experiences on health problems: evidence from four birth cohorts dating back to 1900. *Prev Med*. 2003;37(3):268–77.
2. Mead N, Bower P. Patient-centredness: a conceptual framework and review of the empirical literature. *Soc Sci Med*. 2000;51(7):1087–110.
3. Walseth L, Schei E. Effecting change through dialogue: Habermas' theory of communicative action as a tool in medical lifestyle interventions. *Med Health Care Philos*. 2011;14(1):81–90.
4. Williams LE, Bargh JA, Nocera CC, Gray JR. The unconscious regulation of emotion: nonconscious reappraisal goals modulate emotional reactivity. *Emotion*. 2009;9(6):847–54.
5. Shapiro J. Perspective: does medical education promote professional alexithymia? A call for attending to the emotions of patients and self in medical training. *Acad Med*. 2011;86(3):326–32.
6. Ekman E, Krasner M. Empathy in medicine: neuroscience, education and challenges. *Med Teacher*. 2017;39(2):164–73.
7. Dornan T, Pearson E, Carson P, Helmich E, Bundy C. Emotions and identity in the figured world of becoming a doctor. *Med Educ*. 2015;49(2):174–85.
8. Ahrweiler F, Scheffer C, Roling G, Goldblatt H, Hahn EG, Neumann M. Clinical practice and self-awareness as determinants of empathy in undergraduate education: a qualitative short survey at three medical schools in Germany. *GMS Zeitschrift Medizinische Ausbildung*. 2014;31(4):Doc46.

9. Grochowski CO, Cartmill M, Reiter J et al. Anxiety in first year medical students taking gross anatomy. *Clin Anat*. 2014;27(6):835–8.

10. Dyrbye L, Shanafelt T. A narrative review on burnout experienced by medical students and residents. *Med Educ*. 2016;50(1):132–49.

11. Agledahl KM, Gulbrandsen P, Førde R, Wifstad Å. Courteous but not curious: how doctors' politeness masks their existential neglect. A qualitative study of video-recorded patient consultations. *J Med Ethics*. 2011;37(11):650–4.

12. Hafferty FW. Beyond curriculum reform: confronting medicine's hidden curriculum. *Acad Med*. 1998;73(4):403–7.

13. Tuckett D, Boulton M, Olson C, Williams A. *Meetings Between Experts: An Approach to Sharing Ideas in Medical Consultations*. London: Tavistock; 1985.

14. Hafferty FW. Socialization, professionalism, and professional identity formation. In: Cruess RL, Cruess SR, Steinert Y, editors. *Teaching Medical Professionalism*. 2nd ed. Cambridge; New York: Cambridge University Press; 2016: 54–67.

15. Balint M. *The Doctor, His Patient, and The Illness*. New York: International Universities Press; 1964.

16. Nessa J. Talk as medical work. Discourse analysis of patient-doctor communication in general practice [Doktoravhandling]: Universitetet i Bergen; 1999.

17. Schei E. Doctoring as leadership: the power to heal. *Perspect Biol Med*. 2006;49(3):393–406.

18. Habermas J. *The Theory of Communicative Action*. Cambridge: Polity Press; 1987.

19. Greenhalgh T, Robb N, Scambler G. Communicative and strategic action in interpreted consultations in primary health care: a Habermasian perspective. *Soc Sci Med*. 2006;63(5):1170–87.

20. Ricks C. *TS Eliot and Prejudice*. London: Faber and Faber; 1988.

21. Vetlesen AJ. Profesjonell og personlig? Legerollen mellom vellykkethet og sårbarhet. *Tidsskr-Nor-Lægeforen*. 2001;121:1118–21.

22. Hutchinson TA. *Whole Person Care: Transforming Healthcare*. Springer; 2017.

23. Sen A. *Inequality Reexamined*. Oxford University Press; 1992.

24. Free CGJ, Bhavnani V, Newman A. Bilingual young people's experiences of interpreting in primary care: a qualitative study. *Br J Gen Pract*. 2003;53:530–5.

25. Robb N, Greenhalgh T. "You have to cover up the words of the doctor": the mediation of trust in interpreted consultations in primary care. *J Health Organ Manag*. 2006;20(5):434–55.

26. O'Grady T, Pike S. *I Could Read the Sky*. London: Harvill Press; 1997.

27. Geertz C. *Available Light: Anthropological Reflections on Philosophical Topic*. Princeton University Press; 2001.

CHAPTER 4

The ethics of migrant health: Power and privilege versus rights and entitlements

Gorik Ooms, Rachel Hammonds and Ines Keygnaert

LEARNING OBJECTIVES

In this chapter, we provide:

- An overview of the ethics of 'just health' (1), or 'health justice' (2), the principles behind the ethics, and the challenges faced when it comes to applying those principles to people who are not fellow citizens
- An overview of the rights and entitlements migrants have – or should have – under international human rights law
- Two clinical vignettes that highlight the realities of political power and powerlessness, which allow non-migrant citizens to exclude – at least to some extent – some migrants from the rights and entitlements they should have
- A conclusion with practical recommendations for health workers

---

INTRODUCTION

In 1958, George Rosen wrote: 'The modern conception that the national government is responsible for the health of the people is but a natural extension of the previous view where the local community provided for such needs' (3). He added: 'Most recently, in fact, this trend has moved beyond the national community to the world community with the creation of the World Health Organization' (3). Almost 60 years later, the question of whether the 'world community' is responsible for the health of 'the people' remains highly pertinent – and, if the answer is yes, the ancillary questions – to what extent and how this responsibility is shared with national governments — remains unanswered. Why should taxpayers of one country make financial contributions for the health care of people living in another country?

This is not a book about global health; this is a book about migrant health. We chose to introduce our chapter with a reference to a fundamental global health challenge because we think that one of the underlying migrant health challenges engages with similar issues. Most people have accepted — voluntarily or because their governments decided so — that they have a responsibility to contribute to the health of their fellow citizens. Many people have not accepted that they have a responsibility to contribute to the health of 'other people' (i.e. non-citizens). Following this logic, migrants — especially refugees — may, in the opinion of many, belong to the other people, for whom they have no responsibility. The corollary of this difference in responsibility is a difference in entitlements: the other people do not have the same legitimate claims or entitlements. It is as if they still live in a different country.

In several countries, the opinion that (some) migrants do not have the same entitlements to societal efforts intended to protect and improve health as 'non-migrant' citizens do has been translated into national law and regulations — law and regulations that do not guarantee the same rights and entitlements to (some categories of) migrants as they do for most citizens. This situation poses a dilemma for general practitioners and other health workers whose personal and professional ethics oblige them to treat all their patients equally, as human beings, regardless of their migration or citizenship status. However, for health workers, providing treatment to migrant patients may lead to bureaucratic, financial, and legal problems. For example, the time, effort, and medicines health workers provide may not be reimbursed by the government or quasigovernmental social protection schemes. One could argue that this is only a minor problem, but for a general practice or a health centre or hospital that receives many such patients, the consequences can be considerable. In some situations, health workers may even be considered as complicit in 'human trafficking' if they treat all patients equally and therefore provide health care to migrant patients who also happen to be victims of human trafficking.

The central question for this chapter is what are the rights and entitlements of migrants to health promotion and health care, from an ethical and human rights perspective, and are they different from the rights and entitlements of non-migrants, including citizens? For clarity, we use, to the extent possible, the International Organization for Migration's definition of migrant (refer to Chapter 1). For our purposes, non-migrants, then, are those who lawfully reside within the borders of the state of their habitual place of residence. They may or may not officially be citizens of the country where their habitual place of residence is. This chapter employs the terms *migrant* and *non-migrant* to examine the challenges posed by the contrast between their entitlements under national and international laws. Where it is appropriate, we replace the term non-migrant with (fellow) citizen, that is, in reference to voting.

HEALTH JUSTICE: WHAT DO WE OWE EACH OTHER REGARDING THE PROTECTION AND PROMOTION OF HEALTH, AND WHY?

We would agree with Rosen that the evolution from the view that the local community is, or was, responsible for the health of its members, to the view that the national government is responsible for the health of the people, was a natural evolution. However, its progress is uneven and incomplete in many states. We would argue that this evolution was not a transfer of responsibility from one political unit to another, a higher and broader one, but rather the extension of what people considered as their 'own community'. So long as people identified with parishes, counties, villages, or cities as their own community, those political units were the ones they expected solutions from: solutions to increase their security and their welfare. As soon as people identified themselves as citizens of a state, the state was expected to solve their security, welfare, and other problems. In many states, this evolution continues to face challenges.

Furthermore, even when the primary political unit was at the local level, living in the locality was not a sufficient condition for inclusion in collective efforts to protect welfare. The division of 'the poor' into 'deserving poor' and 'undeserving poor', existed long before the (in)famous sixteenth century English Elizabethan era Poor Law enshrined such concepts (4). The deserving poor were those who were poor due to no fault of their own – and therefore, they deserved assistance – while the underserving poor were the 'wilfully idle, especially those rogues and vagabonds whose lives of itinerant theft by definition threatened the stability of a social order which was anchored in notions of private property' (5).

Five centuries later, it may seem pointless to refer to the idea of (un)deserving poor. However, the idea that people who are in need of support due to no fault of their own are more deserving of solidarity than those who could have avoided ending up in a situation of need still resonates in contemporary debates about personal or individual responsibility for health. For example, some scholars argue that 'since smoking increases the risk for cancer and cardiovascular disease, people who freely decide to smoke should be held accountable for this choice' (6). More relevant for this book, the idea that a non-migrant has, a priori, a more legitimate claim to our solidarity than a migrant who happens to live in the same country seems to explain that 'increasing ethnic heterogeneity' in countries of Western Europe would 'negatively influence public opinion about the welfare state' (7). Even in some of the world's wealthiest countries, the 'modern conception that the national government is responsible for the health of the people' seems to require a footnote defining who those people really are.

The research finding that increasing ethnic heterogeneity is negatively related with public opinion about the welfare state is a sociological finding, not an ethical one. If one believes that migrants should benefit from the same quality of health services as non-migrants, one could simply conclude that people who feel less positive about the welfare state – and probably the financial contributions they must make – are incorrect, from an ethical perspective. But what exactly is that ethical perspective? Is it different from the sociological willingness to participate or contribute? Does it rest on principles of democracy, e.g. if the majority of the citizens agree to provide equal health services to migrants and citizens, then the minority has to abide? That could be a fragile ethical foundation in the present political climate.

One of the most cited inquiries into the ethics of 'what we owe each other in the protection and promotion of health' (1), is Norman Daniels' book *Just Health: Meeting Health Needs Fairly*. Daniels' account of health justice is a tributary of John Rawls' theory of justice, in general, and to Rawls' principle of fair equality of opportunity, in particular: 'Meeting health needs has the goal of promoting normal functioning: It concentrates on a specific class of obvious disadvantages and tries to eliminate them' (1). This principle can be applied to migrants on one condition, namely that society accepts they have the same rights as citizens, who *ought* to enjoy fair equality of opportunity. Daniels does not discuss the topic of migrant health specifically. However, in his chapter on 'International Health Inequalities and Global Justice', Daniels acknowledges that his account of health justice provides 'no simple or straightforward answers' to questions about international health inequalities, and one of the problems he mentions is 'the absence of the kinds of human relationships that ordinarily give rise to the claims of egalitarian justice that we make on each other — for example, being fellow citizens or even interacting in a cooperative scheme' (1). In other words, if migrants are not (yet) considered as fellow citizens, Daniels' theory of health justice may not apply to them.

Shlomi Segall provides an alternative account of health justice, one based on 'luck egalitarianism', in his book *Health, Luck and Justice*. Segall starts from a simple principle: 'Differences in health and health care are unjust if they reflect differences in brute luck' (8). At first sight, this principle does provide straightforward answers to questions of migrant health: while Daniels' account rests on fair equality of opportunity, on collective efforts in the promotion and protection of health as instrumental for fair equality of opportunity, and therefore on the a priori acceptance of migrants as fellow citizens who ought to enjoy fair equality of opportunity, Segall's account only requires differences in health, or health care, that cannot be attributed to individual choices. While Segall, like Daniels, does not discuss migrants' health entitlements in particular, his account of global health justice is far more demanding than Daniels'. We can safely assume that, for Segall, there is no reasonable justification for discriminating against migrants. Unfortunately, we can also safely assume that Segall's account of (global) health justice is not endorsed by the majority, and even that many people who agree with Segall's principle when it comes to migrants would find it hard to accept the consequences of applying that principle to all people worldwide.

PRIVILEGES, POWER (AND LACK THEREOF)

One can open a European or North American newspaper on almost any day and read a story related to the huge gap between the legitimate entitlements of migrants on the one hand, and the health services they are truly receiving on the other. The two clinical vignettes here highlight some of the issues faced by migrants and health professionals with whom they interact.

CLINICAL VIGNETTE 1

Hope is a stunning young woman who fled a sub-Saharan country after being raped. Arriving in Belgium, she does not feel very well and coughs regularly. Applying for asylum, she gets a standard prescription to screen for tuberculosis (TB). At the city reception initiative she is referred to, she eventually gets the news that she does not have TB, but that she is pregnant and HIV positive. 'So he ensured me never to forget that he owned my body'. The asylum care workers assure her that the Belgian government pays for pregnancy-related as well as newborn care and HIV-treatment for all asylum seekers, so she should not worry. Both mother and baby are given antiretroviral treatment (ART) and the baby is given milk powder, all covered within the asylum-related costs. She recovers day by day, and her baby boy brings new hope to her life. However, 2 years later Hope's asylum claim gets rejected. At this point, Hope has met a man whom she likes but does not want to marry (yet) as she is still afraid of becoming too dependent on a man. However, she gets pregnant again. Her appeal of the asylum decision is also refused; she is 34 weeks pregnant and becomes an undocumented migrant in Belgium. Under Belgian law, she is expected to leave the asylum reception centre as well as the country. This change in status creates huge stress for Hope. Returning to her 'country of rape' is no option, as she would be chased and possibly murdered. Therefore staying undocumented in Belgium is the only option she can think of. But that means she is depending on the 'urgent medical care' procedure which is applicable to undocumented migrants in Belgium. She is told she can continue her treatment provided three criteria are fulfilled: the doctor considers it to be necessary care, the social assistant of the city's welfare service approves the doctor's decision, and finally, she fulfils all of the eligibility criteria. Satisfying these criteria requires extensive investigation and thus time. Hope is having contractions and wonders whether the hospital staff will report her to the authorities. The midwife at the hospital assures her that until the delivery she will be taken care of, and upon birth her baby will get the antiretroviral syrup, and probably the full doses for 6 weeks. But then what? The 'Urgent Medical Care' law does not cover provision of powder milk, so Hope is caught between the risks of breastfeeding the new baby while being HIV-positive and no longer on ART and the financial burden of purchasing powder milk every week. She is told that some NGOs have a limited stock of such supplies, but then she is dependent on charity and the availability of stock. She considers moving to another city where the social welfare organization that decides on reimbursement is reputed to be more generous. But how can she be sure? She does not know where to turn to get answers to these questions.

Based on an interview carried out for the study 'What health care for undocumented migrants in Belgium?' (9)

Hope's story demonstrates how migrant women around the globe face a myriad of barriers when trying to access sexual and reproductive health (SRH) care. Accessibility is a complex and multifaceted concept that includes familiarity, comprehensibility, affordability, availability, acceptability, and physical accessibility issues, as well as navigating regulations that are often not understood by either the service user or the service provider (10). Hope's story also exemplifies how the diminished legal status of a migrant has fuelled the speed of the 'othering' practices in their entitlement to care (11). This practice has dual consequences. It not only 'others' migrant patients, as their need for care is perceived to be generated predominantly, if not solely, by their culture, traditions, or the conflict in their country of origin; it also ignores how their legal and socioeconomic situation, as well as their entitlement to health care in the host country, might engender ill health (12,13).

In most European countries, migrant access to maternal and newborn health care has long been treated as an entitlement. Since the 2008 economic crises, many European countries have started to restrict their national laws concerning access, linking entitlements to only the emergency level of care. Some have gone as far as to openly question the emergency classification of a delivery, as it is quite probable that a pregnancy will eventually lead to a delivery (10) and thus cannot be classified as an emergency. At the same time, many of these countries emphasize publicly how generous they are to migrants, yet require them to line up at NGOs or charitable organizations for 'necessary (non-emergency) care' (10). This interpretation is in contravention to the Committee on Economic, Social and Cultural Rights (CESCRs) authoritative interpretation of the obligations under the International Covenant on Economic, Social and Cultural Rights (14), which Belgium has ratified and is legally bound to comply with, and which specifies that accessibility is core to the right to health and thus a 'legal obligation and not a matter of charity or political choice' (15).

Can migrants effectively use international human rights law to obtain what they are entitled to? At this point, we have to make a distinction between different groups of migrants. Remember the definition of migrant of the IOM (refer to Chapter 1). This includes migrants who have obtained 'papers' allowing them to stay in the country where they are, and migrants who did not obtain such papers, or undocumented migrants. As explained previously, according to international human rights law, the difference between having or not having such papers makes no difference when it comes to the right to health. In practice, however, this difference allows states — and the citizens they represent — to violate the right to health in a structural way: to set up health services in such a way that undocumented migrants are excluded. Further, if they use legal remedies, like litigation, to access their rights, they must identify themselves and where they live, which puts them at risk of being deported while a court examines their claim.

CLINICAL VIGNETTE 2

Saffi's family has paid people   smugglers — to help him travel to his uncle in the Netherlands from his West African village, where members of his ethnic group are subject to discrimination. Saffi suffered trauma and physical abuse while traversing the Sahara. His crossing from Libya to Italy took twice as long as expected, and several people died. Saffi helped to throw the bodies into the sea. These experiences have marked him psychologically and physically. He has traversed Europe without presenting his papers to authorities and has arrived in Brussels exhausted. He has heard that if he goes into one of the city's shelters, he risks being taken to a locked detention centre and required to claim asylum in Belgium. He does not know what this means but knows he needs to reach the Netherlands. While sleeping outdoors he is bitten by a dog and as the days pass his leg swells. Saffi is afraid to seek medical care and tries to continue his journey to the Netherlands. He is running a high fever and collapses while walking to the Dutch border. His friends take him to the emergency room of the closest hospital and leave him. The admissions staff asks for payment, documents, and insurance, none of which he can provide. The emergency room staff decides to treat him and insist that he is hospitalized until his infection is under control. In the meantime, tests show Saffi is suffering from TB and he exhibits signs of post-traumatic stress disorder. Hospital staff risk disciplinary action for exposing the hospital to the risk and cost of treating Saffi but feel morally and professionally obliged to help him access the full treatment he needs to address his mental and physical health needs.

Saffi's story highlights several key interrelated legal barriers migrants face in claiming access to health services. Firstly, the legal status hurdles. Depending on how Saffi is classified under Belgian migration law — namely, as an asylum seeker, a refugee, or an undocumented migrant — he has access to different health and social services (9).

The second hurdle is tied to the first — the contents of the health care package to which an individual is entitled is related to their migration status and not their medical needs. Under Belgian national law, undocumented migrants have few legal entitlements with respect to health care. Like all people on Belgian territory, they are entitled to access emergency care; for example, in Saffi's case to treat his life-threatening infection. However, they cannot join the national mutual health insurance fund, which entitles members to a wide range of services, including access to mental health services. They are entitled to receive Urgent Medical Aid (which, importantly, includes preventative and curative treatment) if they receive permission from a medical doctor and the relevant public social services authority (16). The Urgent Medical Aid procedure is time consuming and vests a high degree of discretion in both the medical doctor and the public social services authority, and appealing either of their decisions means involving the local public welfare system and its budgetary constraints (17).

The third hurdle relates to the legal complexity inherent in claiming health rights. The legal requirements for claiming rights require that a migrant has the ability (which includes financial, geographic, gender, and cultural dimensions) to access the legal system, the necessary language skills, and the requisite documents (18). However, very few migrants are aware of their rights or how to navigate the system to obtain their rights. Assistance in accessing the Belgian legal system is provided by NGOs and legal clinics, but demand exceeds supply. For Saffi, as for most migrants, remaining below the legal radar is the typical strategy. The consequences of interaction with the authorities are unknown, so keeping a low profile is best.

The fourth hurdle to claiming health rights is the time-consuming nature of the legal process. Given the sheer number of applicants, the processing of claims for refugee status takes time. For people on the move, like Saffi, becoming entwined in a lengthy, uncertain legal process is to be avoided until, perhaps, you reach your destination. But, in the meantime, if you fall sick en route, the choice is out of your hands. The migration, and to a lesser extent, the health system in the country in which you fall ill serves as a gatekeeper to your health rights.

HEALTH RIGHTS AND ENTITLEMENTS OF MIGRANTS
UNDER INTERNATIONAL HUMAN RIGHTS LAW

In a famous comment on the drafting of the Universal Declaration of Human Rights, Jacques Maritain reports how one of the committees agreed on the list of human rights to be included, on the condition that 'no one asks us why' (19). That was but one episode in the long-running debate between philosophers and lawyers, as to whether a convincing ethical foundation for human rights is essential. The proponents on one side argue that there will never be a consensus on any ethical foundation for human rights, and therefore trying to find one will merely cause disagreement about 'real' human rights and 'questionable' human rights, so we had better stick to the legal texts (20). The proponents on the other side argue that the legal texts are not clear enough, will often require interpretation, and a strong ethical foundation is required to formulate convincing interpretations (1).

In the case of the rights and entitlements that migrants can claim, the international legal texts seem to be clearer than the ethical accounts. The answer to this question can be found by using the interpretative principle of the exception that confirms the general rule on an often-disregarded section of the Covenant (22); namely, article 2(3): 'Developing countries, with due regard to human rights and their national economy, may determine to what extent they would guarantee the economic rights recognized in the present Covenant to non-nationals'.

Like many other scholars, we have reservations about this section, as it seems to undermine the very idea of human rights as 'rights held by individuals simply because they are part of the human species' (21). This section explicitly allows governments of 'developing' countries to discriminate against non-nationals, which we find questionable on ethical grounds, especially in situations when governments question the nationality of people living under their jurisdictions for decades and generations — the Rohingya people in Myanmar come to mind. But it removes all reasonable doubts about the rights and entitlements of migrants in 'developed' countries: they fall under article 2(2) of the Covenant, according to which 'States Parties to the present Covenant undertake to guarantee that the rights enunciated in the present Covenant will be exercised without discrimination of any kind as to race, colour, sex, language, religion, political or other opinion, national or social origin, property, birth or other status (14)'.

To know what that means for health, we need to explore article 12 of the Covenant on the right to health. According to article 12(1), 'States Parties to the present Covenant recognize the right of everyone to the enjoyment of the highest attainable standard of physical and mental health'. This aspirational formulation may unfortunately be responsible for one of the most persistent misconceptions about the right to health, namely that everyone can legitimately claim any health-promoting or health-protecting effort from the government of the country they live in, as long as that effort (health care, for example, but also efforts to provide healthier living conditions) brings them closer to their highest attainable level of health. Article 12(2), however, clarifies the obligations of states: they should take steps 'to achieve the full realization' of the right to health, including:

a. The provision for the reduction of the stillbirth rate and of infant mortality and for the healthy development of the child
b. The improvement of all aspects of environmental and industrial hygiene
c. The prevention, treatment, and control of epidemic, endemic, occupational, and other diseases
d. The creation of conditions which would assure to all medical service and medical attention in the event of sickness

This obligation to take steps to achieve — rather than to *immediately* achieve — the Covenant rights, is the cornerstone of the Covenant, and explained in article 2(1):

> Each State Party to the present Covenant undertakes to take steps, individually and through international assistance and co-operation, especially economic and technical, to the maximum of its available resources, with a view to achieving progressively the full realization of the rights recognized in the present Covenant by all appropriate means, including particularly the adoption of legislative measures.

The steps states should take are thus limited by their available resources, which means that the entitlements of people are affected by the relative poverty or wealth of the states they happen to live in. Again, we would argue that this is somewhat contradictory to the idea of human rights as rights one has by virtue of being a human being, and that contradiction is only partially resolved by the reference to international assistance. The controversy about the obligation to provide assistance is directly related to the question at the beginning of this chapter: to what extent is the 'world community' responsible for the health of 'the people' of the world? But it is not the central question for this chapter. The central question for this chapter is about the responsibility of governments for the health of migrants who live within their borders. And the answer is simple: governments of 'developed' countries have the same responsibility for the health of migrants as for anyone else living within their borders. Discrimination 'of any kind as to race, colour, sex, language, religion, political or other opinion, national or social origin, property, birth or other status' is simply not allowed. Whether a person is a refugee who arrived yesterday without any documents or someone who has paid taxes and social security contributions for decades (and may be able to draw a family tree of eleven generations of tax and social security contributions paying ascendants), they have the same rights under the Covenant — in 'developed' countries.

Furthermore, the right to health does not imply that all people should receive all available health care (or other efforts that would contribute to their health); it implies that people should receive the efforts they need. As the CESCR — the body tasked with monitoring states' compliance with the Covenant — explains, public services needed to improve people's health should not only be available and accessible, they should also be of good quality and acceptable, 'respectful of medical ethics and culturally appropriate, i.e. respectful of the culture of individuals, minorities, peoples and communities, sensitive to gender and life-cycle requirements, as well as being designed to respect confidentiality and improve the health status of those concerned' (22). This means that the entitlements of refugees and migrants (especially newly arrived migrants) will often be more demanding than the entitlements of the general population. Public efforts to protect and improve the health of migrants should address their often precarious living conditions and include health care that is provided in ways that are adapted to needs.

RECOMMENDATIONS FOR HEALTH WORKERS

In an ideal world, we would conclude this chapter with one recommendation: states should comply with the international treaties that they negotiated, signed, and ratified. With respect to health, this means that migrants, like all people found within the borders of a given country, are entitled to accessible, quality, appropriate health care. Thus, in an ideal world, health workers would face no ethical dilemmas as to whom they can treat — they would simply apply their professional skills to treating a patient. However, the previous two clinical vignettes reflect the challenging reality that health workers and migrants face around the globe. So, our recommendations engage with the realities of legal uncertainty, ethical dilemmas, political power, and powerlessness, in which both migrants and health workers operate.

1. **Inform yourself regarding the international legal commitments of the country in which you work and check how these are translated in national laws and practices.** If the national laws in your country of employment prevent you from providing treatment to migrants, inform yourself as to the country's international legal commitments. Under international human rights law, discrimination on the grounds of migration status is prohibited. You can see which treaties your country of employment is bound by and use this as an argument for providing care and informing colleagues who do not know the law. The ratification status for each country can be found at http://indicators.ohchr.org/. Signature (as is the case for the United States) is not sufficient.

2. **Ensure your fellow medical workers are accurately informed regarding the national legislation that governs providing medical treatment to migrants.** Medical professionals need to be certified to continue practicing. Push for regular updates from your national professional body on the national legislation that governs treating migrants and call for making accurate up-to-date knowledge of the national legal situation part of the professional recertification process.

3. **Actively oppose laws and bureaucratic procedures that force you to discriminate.** As noted under Recommendation 1, inform yourself as to the international legal status of your country of employment. You may also want to use moral or

professional arguments. You can channel your discontent to elected officials and your professional body. If your employer introduces discriminatory bureaucratic procedures, work with colleagues and your professional body to remove or mitigate them (see Recommendation 5).

4. **Ensure that migrants receive access to health care by actively engaging with networks that provide such care.**

   In many countries, national and international NGOs (e.g. Médicins du Monde) provide health care to migrants. Offering support to such organizations allows for migrants to receive health care and mitigates the risk of legal consequences for health workers.

5. **Push for a humane policy towards migrants in your place of employment.**

   You may not be able to change the law on your own, but you can push to ensure that the medical institution (e.g. clinic, hospital) where you work has a humane policy regarding providing treatment to migrants. This may include implementing administrative tools (e.g. vouchers) to ensure all people have timely access to an initial consultation.

6. **Push for your national health care budget to take account of the financial cost of providing access to health services for all.**

   Increasing access to health services has financial implications. Ensuring access for all should not result in cuts to services, which could result in further hostility to migrants.

CONCLUSION

If international human rights laws were respected globally, health workers would face no ethical dilemmas as to whom they can treat — they would simply apply their professional skills to treating a patient, regardless of migration status. However, in wealthy states, (including European Union members), recent years have seen a growth in national legislation that encroaches on the health-related entitlements that migrants are legally guaranteed under international human rights law. These national laws violate international legal commitments and create profound ethical dilemmas for front-line health workers who are required to implement them.

This chapter has outlined the ethical and legal basis for ensuring health rights to all, while acknowledging that in the current political climate much work remains to be done to ensure access to health for all. It provides practical recommendations for health workers, grounded in international human rights law, in the hope that this information empowers them to contribute to combating discrimination on the basis of migration status.

REFERENCES

1. Daniels N. *Just Health: Meeting Health Needs Fairly.* Cambridge University Press; 2007.
2. Venkatapuram S. *Health Justice: An Argument from the Capabilities Approach.* Polity. 2012.
3. Rosen G. *A History of Public Health.* Expanded edition. Baltimore, MD: Johns Hopkins University Press; 1993.
4. McIntosh MK. Local responses to the poor in late medieval and Tudor England. *Continuity Change.* 1988;3(2):209–45.
5. Hindle S. Civility, Honesty and the identification of the deserving poor in seventeenth-century England. In: *Identity and Agency in England, 1500–1800,* edited by J. Barry and H. French. London: Palgrave Macmillan; 2004: pp. 38–59.

6. Cappelen AW, Norheim OF. Responsibility in health care: a liberal egalitarian approach. *J Med Ethics*. 2005;31(8):476–80.
7. Mau S, Burkhardt C. Migration and welfare state solidarity in Western Europe. *J European Social Policy*. 2009;19(3):213–29.
8. Segall S. *Health, Luck, and Justice*. Princeton University Press; 2009.
9. Roberfroid D, Dauvrin M, Keygnaert I, Desomer A, Kerstens B, Camberlin C et al. *What Health Care for Undocumented Migrants in Belgium?* Brussels: Belgian Health Care Knowledge Centre (KCE); 2015. Report No.: D/2015/10.273/111.
10. Keygnaert I, Ivanova O, Guieu A, Van Parys AS, Leye E, Roelens K. *What is the evidence on the reduction of inequalities in accessibility and quality of maternal health care delivery for migrants. A review of the existing evidence in the WHO European region [Internet]*. Copenhagen: WHO Regional Office for Europe; 2016.
11. Grove NJ, Zwi AB. Our health and theirs: forced migration, othering, and public health. *Social Sci Med* 2006;62(8):1931–42.
12. Keygnaert I, Guieu A. What the eye does not see: a critical interpretive synthesis of European Union policies addressing sexual violence in vulnerable migrants. *Reprod Health Matters*. 2015;23(46):45–55.
13. Keygnaert I, Guieu A, Ooms G, Vettenburg N, Temmerman M, Roelens K. Sexual and reproductive health of migrants: does the EU care? *Health Policy*. 2014;114(2):215–25.
14. General Assembly of the United Nations. International Covenant on Economic, Social and Cultural Rights, G.A. Res. 21/2200A, 993U.N.T.S. 3; 1966.
15. Hammonds R, Ooms G, Vandenhole W. Under the (legal) radar screen: global health initiatives and international human rights obligations. *BMC Int Health Hum Rights*. 2012;12(1):31.
16. Belgian Federal Government. *Arrêté royal relatif à l'aide médicale urgente octroyée par les centres publics d'aide sociale aux étrangers qui séjournent illégalement dans le Royaume. (Royal Decree on Urgent Medical Aid provided by public social welfare centres to foreigners residing irregularly in the Belgian kingdom.)* Moniteur Belge; 12 December 1996.
17. Belgian Federal Government. *Loi organique des centres publics d'action sociale. Organieke wet betreffende de openbarecentra voor maatschappelijk welzijn*. Moniteur Belge-Belgisch Staatsblad: 8 July 1976.
18. Médecins du Monde-Dokter van de Wereld. Livre vert sur l'accès aux soins en Belgique-Groenboek over de toegankelijkheid van de gezondheidszorg in België. 2014.
19. United Nations Educational, Scientific and Cultural Organisation. Human rights. Comments and interpretations. *A Symposium Edited by UNESCO, with an Introduction by Jacques Maritain*. Paris: UNESCO; 1948.
20. Donnelly J. *Universal Human Rights in Theory and Practice*. 3rd ed. Cornell University Press; 2013.
21. Ishay M. *The History of Human Rights: From Ancient Times to the Globalization Era*. University of California Press; 2008.
22. Committee on Economic, Social and Cultural Rights. General Comment No. 14, The Right to the Highest Attainable Standard of Health, UN Doc. No. E/C.12/2000/4; 2000.

CHAPTER 5

Discrimination and health

Jeanette H. Magnus

LEARNING OBJECTIVES

This chapter will:

- Present and discuss the relevance of discrimination to health inequity in migrant health
- Explore discrimination and the concept of implicit bias in primary health care

---

INTRODUCTION

Migration is one of the key drivers of diversity. Diversity and super-diversity imply differences (1). These differences often manifest in the unequal treatment of individuals or a socially defined group; in other words, unjust treatment (2). Racism and racial discrimination are increasingly receiving attention as determinants of racial/ethnic inequalities in health (3). The social and economic inequalities faced by ethnic minority groups are fundamental explanations for some of the disparity demonstrated between groups (4). We need to place ethnic inequalities in health within a wider social context. The lived experience as a minority is perhaps a more important determinant of differentials in mortality in multi-ethnic populations than biological markers of risk and behavioural factors, such as cigarette smoking or diet.

There is growing evidence of the experiences of discrimination and how these contribute to ethnic health inequalities (5). Discrimination can occur based on social identity characteristics such as age, gender, socioeconomic status, national origin, sexual orientation, gender identity, religious orientation, and disability status, in addition to race/ethnicity (6). Racial or race-based discrimination is behaviours, actions, situations, practices, legislation, or policies that result in avoidable and unfair inequalities in power, resources, and opportunities across racial or ethnic groups (7). The harmful health effects of discrimination across a range of mental health outcomes including depression, psychological distress, anxiety, and well-being have been well documented (8). Perceived discrimination has also been linked to specific types of physical health problems, such as hypertension, self-reported poor health, and breast cancer, as well as for potential risk factors for disease, such as obesity, high blood pressure, and substance use (9). There are, however, few studies on the impact of discrimination on migrant health. In addition to the usual discriminatory characteristics such as age, gender, religion, race/ethnicity, or culture, migrants carry the additional characteristics of being a migrant, and therefore might be more prone to discrimination. In the following we explore the relevant literature with a special emphasis on the primary health care setting.

DISCRIMINATION: THE LAYERS AND COMPLEXITIES

In using the term 'racial discrimination', we include discrimination due to race, ethnicity, culture, and religion, acknowledging the overlapping nature of these categories within popular and academic discourse, rather than as an endorsement of 'race' as an essentialist biological category. While the inclusion of religion in such definitions is debated, we do so in recognition that religion is often conflated with ethnicity and culture in popular culture. Scholars are also increasingly describing the racialized nature of religious identity, thus making it difficult to disentangle. Priest and colleagues offer the following: 'Racism can be expressed through beliefs (e.g. negative and inaccurate stereotypes), emotions (e.g. fear/hatred) or behaviours/ practices (e.g. unfair treatment), ranging from open threats and insults (including physical violence) to phenomena deeply embedded in social systems and structures' (10). Experiences of racial discrimination can be subtle, unintentional, unwitting, and even unconscious. In the health literature there is little recognition of racism and racial discrimination as an ideology of both inferiority and superiority (white supremacy) (7,11).

In addressing the challenges of explaining interrelated racially linked health disparities, systems theories offer a way to conceptualize racial discrimination as something greater than the sum of race-linked disparities across a set of subsystems. According to a systems perspective, a system is an entity that comprises a set of dynamically related components or subsystems. When looking at challenges related to discrimination, it is important to look at the smaller components of the system within the context of the larger system (7).

Racism and discrimination

Racism can occur at three levels (Figure 5.1): internalized (i.e. the incorporation of racist attitudes, beliefs, or ideologies into one's worldview), interpersonal (interactions between individuals), and systemic or institutionalized (production, control and access to labour, material, and symbolic resources within a society) (11). One way to understand the experience of discrimination is that it is a stressor that can broadly impact health (12). The most obvious is direct physical injury caused by racist violence. Another could be reduced uptake of healthy behaviours and/or increased adoption of unhealthy behaviours either directly as stress-coping, or indirectly via reduced self-regulation closely linked to other social determinants of health.

Although most stressful experiences do not increase vulnerability to illness, certain kinds of stressors — those that are uncontrollable and unpredictable — are particularly harmful to health, and these characteristics are common to discrimination experiences. Various models conceptualize discrimination as a social stressor that sets into motion a process of

Racism and discrimination

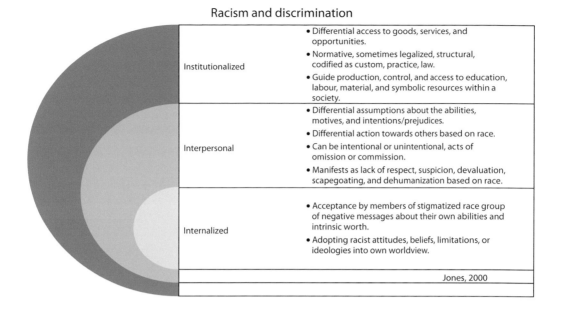

Institutionalized	• Differential access to goods, services, and opportunities. • Normative, sometimes legalized, structural, codified as custom, practice, law. • Guide production, control, and access to education, labour, material, and symbolic resources within a society.
Interpersonal	• Differential assumptions about the abilities, motives, and intentions/prejudices. • Differential action towards others based on race. • Can be intentional or unintentional, acts of omission or commission. • Manifests as lack of respect, suspicion, devaluation, scapegoating, and dehumanization based on race.
Internalized	• Acceptance by members of stigmatized race group of negative messages about their own abilities and intrinsic worth. • Adopting racist attitudes, beliefs, limitations, or ideologies into own worldview.

Jones, 2000

FIGURE 5.1   Levels of racism and discrimination.

physiological responses (e.g. elevated blood pressure, heart rate, cortisol secretions), and these heightened physiological responses can have downstream effects on health over time (13). Routine discrimination can become a chronic stressor that may erode an individual's protective resources and increase vulnerability to physical illness (14). As with other forms of cumulative stress, perceived discrimination may lead to chronic over- or underactivity of allostatic systems impacting allostatic load and other pathophysiological processes (15). Allostatic load (Chapter 2) is the sum of 'the wear and tear on the body' accumulating over time with exposure to chronic or repetitive stress. In addition, negative affective/cognitive and other pathopsychological processes alone or in combination with restricted access to social resources such as employment, housing, and education, and/or increased exposure to risk factors (such as unnecessary contact with the criminal justice system) can create and perpetuate ill health.

Discrimination also impacts children's health status (16). A direct effect of the maternal and family experiences of racial discrimination was found among women of Arab descent living in California, who were significantly more likely to give birth to a low-birth-weight or preterm baby in the 6-month period following September 11, 2001 than in the 6-month period before this date (17). This result is particularly noteworthy since Arab and Arab American women typically have very healthy pregnancies and consistently low rates of low-birth-weight or preterm babies. Similar increases were not noted among any other racial/ethnic group during the same time period. Additional studies are warranted to see how vicarious discrimination, direct or transmitted by various media, impacts migrant health.

Health providers and discrimination

Social psychology scholars have conceptualized prejudicial attitudes or bias as implicit and explicit (18). Explicit attitudes are thoughts and feelings that people deliberately think about and can make conscious reports about. On the other hand, implicit attitudes often exist outside of conscious awareness, and thus are difficult to consciously acknowledge and control. These attitudes are often automatically activated and can influence human behaviour without conscious volition. Such notions are applied most often when people are busy, distracted, tired, and under pressure.

Despite the interest and importance of health care provider racism, we have limited knowledge of the extent and how to best capture it (19). Higher physician implicit bias has been linked to greater physician verbal dominance, giving less time to the patient's statements (20). Unintentional bias on the part of physicians can influence the way they treat patients from certain racial and ethnic groups (18). Most physicians are unaware that they hold such biases, which can unknowingly contribute to inequalities in health care delivery (21). People's ability to self-regulate the expression of bias in their behaviours depends on how aware they are of their racial bias, and how easy or hard the behaviours are to self-regulate (20). Virtually absent in the literature, however, is evidence-based information on how to reduce an individual health care provider's bias (21). Women, regardless of ethnicity, are more likely than men to experience biased interactions and treatment in care. Bias can exist on multiple social dimensions, and patients with multiple minority identities may be particularly affected. Interestingly, no study investigating implicit bias towards migrants was identified (18).

System discrimination

A race discrimination system is the product of both a system of race-linked disparities and a belief system that perpetuates them (7,22). It appears that bias and discrimination at a societal level create psychological environments that can also produce health care disparities among members of a stigmatized target group. A system's perspective gives understanding for how race-linked disparities affect the social and cultural milieu by creating a system that makes race salient in a way that distorts our perceptions and feelings (22). We need to come to a paradigm shift when discussing racial health disparity and focus on when discrimination is not at the root of health inequity. As soon as the concept of the 'others' is introduced we reinforce a system of discrimination. This will also impact how we teach science and train the future cadres of health professionals. Dr CP Jones, an American family physician, presented an allegory, 'A Gardener's Tale', in 2000 in the *American Journal of Public Health*, illustrating the concepts addressed previously. Readers are advised to take time to see presentations at TeDx from 2014, or 'Racism and the Social Determinants of Equity' at Beyond Flexner 2015, worth watching. Box 5.1 presents an abbreviated version of 'A Gardener's Tale' (11).

RACISM AND HEALTH IMPACTS

Exposure to interpersonal discrimination has been posited as an explanation, at least in part, for the stark and consistent racial disparities in health. A dose-response association between health outcomes and degrees of self-reported experience of racial discrimination has been observed (23). A rapidly growing body of literature links experiences of unfair treatment, discrimination, and racism to subsequent morbidity and even mortality. Reporting experiences of discrimination is independently related to the likelihood of reporting fair or poor health independent of socioeconomic status. Interestingly, young people are more likely to report race discrimination than older individuals, but the impact on health does not vary by age, gender, or socioeconomic status. The association between unfair treatment and

BOX 5.1   A GARDENER'S TALE

(Emerging from personal experience at their first house.) In spring, they discovered that only a few of the flower boxes had soil, so they bought potting soil to fill these, and planted marigolds in all of them. Weeks later some plants were doing great, others were struggling; it was clear that those in the old rocky soil were not on par with those in the new soil. Some seeds in each box were stronger and doing better than others, but the strongest flowers in the poor soil could barely keep up with the weakest in the good soil.

An analogy would be: what if a gardener decides to plant red and pink flowers, but likes red better, and plants them in the good soil? And when they do better, s/he would say, 'See? I knew red was better!' And, if the flowers were perennials and went to seed and regrew each year, this would perpetuate, if not worsen, the difference, the inequity.

And what if the gardener said, 'These pink flowers are going to do poorly anyway', and deadheaded the weakest, allowing them no chance at all? And in future generations if the gardener's children and grandchildren always grew up knowing that red flowers did better than pink?

What if the gardener does not redistribute the soil, then the flowers do not have an equal chance to grow? If s/he did, maybe generations of selection would take a few years to compensate for, or maybe because only the stronger pink seeds survived, they would do even better than the red if given a chance to have the same opportunity to grow in fertile soil. We cannot be sure until that opportunity is comprehensively and completely available.

well-being might be more pronounced for mental, as opposed to physical, health outcomes among migrants (24). Thus, with respect to the production of racial disparities in health, the chronicity rather than the severity of exposure to discrimination is often considered to be a stronger predictor of worse outcomes, either across subgroups or over time (5). Furthermore, everyday discrimination is more consistently associated with higher rates of morbidity and mortality than acute instances of unfair treatment. The extent to which exposure to unfair treatment is a key mechanism through which racial disparities in health are produced remains unclear (6). A recent systematic review assesses the limitations of current studies on racism and health service utilization demonstrating the need for more longitudinal studies (25).

There are hormonal consequences of experiencing or just visualizing racial discrimination that can be measured in a laboratory setting as a peripheral stress response, characterized by an increase in blood pressure and cortisol (13). Long-term exposure to discrimination and anxiety repeat episodes, perpetuate a vicious cycle, increasing the stress, and engages neural stress in regulatory circuits in the brain as well as inflammatory markers (12,13). Discrimination is fuelling processes related to mental and non-inflammatory chronic diseases, and science has just started exploring the complexity (26).

A life-course approach is also advocated to understand the influence of racial discrimination on children and young people across the lifespan regardless of the source of exposure (27). Childhood exposure to either direct and/or vicarious racial discrimination has been linked to poor child health, well-being, and development (10). Further exploration of the differential effects of racial discrimination experienced by caregivers, family, and peers, compared to experiences of racial discrimination by the children and young people themselves is needed (28). Mustillo et al. demonstrated that perceived racial discrimination explains as much or more of the black/white disparity in poor birth outcomes (low birth weight and preterm birth) as maternal education, income, cigarette smoking, alcohol consumption, and depressive symptomatology taken together (29). The association between socioeconomic status (SES) and health is typically thought to be remarkably consistent, whether it is across time, place, or health outcome. However, more recent research has begun to call this seemingly evident 'truth' into question. As more evidence comes to light, it appears that the shape of the SES/health gradient might differ according to experience of racial discrimination.

Several studies have linked telomere length to health disparity. Telomeres are a stretch of DNA at each end of a chromosome that protects the protein-encoding part of the DNA. They become shorter each time a cell divides. When a telomere becomes too short, it can no longer protect the cell's DNA, leaving the cell at risk for serious damage. Leukocyte telomere length (LTL) is an indicator of biological ageing; shorter LTL is associated with earlier mortality. It also has been tied to many age-related health issues, such as heart disease, diabetes, dementia, Alzheimer's disease, and arthritis (30). Shorter telomeres have been associated with experiences of heightened psychosocial stress and exposure to adverse social conditions. Studies have found that LTL may exhibit accelerated shortening due not only to physiologic conditions, but also psychosocial stress, and therefore may be a pathway generating racial disparities in health. Experiencing everyday discrimination was associated with shortened telomere length among older black adults and associated with mental health (31). This gives us an understanding that discrimination might generate greater disease vulnerability and possibly premature death.

SOCIETAL IMPACT OF DISCRIMINATION

The societal impact of discrimination, as indicated by the findings of Elias and Paradies, is shown in a substantial loss in disability-adjusted life years (DALYs) due to discrimination. On average, Australia loses up to 3.02% of its GDP ($37.9 billion) per annum as a result of individuals being exposed to some form of racial discrimination. Another important cost component, not included in their study, was the pain and suffering involved due to illness that can be attributed to racial discrimination. These findings also indicate that some of the costs resulting from discrimination are avoidable if measures are taken by governmental and nongovernmental institutions to curb racial discrimination. Countries with racially and ethnically diverse populations can therefore realize substantial savings by enforcing effective antidiscrimination measures. Not addressing, preventing, or combatting discrimination is costly not only for the individual, but for society at large (32).

MIGRANT HEALTH AND DISCRIMINATION

Studies on ethnic discrimination and health controlling for various predictors of disease as well as relevant migration-specific factors are few (33). However, some of the laboratory biological hormone studies have been replicated, and the impact of racial discrimination on psychological and physiological stress responses confirmed in migrant populations (14).

A recent study from Canada highlights that limiting discrimination increases a sense of belonging, supporting good mental health of refugees and increasing the probability of successfully identifying with the national culture (34). Clustering of migrants and minorities in certain geographic areas is common across the globe. Part of this can be due to structural discrimination and legislations that confine the minorities to certain areas, part could be that living in areas where the majority are like you reduces the daily risk of exposure to racism and discrimination. However, the Canadian study on refugees contradicted this, reporting no benefit on mental health if clustered in geographic areas (34). Although some new studies are being produced on the impact of discrimination on health, longitudinal studies are warranted that assess the effects of social contexts and discussions on the openness of the host society, exclusion and separation of migrant communities, and the respective effect on discrimination and distress (35).

DECREASING DISCRIMINATION AND IMPROVING MIGRANT HEALTH

Antonovsky's Salutogenesis and Sense of Coherence (SOC) as a global orientation in which the world is seen, to a greater or lesser extent, as comprehensible, manageable, and meaningful is worth exploring related to discrimination (36). According to Antonovsky, the meaningfulness component is strengthened through participation in shaping outcomes in socially valued contexts. 'When others decide everything for us — when they set the task, formulate the rules, and manage the outcome — and we have no say in the matter, we are reduced to being objects. A world thus experienced as being indifferent to what we do, comes to be seen as a world devoid of meaning' (36). One can speculate that living a life where you are surrounded by various forms of discrimination challenges you and diminishes your SOC. This is interestingly described in a recent study on differences in health and SOC between first- and second-generation migrants in Holland and contributes to the discussion on the healthy migrant effect of the first-generation migrants (37).

To reduce racial and ethnic disparities in health care, we must ascertain the prevalence of biased attitudes among health care providers and whether bias contributes to problems in patient-provider interactions and relationships, quality of care, continuity of care, treatment adherence, and patient health status. European health care and society at large should learn from the history of discrimination as well as the current system of racial discrimination in the United States, and avoid copying them. We must include this in education at all levels and also increase the awareness about implicit bias across the European health care system. Using an intersectionality approach, addressing political and social determinants of health is imperative when addressing migrant health (38). Interestingly, the rigor of methodological studies aimed at improving cultural competency in health care has been challenged (38). Most of the training interventions measured changes in professional attitudes towards the population of interest but did not measure the downstream effect of changing provider beliefs on the care delivered to patients. A limited number of studies have been published on interventions to improve migrant health.

We are socialized into discrimination of 'the other'. Small children are colour-blind until taught otherwise. Systems, group, and individual aspects all have to be taken into account when we now understand the complexity of health inequity and discrimination as a system of power. Health equity is a process not to be perceived as an attainment (39). 'Achieving health equity requires valuing all individuals and populations equally, recognizing and rectifying historical injustices, and providing resources according to need. It requires dismantling systems or structure inequity and putting in their place systems in which all people can know and develop their full potentials' (39, page S75).

SUMMARY

The increasing complexity of our societies and the challenges short- and long-term migration present to all aspects of society call for change. Change in how we think about health, about what creates health, and how we as health care providers must participate in the shaping of a new paradigm. Discrimination, in all shapes and forms, fosters ill health and impacts the individual, young and old, the community, rich and poor, and the society at large, finanically and culturally. Addressing, preventing, and combatting discrimination is an important health and public health challenge for all, not only for migrant health.

REFERENCES

1. Vertovec S. Super-diversity and its implications. *Ethn Racial Stud.* 2007;30(6):1024–54.
2. Krieger N. Refiguring 'race': epidemiology, racialized biology, and biological expressions of race relations. *Int J Health Serv.* 2000;30(1):211–6.
3. Paradies Y, Ben J, Denson N, Elias A, Priest N, Pieterse A et al. Racism as a determinant of health: a systematic review and meta-analysis. *PLOS ONE.* 2015;10(9):e0138511.
4. Nazroo JY. The structuring of ethnic inequalities in health: economic position, racial discrimination, and racism. *Am J Public Health.* 2003;93(2):277–84.
5. Colen CG, Ramey DM, Cooksey EC, Williams DR. Racial disparities in health among nonpoor African Americans and Hispanics: the role of acute and chronic discrimination. *Soc Sci Med.* 2018;199:167–80.
6. Hicken M, Durkee M, Kravitz-Wurtz N, Jackson J. The role of racism in health inequalities: integrating approaches from across disciplines. *Soc Sci Med.* 2018;199(1):11–240.
7. Jones CP. Confronting institutionalized racism. *Phylon.* 2003;50(1):7–22.
8. Khan M, Ilcisin M, Saxton K. Multifactorial discrimination as a fundamental cause of mental health inequities. *Int J Equity Health.* 2017;16(1):43.
9. Pascoe EA, Smart Richman L. Perceived discrimination and health: a meta-analytic review. *Psychol Bull.* 2009;135(4):531–54.
10. Priest N, Paradies Y, Trenerry B, Truong M, Karlsen S, Kelly Y. A systematic review of studies examining the relationship between reported racism and health and wellbeing for children and young people. *Soc Sci Med.* 2013;95(1):115–27.
11. Jones CP. Levels of racism: a theoretic framework and a gardener's tale. *Am J Public Health.* 2000;90(8):1212–5.
12. Brody GH, Yu T, Beach SR. Resilience to adversity and the early origins of disease. *Dev Psychopathol.* 2016;28(4 Pt2):1347–65.
13. Berger M, Sarnyai Z. 'More than skin deep': Stress neurobiology and mental health consequences of racial discrimination. *Stress.* 2015;18(1):1–10.
14. Fischer S, Nater UM, Strahler J, Skoluda N, Dieterich L, Oezcan O, Mewes R. Psychobiological impact of ethnic discrimination in Turkish immigrants living in Germany. *Stress.* 2017;20(2):167–74.
15. Tomfohr LM, Pung MA, Dimsdale JE. Mediators of the relationship between race and allostatic load in African and White Americans. *Health Psychol.* 2016;35(4):322–32.
16. Bécares L, Nazroo J, Kelly Y. A longitudinal examination of maternal, family, and area-level experiences of racism on children's socioemotional development: patterns and possible explanations. *Soc Sci Med.* 2015;142:128–35.
17. Lauderdale DS. Birth outcomes for Arabic-named women in California before and after September 11. *Demography.* 2006;43(2):185–201.
18. Hall WJ, Chapman MV, Lee KM, Merino YM, Thomas TW, Payne BK et al. Implicit racial/ethnic bias among health care professionals and its influence on health care outcomes: a systematic review. *Am J Public Health.* 2015;105:e60–76.
19. Paradies Y, Truong M, Priest N. A systematic review of the extent and measurement of healthcare provider racism. *J Gen Intern Med.* 2014;29(2):364–87.
20. Hagiwara N, Penner LA, Gonzalez R, Eggly S, Dovidio JF, Gaertner SL et al. Racial attitudes, physician-patient talk time ratio, and adherence in racially discordant medical interactions. *Soc Sci Med.* 2013;87:123–31.
21. Van Ryn M. Avoiding unintended bias: strategies for providing more equitable health care. *Minn Med.* 2016;99(1):40–3.

22. Reskin B. The race discrimination system. *Annu Rev Sociol.* 2012;38(1):17–35.
23. Harris R, Tobias M, Jeffreys M, Waldegrave K, Karlsen S, Nazroo J. Racism and health: the relationship between experience of racial discrimination and health in New Zealand. *Soc Sci Med.* 2006;63:1428–41.
24. Hatch SL, Gazard B, Williams DR, Frissa S, Goodwin L, SELCoH Study Team, Hotopf M. Discrimination and common mental disorder among migrant and ethnic groups: findings from a South East London Community sample. *Soc Psychiatry Psychiatr Epidemiol.* 2016;51:689–701.
25. Ben J, Cormack D, Harris R, Paradies Y. Racism and health service utilisation: a systematic review and meta-analysis. *PLOS ONE.* 2017;12(12):e0189900.
26. Busse D, Yim IS, Campos B. Social context matters: ethnicity, discrimination and stress reactivity. *Psychoneuroendocrinology.* 2017;83:187–93.
27. Gee GC, Walsemann KM, Brondolo E. A life course perspective on how racism may be related to health inequities. *Am J Public Health.* 2012;102(5): 967–74.
28. Heard-Garris NJ, Cale M, Camaj L, Hamati MC, Dominguez TP. Transmitting trauma: a systematic review of vicarious racism and child health. *Soc Sci Med.* 2018;199:230–40.
29. Mustillo S, Krieger N, Gunderson EP, Sidney S, McCreath H, Kiefe CI. Self-reported experiences of racial discrimination and Black-White differences in preterm and low-birthweight deliveries: The CARDIA Study. *Am J Public Health.* 2004;94(12):2125–31.
30. Rizvi S, Raza ST, Mahdi F. Telomere length variations in aging and age-related diseases. *Curr Aging Sci.* 2014;7(2):161–7.
31. Chae DH, Nuru-Jeter AM, Adler NE, Brody GH, Lin J, Blackburn EH, Epel ES. Discrimination, racial bias, and telomere length in African-American men. *Am J Prev Med.* 2014;46(2):103–11.
32. Elias A, Paradies Y. Estimating the mental health costs of racial discrimination. *BMC Public Health.* 2016;16:1205–10.
33. Aichberger MC, Bromand Z, Rapp MA, Yesil R, Montesinos AH, Temur-Erman S et al. Perceived ethnic discrimination, acculturation, and psychological distress in women of Turkish origin in Germany. *Soc Psychiatry Psychiatr Epidemiol.* 2015;50:1691–700.
34. Beiser M, Hou F. Predictors of positive mental health among refugees: results from Canada's General Social Survey. *Transcult Psychiatry.* 2017;54(5–6):675–95.
35. Edge S, Newbold B. Discrimination and the health of immigrants and refugees: exploring Canada's evidence base and directions for future research in newcomer receiving countries. *J Immigr Minor Health.* 2013;15:141–8.
36. Antonovsky, A. *Unraveling the Mystery of Health.* San Francisco, CA: Jossey-Bass; 1987.
37. Slootjes J, Keuzenkamp S, Saharso S. The mechanisms behind the formation of a strong Sense of Coherence (SOC): the role of migration and integration. *Scand J Psychol.* 2017;58:571–80.
38. Truong M, Paradies Y, Priest N. Interventions to improve cultural competency in healthcare: a systematic review of reviews. *BMC Health Serv Res.* 2014;14:99.
39. Jones CP. Systems of power, axes of inequity. Parallels, intersections, braiding the strands. *Med Care.* 2014;52:S71–75.

CHAPTER 6

Migrants' use of primary health care services: Overuse, underuse, or both?

Esperanza Diaz and Bernadette N. Kumar

LEARNING OBJECTIVES

In this chapter, we will:

- Give an overview of migrants' use of primary health care
- Provide explanations and outline factors for the differences in the utilization of health services
- Describe general barriers associated with the use of health care services for migrants
- Suggest tools to improve access to health care services for migrants

---

CLINICAL VIGNETTE

It is 5:30 am Thursday early morning and the emergency room (ER) is finally quiet. After working for several hours, the emergency doctor retires for a break, but this does not last long, and he is called back to surgery. A woman from Somalia complains of pain in her abdomen and her family insists that she cannot wait until the general practitioner (GP) shift at 7:00 am. Upon arrival, the emergency doctor observes a group of Somalis surrounding a 45-year-old woman who is crying. It crosses his mind that this is an over exaggeration of symptoms. He wonders why patients from Somalia use the ER when they should use their GP and always come in the middle of the night. He is soon overcome with shame regarding his prejudices. He then determines that he will undertake a thorough anamnesis and a battery of blood tests to ensure that he does not miss anything important.

A recent systematic review, including 36 publications on use of primary care, mental health services, hospitalizations, and emergency care, concluded that, as a group, migrants use health services less than or equal to the majority population (1). Despite the existing evidence, also recently confirmed by the Lancet Commission, the myth that migrants are a heavy burden for health care services is well spread among the majority populations, the media, and even many health professionals (2). Although it is important to have the evidence to fight stereotypes among the public in general, in the case of health professionals it is also vital to understand the underlying mechanisms by which migrants are often perceived as a burden. Besides populist discourses in high-income societies that may affect health care providers, a large body of literature describes that health professionals actually experience challenges in delivering health care across cultures (3,4) and that they are not at ease providing adequate health care in multicultural societies (5). This might not be a surprise, since most medical curricula do not include cultural awareness, competence, or specific migrant health knowledge (6). Correspondingly, migrants from low- and middle-income countries in Europe seem to be less satisfied with health care services than the majority population (7,8). In this chapter, we will try to clarify this apparent discordance between the evidence and the professionals' and patients' experiences and feelings.

FACTORS RELATED TO USE OF PRIMARY HEALTH CARE SERVICES

Is it good or bad that migrants' utilization of health care services differs from the majority? Using health care services is not a means in itself, but use should be directly related to the need of the patient. From that point of view, knowing if migrants use health care services more or less than the majority population does not give us an answer to the important question: do patients, disregarding their background, get the health care services they need? In order to shed some light on this subject, we will discuss factors that are associated with the use of health care services.

Burden of disease

The main factor that should predict use of health services is the burden of disease in a given population: sicker patients should use the services more often than healthy people should. The end outcome to measure disease and thus need for health care is mortality. Lower mortality rates for a given group indicate better health than those with higher rates. Several studies observe lower mortality among most groups of migrants (2). The patterns of mortality differ by *country of origin* (9) and *reason for migration*, with refugees having the worst outcomes among migrants (10). *Length of stay in the new country* is another important factor that explains mortality rates. A convergence in mortality with increasing duration of residence is observed, suggesting that 'healthy migrant' and 'acculturation' effects counteract each other over time (11). Most diseases studied in migrants follow a similar pattern as mortality. Low burden of disease to begin with, varying according to country of origin and reason for migration, worsening quicker for migrants than the majority population. The burden of disease among migrants reaches approximately the same levels after some years in the host country, explained chiefly by allostatic overload theory as described in Chapter 2. Taking all these factors into consideration, the use of services should be proportional to burden of disease. Among migrants we should expect utilization of heath care services to be related to the patients' *area of origin*, their *reasons for migration*, and *duration of stay in the new country*.

This is in accordance with the findings from several countries in Europe; patients from the Middle East, Africa, and some parts of Asia use services more often than those from other geographical areas, and refugee patients use the services more often than other migrants. A convergence with the majority in use of services is seen with increasing duration of residence (12,13). Therefore, we can conclude that migrants' use of primary health care in reality reflects their lower burden of disease.

Life-course perspective

The life-course perspective is relevant for understanding migrants' use of services as compared to majority populations. Children of migrants might use health care services differently for various reasons apart from their burden of disease. Migrant parents might lack informal networks, e.g. neighbours or family members, to seek advice from regarding common diseases. Their experiences regarding the consequences of symptoms like fever or diarrhoea might be much more devastating than what a European-born person is used to, prompting them to use the services more often. For those who are used to different health care systems, it takes some years to understand the different roles of GPs and ERs. These factors might explain why migrant children under the age of 5 years used the ERs more often than Norwegian-born children (14). On the other side, some migrant parents might lack information about available services or the necessary tools or help to access them due to language or other barriers. In Norway, migrant children, particularly those in late adolescence, seem to be healthier and use both primary health care and prescribed medication less than non-migrant children (15). However, the differences in use of medication are minimal for Norwegian-born children of migrants. This indicates a more 'normalized' use of services after parents have lived for a while in the new country. This could be attributed to better information, improved access to health care services, integration in society, and improved language skills (15).

Continuing with a life-course perspective, not much attention has been paid to elderly patients with migrant backgrounds. Both ageing and migration are in themselves complex, multidimensional processes. The trajectories will differ for migrants who migrated as young persons and have lived most of their lives in the host country versus those who have migrated as older persons, as the disease profiles and personal resources are probably very different (16). These differences should have been reflected in the use of health services by frequency, type of services, and complexity of needs; however, disaggregated data by these groups is lacking. As migration to high-income countries began a few decades ago with young migrants, the number of elderly with migrant backgrounds who have lived in the country for a long time is expected to double by 2050 (17). Elderly migrants in Northern, Western and Eastern Europe seem to be frailer than the majority populations, although differences tend to disappear by 80–90 years of age (18). Though the evidence is not consistent, some studies show lower use of primary health care services among the elderly, especially for those from low-income countries. This underuse of services could be due to barriers to access (19), like lack of language skills, lack of knowledge of own rights to interpreter or home care services, reliance on already overburdened family members for appointments, or lack of health insurance (20). Knowledge about the use and need of home care services for elderly patients with migrant backgrounds is limited. However, we should be aware that their relatives and caregivers, many of whom are now highly acculturated in their new country, might not share the traditional expectations of the elderly, of being taken care of by family members.

Socioeconomic factors

Socioeconomic factors like gender, income, or education are associated with both disease burden and use of health services for all groups. Migrants, depending on their origins and reasons for migration, might have higher or lower education and income as compared to the majority populations, and until recently migration was male dominated. Consequently, part of the differences in use of health care services between migrants and non-migrants could be explained by these factors (12).

In the host population, those with low income and education use the health system more than educated, better off groups. Conversely, in some studies migrants with lower levels of income or education tend to have relatively lower use as compared to other migrants, while higher education or income levels do not seem to prevent use for migrants to the same extent as they do for the majority population (21). Although the lower use of health care systems is often interpreted as part of the healthy migrant effect described in Chapter 2, other interpretations must also be considered. One such explanation might be that less-educated migrants have poorer language skills and health literacy, and that only the most educated or integrated migrants get enough information to be able to use the services in accordance with their needs. In addition, migrants closely attached to their communities get most of their social support from them and may lack sources of information regarding health care services. Migrants with higher education have more contact with the majority population, which might increase the possibility of receiving relevant health service-related information and thus lead to a higher utilization of health care services (22).

Another issue is related to our classifications and categories, as explained in Chapter 1, which do not necessarily reflect the subtle differences within groups classified under the same category. A physician from Latin America, for example, might not be able to validate his doctor licence in Europe and have to work, and will be thus classified as a bus driver. A woman from Vietnam who spends the whole day working in the family business might never be registered as a worker. In these two examples, the education or income registered would not adequately capture resources and challenges for the individuals as compared to majority persons within the same categories.

DIFFERENCES IN UTILIZATION OF THE HEALTH CARE SYSTEM: STEREOTYPES, FACTS, OR BOTH?

Notwithstanding the results presented, classifying all migrants as one group makes no real sense, as continents are huge areas with extremely heterogeneous populations. As an illustration of this, putting Japan and China in the same group is as meaningless as Norway and Greece. To further document these within-region differences, we conducted a study of the use of primary health care among four sub-Saharan African migrant groups in Norway. Despite the similarities in diagnoses among the groups, their use of health care services differed by country of origin and length of stay. Compared to migrants from Somalia, the use of both GP and ER were significantly lower for Ethiopians, Eritreans, and Gambians (23). We should bear this in mind when we far too quickly generalize our knowledge or assumptions from one group to another within one continent, or even worse 'for all migrants'.

In our vignette, a woman from Somalia came to the ER in the middle of the night. This type of situation has been also documented by a study in Norway that showed that patients from some countries (Somalia and Iraq, for example) more often use the ER at night and get a nonspecific diagnosis (14). While this is not necessarily the case for all patients from Somalia or Iraq, health professionals might far too quickly generalize this pattern, not only to all patients from Somalia, but to all African or even all migrant patients. This then leads to the impression that 'all migrants' misuse the health care system. We should be aware of this unconscious mechanism of generalization that leads to stereotyping. The mechanisms by which migrants more often can end up with 'nonspecific' diagnoses are further discussed in Chapter 20. The nonspecific diagnoses are not only generated due to the patient, but through the interaction with the GP as well as a system that may not be adequately equipped for dealing with other languages and cultures.

Migrants on the whole use the ER less than the host population, although differences exist depending on the groups, as explained previously (14). Another common idea related to the use of the health care services is that migrants' use of the system is incorrect, i.e. they use the ER instead of going to their GP. While this is true for some groups, especially those with lack of entitlements or those who are new in the country, an American study shows that migrants less often have preventable visits at the ER (24). A study in Norway shows that the groups of migrants that use the ER more often than the host population do so in addition to, and not instead of, visiting their GPs (25). Both studies suggest that either migrants do not get the help they need, or their expectations are not fulfilled at the mainstream services and they therefore look for other solutions to their problems, rather than 'misusing' the system. In our vignette, we should not take for granted that the woman for Somalia has not visited her GP, but rather ask her if she has done so, and if that is the case, what happened there so that she bothers to come to the ER in the middle of the night. Most people, including those from Somalia, actually prefer not to be at the ER at 5:30 am.

For some health care services, there is clear evidence of underuse among migrants. Migrants, regardless of origin, use preventive health care programs such as the cervical cancer screening program less often than the non-migrant populations (26). Barriers for attending these programs are complex, and not only at the user level. A study in Norway among women from Pakistan and Somalia regarding attendance to cervical cancer screening showed that women lacked understanding of the benefits of the screening. Besides the stigma attached to the disease, there was the belief that unmarried women are sexually inactive and therefore do not need to undertake the test. In addition, the lack of general trust towards the health care system constituted a clear barrier for many women. When women were properly informed, they said they wished their GP had informed them about the importance of this test earlier (27). On the other hand, when GPs were asked about their perceptions of the attendance of migrant women to cervical cancer screening, they acknowledged that they relied largely on the women to request the test. While they might raise the issue with non-migrant women, most often they assumed that migrant women were not interested in the test (28).

The underutilization of preventive services has serious health consequences: migrants from Asia and Africa in Norway are often diagnosed with a more advanced stage of breast cancer, partly due to low participation in mammography screening (29).

CULTURAL HUMILITY

An important part of what we call cultural humility is to acknowledge that all of us have preconceived ideas, most of all when the other person is different from us. In cross-cultural consultations, the GP can have prejudices more often than in consultations with patients of the same background and culture. Stereotypes are often, but not always, based on personal experiences about the patients' higher or different expectations. These include preferences for a more paternalistic provider, broader diagnostic procedures, more prescription of medications – specifically antibiotics, quicker referrals to specialists, or lower compliance, to name a few. On the other hand, patients too have preconceived ideas about the system and the GPs. In Norway, for example, GPs are not considered very competent among some migrant groups. This may be due to perceptions such as lacking knowledge based on lack of check-ups for healthy patients, or low prescription rates for some drugs, like inhibitors of gastric acid secretion or antibiotics. Some patients travel back to the country of origin for check-ups with doctors, when there is a serious illness like cancer, or when the patient feels that he or she has not been taken seriously. Some groups have even their favourite countries to travel to in search of good health care: Somali patients living in Norway travel to Germany to get a second opinion, while Indian patients travel to England. Although it is not the task of this book to confirm or discard such preconceived ideas, it is the GP's obligation to address and acknowledge these issues in order to further understand the patient. A better understanding of the patients' perspectives can be useful in negotiating the way forward with the patient and overcoming further barriers.

BARRIERS FOR USE OF HEALTH CARE SERVICES AND SUGGESTIONS TO OVERCOME THEM

CLINICAL VIGNETTE

Phuong is a 45-year-old woman from Vietnam. She moved to Europe 1 year ago to join her sister after being widowed. She speaks only a few words in her host country's language and has never visited her GP before today. She comes with her sister, Linh, who made the appointment for her. Phuong has not left her house for weeks, she has no appetite, has neglected her personal hygiene, and only wants to lie in bed. The family is very worried, and her sister has taken a few weeks off from work to be able to be with her and cheer her up, but it has not helped so she has returned to work. Phuong does not want to go to the GP, as she is scared of being diagnosed as 'crazy' and that her situation will become known among the local Vietnamese community. She has been trying 'coining' and prayers to get rid of the negative energy, but without improvement.

Dr Europe listens to Linh and acknowledges her for her efforts in helping Phuong. Though Phuong does not want to talk herself, Dr Europe asks Linh if she can translate everything she says for her sister. Dr Europe has heard of coining, but does not know what it is, and asks the sisters if they can explain the procedure, which they do. Phuong seems to smile a little when the GP wants to know more about this practice without judging it as wrong or getting angry. Then, Dr Europe asks why they think Phuong is in this situation, and Linh talks about Phuong's sorrow for her late husband and punishment for not conducting the annual ritual after his death. Dr Europe asks some more questions that lead her to suspect that Phuong suffers from depression. She confirms to both sisters that it was right to come to the GP. She also asks if there is anything that Phuong liked to do before she became apathetic or that has helped her in difficult times. She learns that the patient loves drawing, but she does not have the materials she needs here. Dr Europe needs to take some tests and prefers using a professional interpreter for that, so she suggests a new consultation just a couple of days afterwards with a professional interpreter, after making it clear that it is mandatory for interpreters to maintain confidentiality. Phuong, who responds with few words, expresses her dissatisfaction, and they finally agree upon a telephone interpreter, so that Phuong is sure she will not be recognized. In the meantime, they agree that Phuong's sister will buy what is needed for basic drawing and that they will explore the possibility of engaging somebody who can help them with the ritual to be conducted one year after her husband's death.

Potential barriers for use of health care services are often described at three different levels: patient level, provider level, and system level (30); however, it is important to remember that overcoming these barriers often lies at the interaction between levels. Barriers at the patient level are related to the patient's characteristics, some of which, like age, income, education level, and migration background are described in the previous section. Language as a barrier is assessed in Chapter 17 and is often a necessary key to communication. In our example, Dr Europe not only recognizes the barrier but also involves the patient in deciding how it should be bridged. However, if the system does not have accessible, available, and affordable interpreters of good quality or if the GP does not have the skills to use an interpreter, the barrier will remain, despite the efforts of the GP.

Other potential barriers are the patient's health beliefs and attitudes, perceived illness, and personal health practices, when these are not the same as the majority population. Shame and stigma for mental health compounded with the fear and mistrust of services can result in delays in seeking help (31). However, most of these barriers can be bridged in the interaction with a doctor who is non-judgmental and recognizes these issues, in order to find common ground based on the patient's resources and possibilities. In our case, Dr Europe confirms to both the patient and her sister that it is correct to seek help. She asks about 'coining' with an open mind not because she believes that coining is an appropriate treatment, but to try to understand the patient's perspective, in order to be able to negotiate thereafter a solution that suits both parties without compromising what the doctor believes has to be done. In other words, by asking the patient openly about a treatment not recognized in Western medicine, she gains the trust needed that leads to follow-up visit. This subsequent visit provides the GP with the grounds to give a better diagnosis and hopefully begin to help the patient to restore her health. Indeed, once the patient is in contact with the health care system, the provider's role is crucial in assessing and overcoming barriers at the patient level.

The provider characteristics, skills and attitudes, some of them shown by Dr Europe and shown in Chapter 3, are the clue to facilitate adequate use of health care services and improve the quality of services for patients with potential difficulties in special situations. However, this will not help all patients, especially those who do not seek help. Interventions are required to promote mental health awareness and knowledge of services among this specially targeted population to reduce stigma and thereby improve access to services (31).

Despite good doctor-patient relationships and the help of competent interpreters, GPs might still experience obstacles in the care for their migrant patients, including the lack of validated tests for the diagnostic process, early detection, and assessment of care needs (Chapter 20). New validated tools for different groups and knowledge among GPs about these tools are necessary to overcome this problem (32). In addition, for some migrant patients, strong collaborations between primary care, community care organizations, specialized clinics, and municipalities are sometimes needed to optimize health care provision. Access to culturally sensitive facilities and coordination between the GP and specialists about the patient's illness is key to achieving these goals (33,34). In situations when the patient has a very poor network, the continuity of care given by a GP is also crucial.

Health care systems are organized differently in every country. In terms of primary care, most European countries rely on a primary medical care model in which patients seek assistance from their GP when they need health care. The GPs are often the first point of contact for any consultation and will make the necessary referrals to secondary and tertiary level care. As described previously, these systems can constitute a barrier for migrants in terms of preventive medicine. Other countries have more community-oriented or comprehensive primary health care, in which the patients are actively invited to health promotion activities. According to a recent scoping review of primary health care models addressing health equity for migrants, the most commonly identified barriers to care included insurance/eligibility, cultural barriers, language and communication, education and health literacy, social networks and support, patient-provider relationship, organization of services, geographic access, and costs. Although the two models often coexist to varying degrees, the authors concluded that the primary medical care model may be better suited to address social determinants of health and might have more potential capacity to reduce health inequities among migrants. There is acknowledgement that the two models could act synergistically in responding to migrants' health care needs (35).

From another point of view, although migration cannot and should not be viewed as a laboratory experiment, it can be seen as a natural experiment that helps us understand the effect of the different health care systems on the health of the individuals. If two groups of migrants from the same area migrate to two different countries through similar migration journeys, differences in health outcomes for those migrants in the two host countries could be due to factors associated with the receiving country, including their health care systems. Mortality among migrants is indeed associated with their country of destination (9), which points to the importance of health care services and other social and integration services in the host countries.

Within the health system, barriers for migrants include entitlements and bureaucratic obstacles like paperwork and registration schemes that are often too complicated for newcomers with low health literacy to navigate efficiently. The organization of health care systems varies, and the fewer similarities between the country of origin and that of destination, the more challenging it becomes to use the system, especially during the first years as a migrant. Too often, information about the health system is not available in different languages, or only in English as a foreign language, which is not familiar for all migrants. Fragmented structure of services, long waiting lists, co-payments, complex connections of local transportation, shortage of available interpreters, and systematic lack of training in cultural competence for providers can also be barriers at the system level. For undocumented migrants, in addition to the lack of entitlements in many countries, the fear of deportation, stigma, and lack of capital (both social and financial) to obtain services often become barriers that postpone seeking help until it is too late. Recommendations identified in a review for undocumented migrants include advocating for policy change to increase access to health care, providing novel insurance options, expanding safety net services, training providers to better care for migrant populations, and educating undocumented migrants on navigating the system (36). Finally, as explained in Chapter 5, there is ample evidence of discriminatory practices within most health care systems.

CONCLUSION

Migrants do not as a rule overuse or misuse the health care systems. Overall, migrants use health care services less than host populations. However, there are significant differences among groups depending on factors like the area of origin, the reason for migration, and the length of stay in the new country, in addition to other factors. Barriers for use of services can be described at the patient, provider, and system levels. Health care providers can help patients bridge some of the barriers for equity in care, but interventions at the community and the health system levels are also needed. GPs are in a privileged position to detect barriers, and thus advocacy becomes one of their duties, especially when it comes to migrants. In our efforts to deliver equitable health care, we should view migrants as the litmus test for the health care system and not as a problem. Most often, improving the health care system for vulnerable groups will also improve the health of the majority of the population. That is our main goal.

REFERENCES

1. Sarría-Santamera A, Hijas-Gómez AI, Carmona R, Gimeno-Feliú LA. A systematic review of the use of health services by immigrants and native populations. *Public Health Rev.* 2016;37(28).
2. Abubakar I, Aldridge RW, Devakumar D et al. The UCL-Lancet Commission on Migration and Health: the health of a world on the move. *Lancet.* 2018;392(10164)2606−54.
3. Varvin S, Aasland OG. Legers forhold til flyktningpasienten [Physicians' relation to refugees]. *Tidsskrift Norske Legeforening.* 2009;129(15):1488−90.
4. Debesay J, Harslof I, Rechel B, Vike H. Facing diversity under institutional constraints: challenging situations for community nurses when providing care to ethnic minority patients. *J Adv Nurs.* 2014;70(9):2107−16.
5. van den Muijsenbergh M, van Weel-Baumgarten E, Burns N et al. Communication in cross-cultural consultations in primary care in Europe: the case for improvement. The rationale for the RESTORE FP 7 project. *Prim Health Care Res Dev.* 2014;15(2):122−33.
6. Diaz E, Kumar BN. Health care curricula in multicultural societies. *Int J Med Educ.* 2018;9:42−4.
7. Harmsen JA, Bernsen R, Bruijnzeels M, Meeuwesen L. Patients' evaluation of quality of care in general practice: what are the cultural and linguistic barriers? *Patient Educ Couns.* 2008;72:155−62.
8. Suurmond J, Uiters E, de Bruijne MC, Stronks K, Essink-Bot M-L. Negative health care experiences of immigrant patients: a qualitative study. *BMC Health Serv Res.* 2011;11:10.
9. Ikram UZ, Mackenbach JP, Harding S et al. All-cause and cause-specific mortality of different migrant populations in Europe. *Eur J Epidemiol.* 2016;31(7):655−65.
10. Syse A, Strand BH, Naess O, Steingímsdóttir ÓA, Kumar BN. Differences in all-cause mortality: a comparison between immigrants and the host population in Norway 1990–2012. *Demogr Res.* 2016;34(22):615−56.
11. Syse A, Dzamarija MT, Kumar BN, Diaz E. An observational study of immigrant mortality differences in Norway by reason for migration, length of stay and characteristics of sending countries. *BMC Public Health.* 2018;18(1):508.
12. Diaz E, Calderón-Larrañaga A, Prado-Torres A, Poblador-Plou B, Gimeno-Feliu L-A. How do immigrants use primary healthcare services? A register-based study in Norway. *Eur J Public Health.* 2015;25(1):72−8.
13. Diaz E, Kumar BN, Gimeno-Feliu L-A, Calderón-Larrañaga A, Poblador-Pou B, Prados-Torres A. Multimorbidity among registered immigrants in Norway: the role of reason for migration and length of stay. *Trop Med Int Health.* 2015;20(12):1805−14.
14. Sandvik H, Hunskaar S, Diaz E. Immigrants' use of emergency primary health care in Norway: a registry-based observational study. *BMC Health Serv Res.* 2012;12:308.
15. Fadnes L, Diaz E. Primary health care usage and use of medications among immigrant children according to age of arrival to Norway: a population-based study. *BMJ Open.* 2017;7(2):e014641.
16. Kristiansen M. *Health of Older Refugees and Migrants. Technical Guidance.* Copenhagen: World Health Organization. 2018.
17. Ramm J. *Eldres bruk av helse- og omsorgstjenester [The elderly use of health care services].* Oslo; 2013.

18. Walkden GJ, Anderson EL, Vink MP, Tilling K, Howe LD, Ben-Shlomo Y. Frailty in older-age European migrants: cross-sectional and longitudinal analyses of the Survey of Health, Aging and Retirement in Europe (SHARE). *Soc Sci Med*. 2018;213:1–11.
19. Diaz E, Kumar BN. Differential utilization of primary health care services among older immigrants and Norwegians: a register-based comparative study in Norway. *BMC Health Serv Res*. 2014;14:623.
20. Ruspini P. Elderly migrants in Europe: an overview of trends, policies and practices. European Committee on Migration of the Council of Europe 2009.
21. Finnvold JE. How social and geographical backgrounds affect hospital admission with a serious condition: a comparison of 11 immigrant groups with native-born Norwegians. *BMC Health Serv Res*. 2018;18:843.
22. Rapp C, Huijts T, Eikemo TA, Stathopoulou T. Social integration and self-reported health: differences between immigrants and natives in Greece. *Eur J Public Health*. 2018(S5):48–53.
23. Diaz E, Mbanya VN, Gele AA, Kumar B. Differences in primary health care use among sub-Saharan African immigrants in Norway: a register-based study. *BMC Health Serv Res*. 2017;17(1):509.
24. Wang Y, Wilson FA, Stimpson JP et al. Fewer immigrants have preventable ED visits in the United States. *Am J Emerg Med*. 2018;36(3):352–8.
25. Diaz E, Gimeno-Feliu LA, Calderón-Larrañaga A, Prados-Torres A. Frequent attenders in general practice and immigrant status in Norway: a nationwide cross-sectional study. *Scand J Prim Health Care*. 2014;32(4):232–40.
26. Møen KA, Kumar B, Qureshi S, Diaz E. Differences in cervical cancer screening between immigrants and non-immigrants in Norway: a primary health care register-based study. *Eur J Cancer Prev*. 2016;26(6):521–7.
27. Gele AA, Qureshi SA, Kour P, Kumar B, Diaz E. Barriers and facilitators to cervical cancer screening among Pakistani and Somali immigrant women in Oslo: a qualitative study. *Int J Womens Health*. 2017;6(9):487–96.
28. Møen KA, Terragni L, Kumar BN, Diaz E. Cervical cancer screening among immigrant women in Norway- the health care providers' perspectives. *Scand J Prim Health Care*. 2018;36(4):415–22.
29. Thogersen H, Moller B, Robsahm TE, Aaserud S, Babigumira R, Larsen IK. Comparison of cancer stage distribution in the immigrant and host populations of Norway, 1990–2014. *Int J Cancer*. 2017;141(1):52–61.
30. Scheppers E, Dongen Ev, Dekker J, Geertzen J, Dekker J. Potential barriers to the use of health services among ethnic minorities: a review. *Fam Pract* 2006;23:325–48.
31. Posselt M, McDonald K, Procter N, de Crespigny C, Galletly C. Improving the provision of services to young people from refugee backgrounds with comorbid mental health and substance use problems: addressing the barriers. *BMC Public Health*. 2017;17(1):280.
32. Sagbakken M, Spilker RS, Nielsen TR. Dementia and immigrant groups: a qualitative study of challenges related to identifying, assessing, and diagnosing dementia. *BMC Health Serv Res*. 2018;18:910.
33. Vissenberg R, Uysal O, Goudsmit M, Campen Jv, Buurman-van B. Barriers in providing primary care for immigrant patients with dementia: GPs' perspectives. *BJGP Open*. 2018;2(4):bjgpopen18X101610.
34. Khan NA, Saboor HT, Qayyum Z, Khan I, Habib Z, Washeed HT. Barriers to accessing the German health-care system for Pakistani immigrants in Berlin, Germany: a qualitative exploratory study. *Lancet*. 2013;382(Supplement 1).
35. Batista R, Pottie K, Bouchard L, Ng E, Tanuseputro P, Tugwell P. Primary health care models addressing health equity for immigrants: a systematic scoping review. *J Immigr Minor Health*. 2018;20(1):214–30.
36. Hacker K, Anies M, Folb BL, Zallman L. Barriers to health care for undocumented immigrants: a literature review. *Risk Manag Healthc Policy*. 2015;8:175–83.

II

A life-course perspective

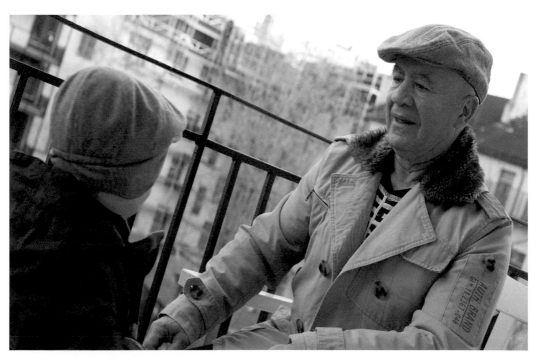

Photo credit: Iffit Querishi/NAKMI.

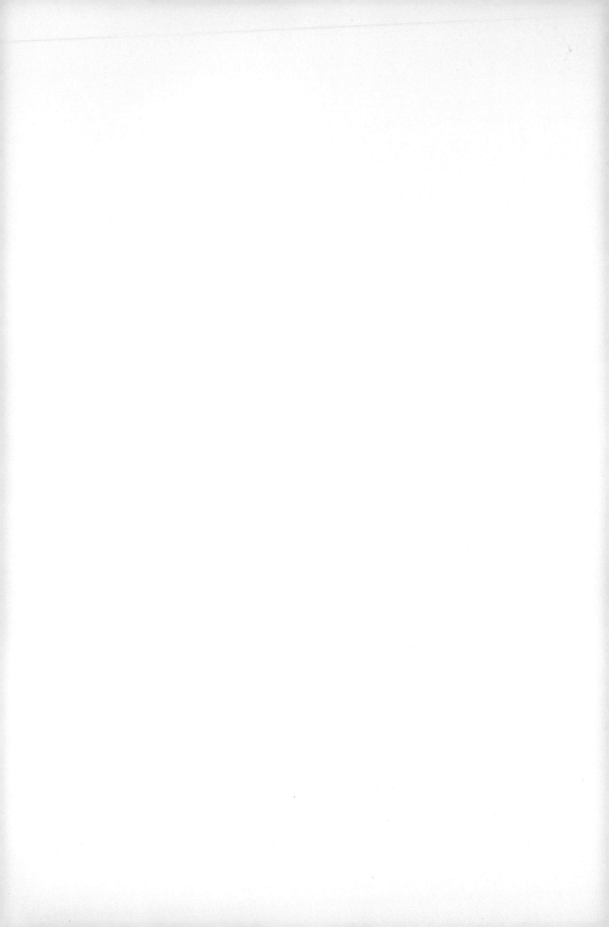

CHAPTER 7

A life-course perspective on migrant health

Yoav Ben-Shlomo, Loubaba Mamluk and Sabi Redwood

LEARNING OBJECTIVES

At the end of this chapter, the reader should be able to:

- Understand and be able to explain what is meant by a life-course approach to disease aetiology
- Consider the different life-course models and how they can operate in an individual scenario
- Appreciate the value of a qualitative approach in understanding a life-course narrative
- Understand the value of migrant health research in trying to determine the role of critical and/or sensitive period or accumulation of risk models

---

CLINICAL VIGNETTE

A Syrian mother presents to her general practitioner about her 9-year-old son. He has been bedwetting since his family migrated from Aleppo 3 months ago. He had witnessed traumatic events due to the war in Syria.

The mother decided not to move to a refugee camp as she feared for their lives if they stayed in Aleppo due to the ongoing war. Before migrating to the UK, the whole family had been subjected to a restricted caloric and nutrient intake during the siege of parts of Aleppo.

The family had been forced to move and were lucky that their grandfather resided in the UK, having done his PhD work there in the 1960s and choosing not to return. He was suffering from coronary heart disease and obesity. The mother is 33 years of age and is pregnant (third trimester). The mother is concerned about the bedwetting and wonders if this is related to her son's past exposure to traumatic events.

HISTORICAL CONTEXT

Interest in the early life origins of chronic disease has a long history. Here we will briefly summarize some of the key ideas (1). The lack of improvement in infant mortality in the second half of the nineteenth century lead to a public health focus on trying to improve infant and child health services with the potential longer-term impact on health in adulthood. George Newman, Chief Medical Officer to the Board of Education in the UK wrote in 1914 'recent progress has shown (a) that the health of the adult is dependent upon the health of the child …[and]… (b) that the health of the child is dependent upon the health of the infant and its mother' (1). Demographic analyses in the early twentieth century highlighted period effects on mortality so that all age groups experienced lower mortality at each period. The implications of this were not clear, as improved survival in early life may have resulted in greater morbidity and mortality in later life. Rheumatic fever, a childhood infection of the heart, was well recognized as a precursor for future cardiac problems due to valvular disease.

The emergence of chronic diseases such as coronary heart disease led to a new focus on mid-life risk factors such as obesity, hypertension, and diabetes, which were supported by the new influential studies such as the Framingham Cohort Study. This 'lifestyle' model of disease aetiology shifted interest away from early life until the late 1970s when interest in social and geographical variations resurrected life-course ideas (2,3). This paradigm shift focussed explicitly on birth weight, as a proxy of fetal development, and weight at 1 year (postnatal growth) as measures of adverse exposures in key developmental windows that may result in lifelong susceptibility to a wide range of conditions and grounded the 'fetal origins of adult disease' movement. In parallel, some researchers took a broader 'life-course' perspective that integrated these new ideas with the existing paradigms around the lifestyle model and social inequalities and suggested different aetiological pathways and models for disease causation (4).

LIFE-COURSE DEFINITIONS AND MODELS

Life-course epidemiology is defined as 'the study of long-term effects on later health or disease risk of physical or social exposures during gestation, childhood, adolescence, young adulthood and later adult life' and has been extended to encompass intergenerational influences (5). A series of different models have been proposed by which adverse exposures could operate:

a. A critical or sensitive period model is when an exposure acting during a critical period of development has effects on the structure or function of organs, tissues, or body systems that are not modified in any dramatic way by later experience, and that precipitate disease later in life ('biological programming'). For example, failure of normal renal development could result in fewer nephrons and later susceptibility to hypertension. A less extreme version operates through a 'sensitive' period whereby exposure has a stronger effect on development and subsequent disease risk but exposure outside this time period may still operate to a lesser degree. So, it has been proposed that women who start to smoke in puberty have a greater risk of breast cancer than if they start after puberty, depending on pack years, as the developing breast may be more susceptible to any carcinogenic effects of smoking during this period (6).

b. Accumulation of risk models propose that rather than key exposure windows, risk is associated with duration of exposure or accumulation of different exposures. Such patterning of exposures could be random (uncorrelated) but are more likely to be correlated due to 'risk clustering'. So, living in poverty will inevitably result in many adverse exposures (infections, poor diet, increased smoking) and result in accumulating adverse exposure years. Two variants of this model exist through a chain of risk metaphor so that one adverse exposure increases the risk of another, e.g. being a refugee increases the risk of maltreatment and abuse, which leads to isolation and loneliness and subsequent poor mental health. There may be a trigger exposure along the chain which is the proximate cause of ill health or mortality, e.g. civil war leading to a decision to flee by boat in hazardous conditions leading to death by drowning. In our case scenario, childhood exposure to stressful experiences is likely to have resulted in psychological distress, and evidence from a large UK-based birth cohort supports the association between multiple stressful events and persistent bedwetting (7).

It is helpful to appreciate that the critical/sensitive period model is a special or embedded case of an accumulation model, and that one needs to explicitly examine each model in relation to the timing as well as duration of any exposure. Figure 7.1 provides a hypothetical example of how post-migration environment (exposure) could impact on risk of ischaemic heart disease (outcome). In our vignette, the risk of type 2 diabetes for migrants is compared to their non-migrant counterparts (baseline risk 1.0). The figure shows that migrants who migrated later in life and have therefore experienced fewer post-migration years (analogous to pack years of smoking) have lower risk than those who migrated at a younger age, but still elevated compared to non-migrants. The pattern of relative risks (1.0, 1.5, 2.2, 4.6) would be consistent with a dose-response effect as predicted from

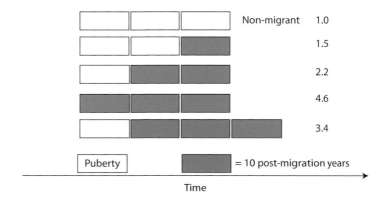

FIGURE 7.1 Migration life years and risk of ischaemic heart disease in relation to accumulation or sensitive period effects.

an accumulation model and would strengthen any causal inference. However, if we compare two groups with equal post-migration exposure (30 years) but one group migrated during puberty and the other migrated as adults, it is clear that the former has a far greater risk (4.6 vs 3.4). This would suggest that while years of post-migration exposure increase risk, probably through an increased obesity pathway, there is a sensitive period effect so that an even greater adverse effect is observed if exposure occurs during puberty, an important developmental phase, where endocrine effects on adiposity may operate. Such a model could apply to the grandfather in the clinical vignette. His migration to the United Kingdom in young adulthood plus his permanent residence there is likely to have exposed him to many years of an obesogenic environment leading to his diabetes and coronary heart disease.

CONCEPTS OF RESILIENCE AND ADAPTATIONS

Despite similar adverse experiences, some individuals seem to do better than others, and psychological and biological researchers have been interested in both 'resilience', a dynamic process of positive adaptation in the face of adversity, as well as 'plasticity', the potential for change in intrinsic characteristics in response to environmental stimuli, e.g. brain recovery after a stroke due to extrinsic stimulation. It is unclear to what degree these traits are genetic, or determined in early life, or can be modified, albeit with difficulty, in later life through methods such as cognitive behavioural therapy (8).

A life-course approach enables a temporal perspective of how resilience may operate (see Figure 7.2). In this hypothetical scenario, we follow a physiological trait such as cognitive ability and how it varies across the life course. This figure could reflect the trajectory of a

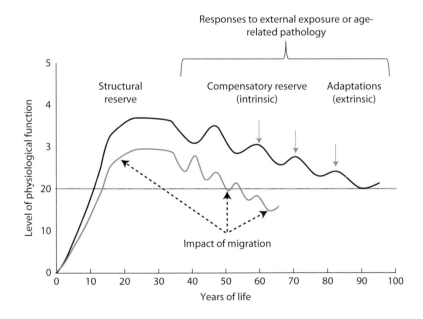

FIGURE 7.2 The impact of migration on the life-course trajectory of a physiological trait.

specific individual or the average trajectory of a group of people, for example, refugee women from Syria. The horizontal line on the figure at 20% indicates a threshold level at which individuals will be clinically apparent as they are aware of cognitive difficulties and decline. In this example, the maximal peak level of cognitive ability, which we have labelled as structural reserve, is determined by early life exposures such as educational opportunities. This peak will also predict the probability of developing mild cognitive impairment (MCI) or dementia, as the higher the maximal level the longer it will take to decline; hence competing causes of death will mean that MCI or dementia is never diagnosed in life. This explains the strong protective association between higher self-reported educational level and genetic variants which can act as an instrumental variable for higher education with reduced dementia risk (9).

It remains more controversial as to whether higher education alters the rate of cognitive decline, but as the figure makes clear, individuals can recover function either through intrinsic biological pathways or through external adaptations to their life circumstances with a reduction in the rate of decline. For example, ischaemic brain damage may recover due to plasticity in function and repair mechanisms leading to new synaptic connections. Furthermore, active social engagement in mid-life may have protective effects due to cognitive stimulation and reduced depression, though it remains unclear as to whether these associations reflect reverse causation.

REFUGEE STORIES – CLUES THROUGH A NARRATIVE LIFE-COURSE PERSPECTIVE

In epidemiology, the life-course approach aims to identify the underlying biological, behavioural, and psychosocial processes that operate across the lifespan (10). The focus in the social sciences, especially those concerned with understanding the insider perspective of experiences of health and illness using qualitative research methods, is on how people's individual lives are linked with wider structural conditions and the historical context of opportunities and constraints (11).

Being forced to flee one's home country is a critical event in a person's life. The timing, pacing, and sequencing of life events such as migration are central to understanding their effects on health and well-being, as the clinical vignette illustrates: leaving one's home country to pursue an education and career as a young adult and choosing to stay in a new country differs sharply from a young boy whose family is forced to flee sustained bombings and starvation. While migration meant biographical continuity for the grandfather, the young refugee's migratory experience is characterized by biographical disruption. The boy's pregnant mother and sister are similarly affected because apart from the grief and terror they have suffered, previously taken-for-granted structures and resources have disintegrated, and life has been reframed under conditions of uncertainty due to the unknown regimes of the host country.

Qualitative life-course research offers a window into these experiences. Its theoretical background is interpretive sociology in the tradition of symbolic interactionism (12). Symbolic interactionism foregrounds how people relate to each other and how meaning and identity are generated through interpretation and social action. In relation to health, qualitative studies can contribute to a better understanding of the paths taken by individuals and the events affecting their lives against a backdrop of wider social structures and political events, explain how people experience transitions, why they choose certain actions and reject others, and how they deal with a range of different stressors in their lives. The life-course approach emphasizes the interplay between the individual micro-level experience and the macro-level societal context. Related to the clinical vignette, this means that the micro-level experience of the young patient and his bedwetting is closely linked with his and his family's prolonged exposure to the consequences of a war in Syria targeting civilians. The experiences during their journey from Aleppo to Europe, and the post-migration reception in the UK, will have also been shaped by the global political situation characterized by a widespread reluctance on the part of national governments to help forced migrants, and by restrictions on their access to basic services and humanitarian help. Thus the life-course approach attends to individual need as well as to social justice, and the relationship between the two.

LISTENING TO REFUGEE STORIES

The development of 'narrative medicine' (13) refers to the practice of respectful health care by clinicians who have the capacity to 'recognise, absorb, metabolize, interpret, and be moved by stories of illness. Put simply, it is medicine practiced by someone who knows what to do with stories'. Listening to patients' stories is a key element of medical practice, yet even if encounters take place within a shared cultural context, narratives can be 'chaotic' (14), disjointed, or fragmented. Stories told by refugees may be very hard to listen to, but they provide some access to the way they understand health and illness and the values nested within the wider narratives of their society and culture (15).

Refugees have experienced a profound form of biographical disruption that is often 'written into the body'. A major factor affecting the health of migrants is trauma related to events in their home country precipitating a departure, the migration journey itself, or both. The hope that life will be better and that they will be safe from danger is tempered by many other factors such as the grief for the many losses they have experienced. These losses are likely to be wide-ranging: the loss of family members and friends as a result of violence or bombardments, of property and possessions, and of their job, their status, or their career. Less tangible, but nonetheless profound, are losses such as their hopes and dreams for a future in their home country, the feeling of familiarity and of being at home, and the ability to navigate their own lives with ease and confidence in the face of much uncertainty.

Refugees may also feel a sense of guilt that they are safe and other members of the family are still living in a dangerous place. Experiences of torture and trauma mean that refugees may fear people in authority, the police, and sometimes health professionals because they may have been part of the regime that persecuted them. Not knowing where to turn to for help combined with the practical challenges from a lack of resources and uncertainties, whereas in the past they might have had an extended family and a supportive community, can lead to feelings of dislocation and powerlessness. Not being able to take things for granted such as dealing with the health or welfare system, banks, schools, and transport can also be frustrating, while separation from the extended family can bring loneliness and isolation.

Many refugees suffer from serious illnesses such as tuberculosis and the consequences of malnutrition and physical injury. Many others present with multiple physical complaints, especially pain in various parts of the body, in the absence of objectively verifiable organic dysfunction. Medical practice has no way to interpret such nonspecific pain and complaints, so they become translated into somatization or depression. Both have been reported as prominent in the refugee population (16). However, such symptoms could also be thought of as the distress caused by trauma and loss, expressed through the medium of the body (17), highlighting the interconnection of bodily symptoms and refugee-related trauma. Bedwetting reported by the mother of the boy in the clinical vignette is similarly nonspecific but could be seen as linked to the distress caused by his father's violent death and the loss of all that was familiar to him.

The illness stories told by refugee patients are often articulated in terms of threats and assaults not only on their own bodily and emotional integrity, but also on that of their society, culture, and traditions. Pain needs to be listened to and read for what it communicates about the state of the body and mind, while also bearing witness to what it communicates about the social and cultural reality and the existential crisis related to the wider social and historical context. However, some migrant patients report that their health concerns are not being taken seriously by doctors, while doctors feel overwhelmed by the pressure to 'deal with' presenting problems (18). Listening to refugee narratives is challenging under the constraints of clinical practice, but it can help restore some sense of integrity for the individual. It can also help towards providing some hope, however faint, for peace and return to the home country, and the opportunity to put back together what has been lost.

MIGRANT STUDIES OF DISEASE EPIDEMIOLOGY

Epidemiology has a long history of undertaking migrant studies (19) in order to try and tease out the relative importance of genetics versus environmental factors; the underlying assumption is that any changes in disease risk of migrants compared to their 'source' population following migration is a function of the 'host' environment or a gene-environment interaction (20). If the host environment is of importance, migrants should have disease risk somewhere between that of the source and host populations. Most early studies looked at international migration both because this is likely to incur far greater environmental changes and also because routine mortality statistics could be used to compare mortality rates by country of birth (21). The classic populations that have been studied have been Japanese migrants to the United States (19,22), European migrants to South Africa and Israel (23,24), and South Asian migrants to the United Kingdom (25).

Ideally, the probability of migration would be allocated randomly to avoid selection effects (see below). This is not usually possible, as it would require a randomized controlled trial (RCT) where either individuals or groups (cluster RCT) are randomized, thereby usually eliminating the problem of confounding (though other biases are still possible due to loss to follow-up). However, rare examples can be found in the literature. The island of Tonga in the South Pacific introduced in 2002 a national lottery scheme (Pacific Access Category) whereby any citizen between 18 and 45 years of age can register in a lottery whose prize is to emigrate to New Zealand. By comparing successful and unsuccessful applicants, one can measure the impact of migration unconfounded by selection effects. The evidence from the Tongan migrant study suggests that migration is associated with increases in blood pressure and prevalence of hypertension consistent with other less powerful observational studies (26).

Many studies undertake simple cross-sectional comparisons between the migrant and host populations. This is problematic, as without data on the source population, it is hard to know how much risk has altered secondary to migration. Far better is a cohort study where migrants are ideally measured *before* and *after* migration, and samples of the source and host populations are included. This has the major advantage that differences between migrants and non-migrants can be quantified and adjusted for in the analysis, thereby minimizing the 'healthy migrant' effect (Chapter 2). The obvious problem with such a design is that one would ideally know in advance who will migrate, and this is often not possible unless migration is forced. It is therefore unusual to see specific cohort studies of migrants unless established post-migration. One suggested design that has not been used much is the comparison of the same-source migrant populations across two different host populations (27) who have either very different risk factors or health care environments. In this design, it is assumed that the selection factors are similar across the two populations and any observed differences reflect the post-migration environment.

Another potential issue that needs to be considered in migrant studies is known as the 'salmon bias' (see Chapter 18). For example, a cohort study in China found that worse self-reported health was associated with both a reduced likelihood of internal migration (healthy selection) and predicted returning home (salmon bias) (28). However, this may not be the case for low- to middle-income country migrants residing in high-income countries. In this scenario, access to better health care, including palliative care, may override any desire to be with extended family.

MIGRATION THROUGH A LIFE-COURSE LENS

Relatively little has been written about migration from a life-course perspective (27,29). One of the critical aspects is being able to describe the migrant experience in terms of timing and duration – hence age at migration is frequently used as a key variable to study critical/sensitive periods as well as accumulation in terms of post-migration exposure. We have used the framework proposed by Zimmerman and colleagues to consider how life-course influences could impact the health of migrants (30). We consider the following factors that may be important:

1. Pre-migration characteristics: The degree to which migrants are typical or atypical of the host population. Most measures will include some measure of socioeconomic status, e.g. years of education or some biological measure of development, e.g. adult height, that capture early life exposures.
2. Pre-migration drivers: There is a wide variety of migration drivers that can be classified as (i) environmental, e.g. food security, (ii) political conflict insecurity, (iii) demographic, e.g. population density, (iv) economic, e.g. employment opportunities, and (v) social, e.g. family/kin obligations (31). These drivers are important, as they will partially influence the selection factors and pre-migration characteristics but may also influence the next factor.
3. Migration experience: This will reflect the actual transition process and whether it is legal or illegal, rapid or slow, and may involve repeated attempts to migrate.
4. Post-migration experience: This will include how the host population treats the migrant and whether they integrate or not. It may include new adverse exposures or more beneficial exposure through better education, higher socioeconomic status, and better access to high-quality health care.
5. Pre- and post-migration interactions: It is possible that migrants who experienced an adverse environment in their source population are then further disadvantaged by the host population through a 'double whammy' effect, i.e. an adaptive response to store fat in an energy-deficient environment is exacerbated by moving in later life to an obesogenic environment where there is calorie excess (Figure 7.3).

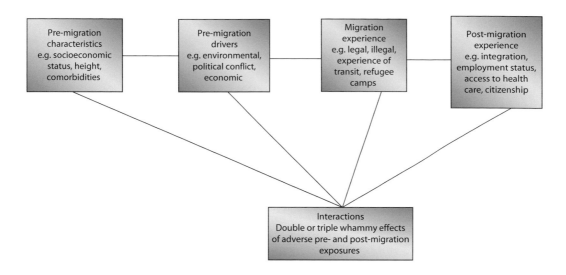

FIGURE 7.3   Illustration of how pre-, peri-, and post-migration exposures can operate to influence health. (Adapted from Zimmerman C et al. *PLOS MED* 2011;8(5).)

ILLUSTRATIVE EXAMPLES

The following section highlights some examples that illustrate the concepts discussed previously. Results from the Hong Kong Cardiovascular Risk Factor Prevalence Study (1995–1996) demonstrate a potential critical or sensitive period effect in relation to migration in early life (32). The research, *a priori*, looked at migrants from mainland China to Hong Kong and differentiated growth phases, potentially mediated by different hormonal influences, into three developmental windows: infant (0–1 years), childhood (2–7 years), and pubertal (8–17 years) periods. Most of the migrants came from the Guangdong province and around a third had migrated before 18 years. For ischaemic heart disease, there was evidence to support a critical period effect so that migration between 0 and 7 years was associated with elevated risk but migration at any other period showed little difference in risk compared to those born in Hong Kong. In contrast, the risk patterns for type 2 diabetes were more consistent with a sensitive period effect for early life, as risks diminished with migration in later life. The results are most likely explained by either pre-migration factors (e.g. worse intrauterine development in mainland China) or a combination of pre- and post-migration influences.

The Indian Migration Study examined cardiometabolic risk factors in relation to urban life years by comparing siblings who were born in a rural area or migrated to an urban area to unrelated urban-born residents. For blood pressure and fasting insulin, they found a simple accumulation effect so that systolic blood pressure and fasting insulin increased for every decade of urban life years (33). In contrast, body fat showed a marked increase in the first decade but after this there was little difference in age-related changes compared to rural residents so that absolute differences tracked over time. In this case, the post-migration experience is most likely to be the main driver and dietary changes associated with urbanization leading to increased adiposity are probably the main factor in increasing cardiometabolic risk.

One way to examine the migration transition is to compare risk across different types of migrants (e.g. economic vs refugee) on the assumption that differences reflect the process of migration rather than selection factors. Recent evidence from a retrospective cohort study in Sweden highlights an almost threefold increased risk of psychotic illness in refugees from all origins (except sub-Saharan Africa) compared to the native population. However, rates are even higher in refugee populations compared to non-refugee migrants from similar regions of origin (34). This cannot differentiate whether the increased risk of psychotic disorders is attributed to pre-migration adversity such as witnessing and experiencing of violence and war or the migration journey to reach Sweden, which may also have been hazardous and traumatic.

GOING BEYOND THE FIRST GENERATION: THE IMPACT ON MIGRANT CHILDREN

Studying the offspring of migrants is another powerful way of trying to unpick whether any adverse effects relate to pre-migration factors, the migration experience, or the post-migration environment. Children may indirectly experience this if their mothers were pregnant with them prior to or during migration, as uterine exposures can have long-term influences, as seen in the Dutch Hunger Winter Study of adults whose mothers were pregnant during the German occupation of the Netherlands (35). For example, in our scenario the mother was in her first trimester of pregnancy while being calorie-restricted in Syria. This may have consequences for her child's future health.

Increased risk of psychotic disorders among migrants can be seen among the second generation, suggesting that post-migration factors may play an important role compared to pre-migration factors (36). Results from a two-year, first-contact incidence study of schizophrenia in the Netherlands showed that the incidence doubled in first-generation migrant groups compared to Dutch natives (37). Furthermore, second-generation migrants from non-Western countries had an even higher age- and gender-adjusted risk compared to first-generation migrants. Such findings may be explained by acculturation difficulties and marginalization.

CONCLUSIONS

We have presented evidence that understanding the health of migrants may be facilitated by taking a life-course approach. This should consider selection, pre-migration experiences, the migration transition, and post-migration life in a new host environment which may enhance or worsen pre-existing health status. Much of what we have discussed is of theoretical interest and may have little immediate impact on how a general practitioner manages their migrant community. However, we hope that this understanding will encourage them to seek aetiological clues beyond immediate triggers, and consider life experience over a longer period. This approach can enhance not only their own understanding, but also help their patients make sense of why they may have developed ill health. A life-course approach to migrant health enriches our understanding of disease aetiology. However, it is also important not to view life-course influences as overly deterministic or unmodifiable. While no one can remove these past exposures, resilience, plasticity, and the human ability to adapt is often underestimated, and interventions may be equally effective even if some patients start off at a lower reserve due to adverse early life exposures.

ACKNOWLEDGEMENTS

Loubaba Mamluk and Sabi Redwood are funded by the National Institute for Health Research Collaboration for Leadership in Applied Health Research and Care West (NIHR CLAHRC West). YBS is the equity appropriateness and sustainability theme lead for the NIHR CLAHRC West. CLAHRC West is part of the NIHR and is a partnership between University Hospitals Bristol NHS Foundation Trust and the University of Bristol. The views expressed in this publication are those of the authors and not necessarily those of the NHS, the National Institute for Health Research, or the Department of Health.

REFERENCES

1. Kuh D, Davey Smith G. The life course and adult chronic disease: an historical perspective with particular reference to coronary heart disease. In: Kuh D, Ben-Shlomo Y, editors. *A Life Course Approach to Chronic Disease Epidemiology*. 2nd ed. Oxford: Oxford University Press; 2004: pp. 15–40.
2. Forsdahl A. Are poor living conditions in childhood and adolescence an important risk factor for arteriosclerotic heart disease? *Br J Prev Soc Med*. 1977;31:91–95.
3. Barker DJP, Osmond C, Golding J et al. Growth in utero, blood pressure in childhood and adult life, and mortality from cardiovascular disease. *Br Med J*. 1989;298:564–67.
4. Ben-Shlomo Y, Kuh D. A life course approach to chronic disease epidemiology: conceptual models, empirical challenges and interdisciplinary perspectives. *Int J Epidemiol*. 2002;31(2):285–93.
5. Kuh D, Ben-Shlomo Y, Lynch J et al. Life course epidemiology. *J Epidemiol Commun Health*. 2003;57(10):778–83.
6. Band PR, Le ND, Fang R et al. Carcinogenic and endocrine disrupting effects of cigarette smoke and risk of breast cancer. *Lancet*. 2002;360:1044–49.
7. Joinson C, Sullivan S, von Gontard A et al. Stressful events in early childhood and developmental trajectories of bedwetting at school age. *J Pediatr Psychol*. 2016;41(9):1002–10.
8. Proudfoot J, Guest D, Carson J et al. Effect of cognitive-behavioural training on job-finding among long-term unemployed people. *Lancet* 1997;350(9071):96–100.
9. Anderson EL, Wade KH, Hemant G et al. The causal effect of educational attainment on Alzheimer's disease: a two-sample Mendelian randomization study. *bioRxiv*. 2017. https://doi.org/10.1101/127993
10. Kuh D, Ben-Shlomo Y. *A Life Course Approach to Chronic Disease Epidemiology*. Oxford: OUP; 1997.
11. Elder GH, Johnson MK, Crosnoe R. The emergence and development of life course theory. In: Mortimer JT, Shanahan MJ, editors. *Handbook of the Life Course*. Springer; 2003: 3–19.
12. Blumer H. *Symbolic Interactionism. Contemporary Sociological Theory, 62*. Berkeley: University of California Press; 1969.
13. Charon R. Narrative medicine: a model for empathy, reflection, profession, and trust. *JAMA* 2001;286(15):1897–902.
14. Frank AW. *The Wounded Storyteller: Body, Illness, and Ethics*. University of Chicago Press; 2013.
15. Greenhalgh T. Cultural contexts of health: the use of narrative research in the health sector [Internet]. WHO; 2016.
16. Rohlof HG, Knipscheer JW, Kleber RJ. Somatization in refugees: a review. *Soc Psychiatry Psychiatr Epidemiol*. 2014;49(11):1793–804.
17. Coker EM. "Traveling pains": embodied metaphors of suffering among Southern Sudanese refugees in Cairo. *Cult Med Psychiatry*. 2004;28(1):15–39.
18. Lindenmeyer A, Redwood S, Griffith L et al. Experiences of primary care professionals providing healthcare to recently arrived migrants: a qualitative study. *BMJ Open*. 2016;6(9):e012561.
19. Haenszel W. Studies of migrant populations. *J Chronic Dis*. 1970;23:289–91.
20. Marmot MG. Changing places changing risks: the study of migrants. *Public Health Rev* 1994;21:184–95.
21. Marmot MG, Adelstein AM, Bulusu L. *Immigrant mortality in England and Wales 1970-1978 OPCS Studies of Medical and Population Subjects no 47*. London: HMSO; 1984.

22. Winkelstein W Jr, Kagan A, Kato H et al. Epidemiologic studies of coronary heart disease and stroke in Japanese men living in Japan, Hawaii and California: blood pressure distributions. *Am J Epidemiol.* 1975;102:502–13.

23. Dean G, Kurtzke JF. On the risk of MS according to age at immigration to South Africa. *BMJ.* 1971;3:725–29.

24. Leibowitz U, Kahana E, Alter M. The changing frequency of multiple sclerosis in Israel. *Arch Neurol.* 1973;29:107–10.

25. McKeigue PM, Miller GJ, Marmot MG. Coronary heart disease in south Asians overseas: a review. *J Clin Epidemiol.* 1989;42(7):597–609.

26. Gibson J, Stillman S, McKenzie D et al. Natural experiment evidence on the effect of migration on blood pressure and hypertension. *Health Econ.* 2013;22(6):655–72.

27. Spallek J, Zeeb H, Razum O. What do we have to know from migrants' past exposures to understand their health status? A life course approach. *Emerg Themes Epidemiol.* 2011;8(6):1–8.

28. Lu Y, Qin LJ. Healthy migrant and salmon bias hypotheses: a study of health and internal migration in China. *Soc Sci Med.* 2014;102:41–48.

29. Kley S. Explaining the stages of migration within a life-course framework. *Eur Sociol Rev.* 2011;27(4):469–86.

30. Zimmerman C, Kiss L, Hossain M. Migration and health: a framework for 21st century policy-making. *PLOS MED* 2011;8(5): e1001034.

31. Foresight. *Migration and Global Environmental Change.* Final Project Report: Executive Summary, The Government Office for Science, London; 2011: 9–236.

32. Schooling M, Leung GM, Janus ED et al. Childhood migration and cardiovascular risk. *Int J Epidemiol.* 2004;33(6):1219–26.

33. Kinra S, Andersen E, Ben-Shlomo Y et al. Association between urban life-years and cardiometabolic risk: the Indian migration study. *Am J Epidemiol.* 2011;174(2):154–64.

34. Hollander A-C, Dal H, Lewis G et al. Refugee migration and risk of schizophrenia and other non-affective psychoses: cohort study of 1.3 million people in Sweden. *BMJ.* 2016;352:i1030.

35. Ravelli ACJ, van der Meulen JHP, Michels RPJ et al. Glucose tolerance in adults after prenatal exposure to famine. *Lancet.* 1998;351:173–77.

36. Bourque F, van der Ven E, Malla A. A meta-analysis of the risk for psychotic disorders among first-and second-generation immigrants. *Psychol Med.* 2011;41(5):897–910.

37. Veling W, Selten J-P, Veen N et al. Incidence of schizophrenia among ethnic minorities in the Netherlands: a four-year first-contact study. *Schizophr Res.* 2006;86(1):189–93.

CHAPTER 8

Promoting the health of migrant children and children of migrants

Krista M. Perreira and Lars T. Fadnes

LEARNING OBJECTIVES

At the end of this chapter, the reader will be able to:

- Define children of migrant populations including first-generation migrants, offspring of migrant parents, refugees and asylum seekers, unauthorized/irregular migrants, and unaccompanied minors

- Explain how the pre-migration, migration, and post-migration experiences of children of migrants and their parents can affect their physical and mental health

- Describe differences in the physical and mental health of children of migrants across population groups

- Discuss factors limiting access to medical care for migrants and strategies to improve migrants' access to medical care

---

CLINICAL VIGNETTE

Mohammed was born in Somalia and is now 17 years of age and living in a small city in Sweden. He arrived in Europe as a refugee at the age of 11. As he lost most of his family in the civil war, he arrived alone and grew up among foster parents. Mohammed is generally healthy and except for some periods with bothersome abdominal pain, he generally expresses that he is happy, and he is active both physically and socially. He has done well in school and he speaks Swedish fluently. Eight months ago, he was hit by a car in busy city traffic, experienced a major concussion, and lost consciousness for several minutes in addition to getting some minor bruises. After a week of hospitalization, he had some remaining sequelae including some memory difficulties, frequent headaches, and some difficulties in expressing more complex matters. Over the subsequent months, he also struggled with abdominal pain as well as feelings of fatigue and mood swing.

INTRODUCTION

A healthy childhood sets the stage for a healthy adulthood (1). Poor nutrition, limited physical activity, and exposure to adverse childhood experiences can directly affect children's cognitive, physical, and socioemotional development (2). In addition, many chronic diseases in adulthood stem from poor health and health behaviours established between early childhood and late adolescence (3). Physical and mental health are also essential for economic well-being (4). Healthy children attend school more regularly, perform better in school, and attain more schooling than children in poor physical or mental health. Consequently, they are better able to work and achieve higher earnings in adulthood.

Though they are a heterogeneous group, many children of migrants grow up in economic and social circumstances that can potentially place them at higher risk of poorer physical and mental health than native-born children with native-born parents (commonly referred to as *third-generation children* or *non-migrants*) (5,45). Children of migrants include those born in a foreign country to foreign-born parents and native born with at least one foreign-born parent. Whereas the former category are referred to as migrants, the latter may or not be referred to as migrants depending on the host country regulations. Children of migrants can be further disaggregated into those who legally migrate to their new homes as economic migrants, refugees, or asylum seekers as well as those commonly labelled *unauthorized* or *irregular* migrants who do not have legal permission to reside in the country and may also have unauthorized/irregular migrant parents. They also include unaccompanied minors who have migrated alone without their families or have become separated from their families during their travels.

Though a child is typically defined as a person under the age of 18 or 21, determining that an unaccompanied minor is indeed a child can be challenging. Many arrive in settlement countries without birth certificates or any other form of identification, and clinical examinations to assess age are not always conclusive. An incorrect assessment can adversely affect a child's care and access to resources. Offspring of migrant parents typically have legal status to live and work in their countries of settlement but may have one or more unauthorized/irregular migrant parents or other family members lacking legal status to live and work in their countries of settlement (6).

Focussing on the children of migrants in Europe and the United States (US), this chapter provides an overview of the health of children of migrants. We highlight the ways in which migration, children's nativity, and parents' nativity can influence physical and mental well-being as well as access to medical care. Though physical and mental health can be closely intertwined and share many of the same risk and protective factors (refer to Chapter 18), for ease of discussion we summarize the literature on these two aspects of health separately. We conclude with a discussion of strategies to promote the health of children of migrants through policies and clinical practices.

A LIFE-COURSE THEORY OF CHILDREN'S MIGRATION AND HEALTH

As the number of international migrants has grown, the presence of children in these migration streams has also increased. According to UNICEF (7), 31 million children are migrants living outside their countries of birth. They include approximately 11 million child refugees and asylum seekers who are fleeing violent conflicts, persecution, and/or natural disasters (7).

The migration and acculturation processes experienced by children of migrants and/or their parents can expose children to a variety of physical, emotional, and social stressors (8,9). It may also inculcate children with resiliencies − internal assets (e.g. coping skills) and external resources (e.g. parental support) that enable children to adapt and overcome stressors (9). The migration process describes all the activities involved with deciding to migrate, preparing for migration, undertaking the migration journey, and settling in a new home. The acculturation process describes the cultural changes and adaptations that occur when two or more cultures come into contact (5). In our increasingly global society, these cross-cultural exchanges and acculturation processes can begin prior to migration but are studied most often in the context of initial settlement in a host country (10).

Viewed from within a life-course framework, migration and acculturation processes are among the many social determinants of health that can affect well-being (10). Life-course theory highlights the dynamic interrelation between contexts and individual agency or decision making as well as the linkages between lives within families and communities and across generations. It also highlights the importance of critical periods in development when specific exposures can lead to sometimes irreversible changes that shape a child's health and development for the rest of their lives. In addition, the theory emphasizes the potential for changes in one stage of life to either add to or interact with changes in another stage of life to shape a child's health and development.

The migration of children and their parents/caregivers fundamentally shifts the structural, social, and cultural contexts of their development. The health effects of these shifts will then depend on the age of the parent at migration and the age of the child at migration, as well as exposures to risk and protective factors prior to migration in their country of origin, during migration as they travel to their new destination, and after migration as they settle into their new home (5).

Prior to migration

Children, especially young children, rarely have the opportunity to participate in the decision to migrate (9). Their migration decisions are inevitably linked to the migration decisions of their parents or family caregivers. They may migrate with their parents/caregivers or, often after a period of separation, migrate to join parents/caregivers. Like their parents/caregivers, they migrate to escape violence and/or poverty in their sending countries and/or they migrate for employment and educational opportunities available in their receiving countries.

Regardless of their reasons for migration, the circumstances surrounding the context of their exits influence their pre-migration health and their health risks during and after migration. Their country of origin and socioeconomic status (SES) within their country prior to migration will affect their exposures to infectious diseases, environmental contaminants (e.g. lead, air pollution, or chemical hazards), and potentially toxic stressors ranging from discrimination or family violence to war. Their age at migration, their gender, and the social circumstances (e.g. family separation) surrounding their migration will also affect their resiliencies. For example, older children and young adult parents with more financial, human, and social capital may begin their migration journeys in better physical and mental health. In addition, males may undertake migration journeys as a rite of passage with more social and institutional supports for their journeys.

During migration

The migration journey itself can vary widely for children and their parents/caregivers. For some, migration involves a short, comfortable plane, train, boat, or car ride across international borders. They are legal migrants allowed to travel safely and freely between countries. For others, migration involves a long, perilous, and clandestine journey exposing them to hazardous physical and emotional circumstances (7,11). They may begin a journey healthy and in the company of friends and family but end the journey alone, dehydrated, and starving or dead. Unauthorized/ irregular migrants can also be subject to the vagaries of human trafficking. In the United States approximately 11 million migrants are considered unauthorized/irregular, 9% of them children (ages 0–17), and this number has held steady (12). In the European Union (EU), estimates during 2011 varied from 1.9 to 3.8 million and appear to be increasing (13). Among irregular migrants detected at an EU border in 2015, approximately 10% were children (ages 0–17) (13).

After migration

After settling in their receiving countries, the health trajectories of children will depend substantially upon their SES within the host country, their own and their parents' legal status, and national or local government policies protecting their human rights and affecting their access to health and social services (10,45). The children of legal economic migrants with relatively high SES in two-parent families and with some fluency in the language of the receiving country may transition seamlessly into their receiving communities with few health concerns. Depending on the country in which they settle, they will likely have access to health insurance through their jobs, access to state-provided health care, and/or can afford to pay for some of the costs associated with their medical care. When children or parents have low incomes or education, little fluency in the language of their receiving countries, and unauthorized/irregular migration status, they can face additional health risks upon settlement into their receiving communities and may have little access to health care (14).

However, the health of all migrants with or without legal residency status can be undermined by acculturative stressors in their receiving communities, at work, and at school (10). These stressors associated with the process of cultural adaptation include family conflicts, language conflicts, and discrimination. Family conflicts occur as parents and their children adjust to changing gender roles, responsibilities, and expectations. Language conflicts occur as family members gain fluency at different rates. Discrimination occurs when migrants experience unfavourable treatment because of their nativity, race/ethnicity, skin colour, or religious background (refer to Chapter 5). They may experience verbal or physical harassment, feel marginalized and threatened in public, and have more limited educational and employment opportunities. They may also experience threats of deportation, internment in detention centres, and forced separation from parents/caregivers (15). These types of acculturative stressors have been repeatedly associated with poor mental health and even physical health, especially cardiovascular health and inflammatory disorders (5). Ethnic heritage maintenance, family cohesion, high parental support, high perceived social support, and a sense of belonging, and safety in schools and communities can partially mitigate the negative consequences of some of these risks (5,8,16).

OFFSPRING OF MIGRANT PARENTS

Though the native-born children of migrant parents do not experience the travails of migration directly, their health can still be influenced by their parents' circumstances prior to, during, and after migration. Health-related risk exposures can affect the reproductive health of both women and men, with implications for fetal development (4). In addition, poor physical and mental health among parents can reduce their capacity to work and to nurture their children (17). Finally, for children with unauthorized/irregular migrant parents, the deportation of a parent as well as the constant fear of a parent's deportation can threaten their physical and emotional well-being (18).

The health of offspring of migrant parents can also be jeopardized by many of the same post-migration acculturative stressors that threaten the health of first-generation migrant children. For these children too, intergenerational family and language conflicts as well as school- and community-based discrimination have been identified as critical risk factors (5,45). These risk factors can be counterbalanced to some extent by a strong sense of ethnic affirmation and belonging, by high levels of parental warmth and positive communication, and by social support and other resources within communities to facilitate integration (5). Governmental policies limiting migrants from access to public services (e.g. education, health, and social services) reduce their integration into their host societies and have negative physical and mental health consequences for both foreign-born and native-born children of migrants (19).

PHYSICAL WELL-BEING AND PATTERNS OF MORBIDITY

The *migrant paradox* or *healthy migrant effect* in children refers to the finding of lower average mortality and morbidity among migrant children in comparison to children of migrants and non-migrant counterparts. However, as discussed later, evidence supporting a migrant paradox in children is mixed. Morbidity patterns vary to some degree between non-migrants and different groups of migrants, as well as across different phases of migration (20,49).

Morbidity

Comparisons of health between migrant children and non-migrants have found both higher and lower rates of health problems, risk factors, accidents, and injuries (46). The distribution of symptoms, risk factors, and health problems also seems to differ between children of migrants and non-migrants (20,46). Initially, morbidity patterns among migrant children are more similar to the patterns in their home countries, and with increasing lengths of residence converge towards non-migrant health patterns in their host countries (46). Comparing morbidity differences across a spectrum of diseases, respiratory tract infections, renal, oral, and gastrointestinal conditions, eczema, and symptoms such as fever and nausea were more frequently presented among native-born children with migrant parents/caregivers compared to non-migrants (20). Only nausea and gastrointestinal conditions were presented more frequently among migrant children compared to third-generation non-migrants (20). Several conditions were less frequently presented among migrants compared to non-migrants, including attention-deficit disorder and anxiety, allergy and asthma, and neurological, musculoskeletal, and rheumatic conditions. Notably, mental suffering sometimes presents through nausea or gastrointestinal symptoms. Often referred to as somatization, these symptoms can have varying forms across ethnic groups (21).

Evidence also indicates a link between racial discrimination and impaired health (22). Experiences of discrimination among older children have been linked with elevated blood pressure, insulin resistance, and in a longer perspective, coronary heart disease and diabetes. Interventions contributing to reducing perceived discrimination could thus be important in promoting health and well-being of children (refer to Chapter 5).

Medication use

Given the observed differences in disease experiences, clinicians and researchers also observe differences in medication usage. A population-based study in Norway showed that migrant children used less than nearly all assessed groups of prescribed medications compared to non-migrants after adjusting for age and sex; native-born children of migrant parents used slightly more antimicrobial medications and less psychoanaleptics and drugs for obstructive airways compared to third-generation non-migrants (23). Among children with asthma, the proportion of children using medications for obstructive airway was lowest among migrant children. The same pattern occurred for other prescription medications. Studies among children in Sweden, Spain, and the Netherlands have shown similar patterns, with lower utilization of prescribed medications among migrant children compared to non-migrants (23).

These differences in prescribed medications could have various explanations. One hypothesis is *healthy migrant selection* (refer to Chapter 2). Another possibility is that there are variations by nativity in health-seeking behaviours, in perceptions and knowledge of use of medications, and financial barriers to access medications. In addition, it is possible that migrants more often buy medications abroad than non-migrants, and that low language comprehension may reduce adherence to medication usage. Studies from the Netherlands and the United States have indicated that language comprehension is a predictor for uncontrolled asthma, with more extensive symptoms among migrant children with limited language comprehension (24).

Lifestyle and nutrition

Lifestyle and nutrition are also important health indicators. As migrants become more acculturated into Western settings, many adopt Western diets typically including larger amounts of unhealthy fats, meats, snack foods, and fast foods than the diets in their countries of origin (25). In the United States, it was found that native-born children of migrant parents had higher rates of overweight and obesity than migrant children or third-generation non-migrants (26). Furthermore, physical inactivity is common among migrant children (26,46). To counteract negative changes in food patterns and inactivity, promoting consumption of more fruits and vegetables and increasing physical activity through interventions aiming for behaviour change (e.g. through motivational interviewing or community-based electronic promotion interventions) could have important public health impacts (27). Such interventions could also benefit academic performances and future achievements of children (28). In addition, interventions can be directed at structural determinants of health (e.g. location of grocery stores, liquor stores, and parks) which can constrain the lifestyle choices and behaviours of migrant parents and their children (29).

PSYCHOLOGICAL WELL-BEING

Pre-migration, migration, and post-migration experiences can lead to a wide spectrum of mental health disorders among the children of migrants (refer to Chapter 17). Internalizing disorders include those associated with withdrawal, sadness, worry, and somatic complaints; externalizing disorders include those associated with overt behaviour problems such as aggressive behaviour, conduct problems, delinquency, and hyperactivity (30). Substance use, which can be associated with both internalizing and externalizing disorders, is also of concern for children of migrants (31). Although we lack comprehensive prevalence data on internalizing and externalizing disorders as well as substance use among children of migrants by migrant ethnicity and location of settlement, many country- and population-specific studies provide insights into the mental health needs of children of migrants and potential strategies to improve their well-being.

Internalizing disorders

Globally, 300 million (4.4% of the world's population) suffer from depression and 265 million (3.6% of the world's population) suffer from anxiety disorders, including post-traumatic stress disorder (PTSD) (32). The prevalence of depressive disorders tends to increase with age, while the prevalence of anxiety disorders remains constant across age groups (32). These two disorders may also co-occur with 25–50% of children and adolescents with depression also reporting anxiety and 10–15% of those with anxiety also reporting depression (32).

Though research on physical health frequently suggests that foreign-born children have better physical health than native-born, non-migrant children, this healthy migrant effect has not been found conclusively with respect to mental health. Studies based in the United States find that foreign-born children in comparison to non-migrant children may have higher or lower internalizing symptoms depending on their race/ethnic backgrounds and age (26,28). However, with some exceptions (e.g. 20), studies of children in Europe find no differences or find that foreign-born children have more symptoms of internalizing disorders than native-born children (45). These differences in findings may partially reflect differences in the populations of migrant children studied.

Among the children of migrants, children seeking refugee or asylum status, those with unauthorized/irregular status or parents with unauthorized/irregular status, and separated and unaccompanied minors have been identified as most at risk for depression and anxiety disorders (18,33). These children experience an accumulation of stressors with exposure to war and violence prior to migration, traumatic experiences during migration, prolonged internment within detention centres, fear of their own or their parents' deportation after migration, and stigmatization or marginalization within their settlement communities (11,22,33). Commonplace acculturative stressors associated with family adjustments, language acquisition, and discrimination are layered upon these. As a result, rates of depression, anxiety, and PTSD in these populations has been as high as 30–55% even years after resettlement (8,33).

Externalizing disorders

Foreign-born children in the United States tend to pre-set fewer externalizing symptoms than native-born children (26,28). Contrary to popular belief, foreign-born adolescents in the United States are also less likely to engage in delinquent acts (e.g. theft or selling drugs) or violence than native-born adolescents (34,18). In fact, migrant adolescents in the United States were more likely to be victims of violence and bullying, especially in school, than perpetrators (35).

By contrast, European-based studies have found comparable or greater rates of externalizing symptoms in foreign-born and native-born children (45). A large, multi-country study in Europe suggested that both migrant children and children of migrant parents were more likely to engage in physical fighting and bullying than children of non-migrants (36). At the same time, a study based in Sweden showed that foreign-born Asian and African children were up to three times more likely to report being bullied than Swedish children when they were enrolled in schools with a predominantly native-born majority (47).

Substance use

Alcohol and illicit drug use among adolescents varies by country of birth and country of residence. US studies have consistently shown lower rates of substance use (e.g. binge drinking, marijuana use, and illicit drug use) among foreign-born adolescent children relative to US-born adolescents (48). However, rates increase with greater exposure to US norms as measured by length of residence in the United States (48).

Studies of alcohol and illicit drug use in Europe show both higher and lower rates of substance use among foreign-born adolescents relative to native-born adolescents, with reported rates varying by gender, host country, and time in the host country (36,37). In Sweden, frequent binge drinking and illicit drug use were more prevalent among foreign-born non-Europeans as compared to native-born Swedes (37). A study of children ages 12–16 in Spain found that foreign-born adolescents reported higher prevalence than native adolescents of recent alcohol use but lower prevalence of marijuana use (38).

PROMOTING HEALTH

Access to health care services is strongly linked to health financing and insurance systems. When there are substantial financial barriers to health care, health care is often sought later when the risk for urgent or life-threatening situations increases. However, health financing systems are not the only factor affecting access to health services. Nonfinancial barriers can compromise the ability of migrants to obtain access to medical care, including lack of public transportation services, working conditions, and rights to leave work to care for sick children (14). Evidence from the United States also demonstrates that hostility towards migrants, discrimination on the basis of race/ethnicity, and laws providing differential access to public services on the basis of migrant legal status can lead to reductions in access to health care (19) (refer to Chapters 4 and 5).

Barriers to accessing health care are reflected in migrants' patterns of health care utilization. Migrant children are less likely to utilize health care than both native-born children of migrant parents and non-migrants (20,23). This is likely due to their lower average SES and rates of health insurance coverage. In addition, consistent with the healthy migrant selection hypothesis, migrant children may be healthier and need fewer health care services. Alternatively, utilization by migrant children may reflect the health-seeking behaviours of their parents and a lack of support services to assist them. Parents facing language barriers, difficulties in expressing health problems, as well as insufficient knowledge of organization and structure of the local health systems (39) may avoid seeking care for their children. With limited utilization of routine and preventive health care, migrants and their children may turn to emergency rooms for care. However, in the United States, migrants tend to have lower emergency room use than non-migrants (40), whereas in Europe, evidence from Italy suggests higher emergency room use, especially among young children (41).

To promote health care utilization and the health of migrant children, health care workers need to be trained to meet the needs of different groups of migrants by understanding cultural differences and using qualified interpreters to reduce language barriers (42) (refer to Chapter 6). Differences in disease patterns and communication barriers by migrant background can lead to more clinical uncertainty among clinicians treating migrant children compared to non-migrant children (23). Moreover, providers often have implicit biases that reduce the quality of care provided to migrants of various ethnic backgrounds (43). Bridging the language gap by using trained interpreters not only makes health services more accessible and useful for migrants, it also prevents medical errors (refer to Chapter 20). Children should, however, not be engaged as interpreters themselves. Implicit biases are more difficult to address but can begin with the adoption of a cultural-humility perspective where health care workers adopt a perspective of lifelong learning of other cultures, recognize and challenge power imbalances, create mutually beneficial partnerships, and create institutional accountability (44).

SUMMARY

The injury of Mohammed presented in the clinical vignette at the beginning of this chapter illustrates a critical phase where management can contribute to define the outcome. Mohammed was provided follow-up by a primary health care team and a rehabilitation unit, and during the subsequent months he gradually recovered and expresses that he is feeling well both mentally and physically. Mohammed is an example of a child with substantial resilience overcoming a major setback with some health care support. However, without health care support in a critical phase, the outcome might not have been similarly positive.

Migrants can go through a range of challenges, including traumas and economic vulnerability, as well as more frequently experiencing stigma and discrimination while adapting to culturally different settings. Experiences before, during, and after migration can lead to a wide spectrum of mental health disorders among migrant children. Despite this, many studies comparing various dimensions of health between migrant and non-migrant children have found lower rates of health problems, risk factors, accidents, and injuries among migrants. The disease spectrum among migrants is initially more similar to the patterns in the home country and then converges over time towards the health patterns of non-migrants in the host country. In addition, migrant children often use fewer prescribed medications, although the opposite has been observed in some studies and clinicians should be cautious about over generalizing. Some groups of migrants, especially refugees and those with undocumented/irregular status, may be particularly vulnerable to illness, missed diagnoses, and limited medical treatment.

Child health is also strongly linked to the family context and the situation of the parents/caregivers. As migrants become more acculturated into high-income settings, many adopt host county – and generally less healthy – diets. Yet even among children who have experienced major traumas during childhood, many have a large degree of resilience and seem to cope well with the life challenges they face.

Most importantly, the health of children of migrants is linked to the sociopolitical context of their reception in host countries. To ensure that migrant children get appropriate health care when needed and can develop into healthy adults, adequate health financing and insurance systems need to be in place. In addition, implicit biases, discriminatory practices, and structural barriers to their care need to be eliminated.

REFERENCES

1. Campbell F, Conti G, Heckman JJ, Moon SH, Pinto R, Pungello E et al. Early childhood investments substantially boost adult health. *Science.* 2014;343(6178):1478–85.
2. Hair NL, Hanson JL, Wolfe BL, Pollak SD. Association of child poverty, brain development, and academic achievement. *JAMA Pediatr.* 2015;169(9):822–9.
3. Blackwell DL, Hayward MD, Crimmins EM. Does childhood health affect chronic morbidity in later life? *Soc Sci Med.* 2001;52(8):1269–84.
4. Currie J. Healthy, wealthy, and wise: socioeconomic status, poor health in childhood, and human capital development. *J Econ Lit.* 2009;47(1):87–122.
5. Perreira KM, Ornelas IJ. The physical and psychological well-being of immigrant children. *Future Child.* 2011;21(1):195–218.
6. Capps R, Fix M, Zong J. *A Profile of U.S. Children with Unauthorized Immigrant Parents.* Washington, DC: Migration Policy Institute; 2016.
7. United Nations Children's Fund (UNICEF). *Uprooted: The Growing Crisis for Refugee and Migrant Children.* New York, NY: UNICEF; 2016.
8. Fazel M, Reed RV, Panter-Brick C, Stein, A. Mental health of displaced and refugee children resettled in high-income countries: risk and protective factors. *Lancet.* 2012;379(9812):266–82.
9. Ko LK, Perreira KM. "It turned my world upside down": Latino youths' perspectives on immigration. *J Adolesc Res.* 2010;25(3):465–93.
10. Acevedo-Garcia D, Sanchez-Vaznaugh EV, Viruell-Fuentes EA, Almeida J. Integrating social epidemiology into immigrant health research: a cross-national framework. *Soc Sci Med.* 2012;75(12):2060–68.
11. Perreira KM, Ornelas IJ. Painful passages: traumatic experiences and post-traumatic stress among US immigrant Latino adolescents and their primary caregivers. *Int Migr Rev.* 2013;47(4):976–1005.
12. Passel JS, Cohn D. *Unauthorized Immigrant Population: National and State Trends, 2010.* Washington, DC: Pew Research Center; 2011.
13. European Parliament Research Service (EPRS). Irregular immigration in the EU: Facts and Figures; 2015. Available from: http://www.europarl.europa.eu/RegData/etudes/BRIE/2015/554202/EPRS_BRI(2015)554202_EN.pdf.
14. Derose KP, Escarce JJ, Lurie N. Immigrants and health care: sources of vulnerability. *Health Aff.* 2007;26(5):1258–68.
15. Dreby J. US immigration policy and family separation: the consequences for children's well-being. *Soc Sci Med.* 2015;132:245–51.
16. Kouider EB, Koglin U, Petermann F. Emotional and behavioral problems in migrant children and adolescents in American countries: a systematic review. *J Immigr Minor Health.* 2015;17(4):1240–58.
17. Goodman SH, Rouse MH, Connell AM, Broth MR, Hall CM, Heyward D. Maternal depression and child psychopathology: a meta-analytic review. *Clin Child Fam Psychol Rev.* 2011;14(1):1–27.
18. Capps R, Koball H, Campetella A, Perreira K, Hooker S, Pedroza JM. *Implications of Immigration Enforcement Activities for the Well-Being of Children in Immigrant Families.* Washington, DC: Urban Institute and Migration Policy Institute; 2015.
19. Philbin MM, Flake M, Hatzenbuehler ML, Hirsch JS. State-level immigration and immigrant-focused policies as drivers of Latino health disparities in the United States. *Soc Sci Med.* 2017;e1–10.
20. Fadnes LT, Moen KA, Diaz E. Primary healthcare usage and morbidity among immigrant children compared with non-immigrant children: a population-based study in Norway. *BMJ Open.* 2016;6(10):e012101.
21. Aragona M, Rovetta, E Pucci, D Spoto J, Villa AM. Somatization in a primary care service for immigrants. *Ethn Health.* 2012;17(5):477–91.
22. Sanders-Phillips K, Settles-Reaves B, Walker D, Brownlow J. Social inequality and racial discrimination: risk factors for health disparities in children of color. *Pediatrics.* 2009;124(Suppl 3):S176–86.
23. Fadnes LT, Diaz E. Primary healthcare usage and use of medications among immigrant children according to age of arrival to Norway: a population-based study. *BMJ Open.* 2017;7(2):e014641.

24. van Dellen QM, Stronks K, Bindels PJ, Ory FG, Bruil J, van Aalderen WM et al. Predictors of asthma control in children from different ethnic origins. *Respir Med.* 2007;101(4):779–85.
25. Chan KS, Keeler E, Schonlau M, Rosen M, Mangione-Smith R. How do ethnicity and primary language spoken at home affect management practices and outcomes in children and adolescents with asthma? *Arch Pediatr Adolesc Med.* 2005;159(3):283–9.
26. Gordon-Larsen P, Harris KM, Ward DS, Popkin BM, National Longitudinal Study of Adolescent Health Acculturation and overweight-related behaviors among Hispanic immigrants to the US: the national longitudinal study of adolescent health. *Soc Sci Med.* 2003;57(11):2023–34.
27. Nour M, Chen J, Allman-Farinelli M. Efficacy and external validity of electronic and mobile phone-based interventions promoting vegetable intake in young adults: systematic review and meta-analysis. *J Med Internet Res.* 2016;18(4): e58.
28. Samdal GB, Eide GE, Barth T, Williams G, Meland E. Effective behaviour change techniques for physical activity and healthy eating in overweight and obese adults: systematic review and meta-regression analyses. *Int J Behav Nutr Phys Act.* 2017;14(1):42.
29. Crosnoe R. Health and the education of children from racial/ethnic minority and immigrant families. *J Health Soc Behav.* 2006;47(1):77–93.
30. Metzl JM, Roberts DE. Structural competency meets structural racism: race, politics, and the structure of medical knowledge. *Virtual Mentor.* 2014;16(9):674.
31. Forns M, Abad J, Kirchner T. Internalizing and externalizing problems. In: Levesque R, editor. *Encyclopedia of Adolescence.* New York: Springer, 2011; 1464–9.
32. King SM, Iacono WG, McGue M. Childhood externalizing and internalizing psychopathology in the prediction of early substance use. *Addiction.* 2004;99(12):1548–59.
33. Kouider EB, Koglin U, Petermann F. Emotional and behavioral problems in migrant children and adolescents in Europe: a systematic review. *Eur Child Adolesc Psychiatr.* 2014;23(6):373–91.
34. Powell D, Perreira KM, Harris KM. Trajectories of delinquency from adolescence to adulthood. *Youth Soc.* 2010;41(4):475–502.
35. Pottie K, Dahal G, Georgiades K, Premji K, Hassan G. Do first generation immigrant adolescents face higher rates of bullying, violence and suicidal behaviours than do third generation and native born? *J Immigr Minor Health.* 2015;17(5):1557–66.
36. Stevens GW, Vollebergh WA. Mental health in migrant children. *J Child Psychol Psychiatr.* 2008;49(3):276–94.
37. Svensson M, Hagquist C. Adolescent alcohol and illicit drug use among first- and second-generation immigrants in Sweden. *Scand J Soc Med.* 2010;38(2):184–91.
38. Bronstein I, Montgomery P. Psychological distress in refugee children: a systematic review. *Clin Child Fam Psychol Rev.* 2011;14(1):44–56.
39. Derose KP, Bahney BW, Lurie N, Escarce JJ. Immigrants and health care access, quality, and cost. *Med Care Res Rev.* 2009;66(4):355–408.
40. Agudelo-Suarez AA, Gil-Gonzalez D, Vives-Cases C, Love JG, Wimpenny P, Ronda-Perez E. A metasynthesis of qualitative studies regarding opinions and perceptions about barriers and determinants of health services' accessibility in economic migrants. *BMC Health Serv Res.* 2012;12:461.
41. Tarraf W, Vega W, González HM. Emergency department services use among immigrant and non-immigrant groups in the United States. *J Immigr Minor Health.* 2014;16(4):595–606.
42. Ballotari P, D'Angelo S, Bonvicini L, Broccoli S, Caranci N, Candela S et al. Effects of immigrant status on Emergency Room (ER) utilisation by children under age one: a population-based study in the province of Reggio Emilia (Italy). *BMC Health Serv Res.* 2013;13(458):e1–10.
43. Karliner LS, Jacobs EA, Chen AH, Mutha S. Do professional interpreters improve clinical care for patients with limited English proficiency? A systematic review of the literature. *Health Serv Res.* 2007;42(2):727–54.
44. Hall WJ, Chapman MV, Lee KM, Merino YM, Thomas TW, Payne BK et al. Implicit racial/ethnic bias among health care professionals and its influence on health care outcomes: a systematic review. *Am J Public Health.* 2015;105(12):e60–76.

45. Dimitrova R, Chasiotis A, van de Vijver F. Adjustment outcomes of immigrant children and youth in Europe. *Eur Psychol.* 2016;21(2):150–62.
46. Kandula NR, Kersey M, Lurie N. Assuring the health of immigrants: what the leading health indicators tell us. *Annu Rev Public Health.* 2004;25:357–76.
47. Gimeno-Feliu LA, Armesto-Gomez J, Macipe-Costa R, Magallon-Botaya R. Comparative study of pediatric prescription drug utilization between the Spanish and immigrant population. *BMC Health Serv Res.* 2009;9(225):e1–9.
48. Salas-Wright CP, Vaughn MG, Schwartz SJ, Córdova D. An "immigrant paradox" for adolescent externalizing behavior? Evidence from a national sample. *Soc Psychiatry Psychiatr Epidemiol.* 2016;51(1):27–37.
49. Rechel B, Mladovsky P, Ingleby D, Mackenbach JP, McKee M. Migration and health in an increasingly diverse Europe. *Lancet.* 2013;381(9873):1235–45.

CHAPTER 9

Adolescent migrant health

Marina Catallozzi, Chelsea A. Kolff,
Rachel A. Fowler and Terry McGovern

LEARNING OBJECTIVES

In this chapter, the reader will be able to:

- Identify the features common to all adolescents seeking health care
- Understand the common medical issues that migrant youth face
- Understand the human-rights-based legal framework that influences health care access and overall health of youth
- Describe and implement youth-friendly services as they apply to migrant youth
- Understand the importance of a strengths-based approach as opposed to a risk-focussed paradigm when caring for migrant youth

---

CLINICAL VIGNETTE

Azizah is a 16-year-old who has travelled from Bangladesh to Kolkata in search of work. Her father died and she, her mother, and younger sister were not able to afford to stay in their flat. Before her father's death, she had been promised to a 32-year-old man who worked with her father. She went to him in desperation with the hope of marriage to save her remaining family. He told her he would marry her and forced her to have sex. After an unprotected sexual encounter, he informed her mother and his family of the encounter and deemed her unfit to marry. Her cousin living in Kolkata learned of her situation and wrote to her of her own success working in a factory. She sent Azizah the funds to be able to join her and to get a job so that she could support her family from afar. She left behind her mother and sister, who suffered from a respiratory condition. Upon arrival to Kolkata, Azizah moved in with her cousin who lived with 12 other young women in a cramped two-room flat. Azizah was able to get work at her cousin's factory quickly. She began sending money home to her family within the month. Azizah has tried not to think about her family back home or of the forced sexual encounter that has left her sad, scared, and tired. She has not noticed that she feels sick all the time. Her cousin is concerned that she may be pregnant. Azizah is not sure what to do.

INTRODUCTION

Adolescence is a period of remarkable development as young people bridge the gap from childhood to adulthood and transition to increased independence. The growth and change that occur in a young person cognitively, physically, emotionally, and socially set the stage for many health behaviours and outcomes through a person's life course (1). Several of the chronic illnesses and issues in adults are established secondary to health behaviours established in adolescence. Migration within countries and internationally creates unique opportunities for young people; with support and protections in place, these young people have the capacity to thrive and contribute to their families and society. Migrant youth who are able to successfully leverage these opportunities can experience social and economic advancement and be influential agents of change in their families, communities, their countries of origin, and globally (2). However, migration also can produce risk and pose dangers to young people. Adults, and specifically providers that care for migrant youth in clinical settings, must be attuned to a young person's past experiences and current situation to best assess how to provide high-quality, youth-friendly care. Due to the immense growth and change adolescents experience, the importance of this stage for establishing health behaviours that persist throughout their lives, and the unique vulnerabilities that adolescents face, access to preventive care remains of central importance for all adolescents, and particularly for migrant youth.

ADOLESCENCE AS AN EMERGING CONCEPT

Adolescence is a fairly new concept that first emerged in high-income countries at the turn of the twentieth century as there was an increased focus on the detrimental effects of child labour and emphasis on universal education (3). The World Health Organization (WHO) defines adolescence as 10–19 years of age. Youth is defined as people ages 15–24 years, and the descriptions young people and 'adolescents and young adults' refer to the period from ages 10–24 years old. The proportion of young people in the global population has been increasing; in 2017, 10- to 24-year-olds accounted for 24% of the world population and 1.81 billion globally (4). Representing a growing segment of the population, young people are increasingly seeking jobs, education, and improved living conditions.

Central components of adolescence include physical growth and maturation, cognitive development, individuation from families, assumption of self-responsibility and independence, and identity development (1). A myriad of factors drive migration among young people, including a desire for increased job availability, higher wages, education, social opportunities, security, and fear of discrimination or violence (2). Migrant youth have particular challenges with their developing identity. The strong influence of the new prevailing social culture where they currently are living may be at odds with their own culture and that of their families, resulting in an internal dissonance (5). Young people must navigate these potentially varying cultural influences and pressures as they strive to develop their own sense of identity.

The scope of the issue is far-reaching. As of 2016, there were close to 50 million migrant children living outside their country of birth or displaced within a State (6). Health care systems and providers must anticipate the needs of migrant youth and be equipped to respond with appropriate support and resources.

LEGAL CONSIDERATIONS FOR MIGRANT YOUTH

Adolescent migrants are vulnerable to human rights violations. The 1989 United Nations Convention on the Rights of the Child (CRC) affirms that persons below the age of 18 are bearers of human rights and are given liberties and responsibilities in accordance to their age and maturity (7). The CRC recognizes evolving capacities; in other words, as adolescents acquire greater competence and maturity with age, the need for adult guidance diminishes (1) (Chapter 4).

Legal frameworks impact adolescent health outcomes and future health risks by governing both access to health resources and protection from hazards (1). Some laws specifically address health (e.g. access to contraception), health risks (e.g. consumption of alcohol, access to tobacco), and the social determinants of health (e.g. age of marriage, protection from hazardous work, decent housing) (1). National legal frameworks commonly rely on fixed age limits for adolescents, stripping many adolescents of their right to make safe and informed decisions that affect their health and well-being (1). Furthermore, countries with plural or multiple legal systems allow various sources of law to govern, including English common law, French civil or other law, statutory law, customary law, and religious law or practice (1). When discriminatory cultural and religious practices enjoy binding status in law, profound health effects are able to persist. Consequently, inadequate and inconsistent legal frameworks can adversely affect adolescents' health and rights.

For migrant adolescents, failing health systems and domestic legal frameworks are significant barriers to health and well-being. There is a paucity of migrant-specific data on sexual and reproductive health service access, maternal mortality, gender-based violence, and child marriage. Poor migrant health outcomes are due in part to the failure of States to comply with international standards, reservations to international treaties and/or binding religious, traditional or customary law, and/or constitution protections, which all allow discrimination to persist. Adolescents are a key target group in the Sustainable Development Goals 1–12 and 16 (1). Developmentally informed legal frameworks and accountability mechanisms that provide both adolescent protection and autonomy are vital.

HEALTH CARE CONSIDERATIONS FOR MIGRANT YOUTH

The health care of adolescents and the training of the providers who care for them remains an under-addressed priority around the world, as adolescent medicine is still a relatively novel specialty (8). In spite of the previously mentioned life-course patterns of either health-promoting or health-damaging behaviours that influence adult health and rates of acute and chronic disease and life expectancy, adolescents tend to be a forgotten population (Chapter 8). They generally receive little attention from the health sector because they are seen as a relatively healthy population with a low burden of disease. Social, racial/ethnic, and socioeconomic disparities impact adolescents' utilization of primary care and mental health services, chronic disease and risk behaviours, and overall health outcomes during adolescence and into adulthood (1). It is essential that providers who care for adolescents, regardless of their specialty designation, feel comfortable addressing the preventive and clinical care needs of adolescents. As it stands, the current system of provision of health care for adolescents is falling short.

HEALTH CARE DELIVERY

The tenets of adolescent medicine extend to health care delivery for all young people, including migrant youth in their various contexts. Providers engaging with migrant youth can leverage these tools to elucidate any situational factors due to migration that may affect a young person's health. Barriers encountered by adolescents seeking care may intersect with or be compounded by a young person's migrant background. This confluence of barriers may increase the difficulty in seeking health care. Effective care for migrant youth reflects cultural humility and an understanding of the varied situational contexts in which these young people live (Chapter 5). For example, the young woman featured in our vignette, Azizah, needs to seek medical care to confirm whether or not she is pregnant or has contracted a sexually transmitted infection in Bangladesh. This young woman, who has experienced trauma, is unlikely to seek out this care in a country that she knows little about. The services that are provided and the manner in which they are delivered can mean the difference between life and death, self-respect and shame, for Azizah.

YOUTH-FRIENDLY SERVICES

Youth-friendly services are central to the provision and utilization of quality health care for adolescents and young adults. The WHO framework for making health services adolescent friendly outlines five key tenets. Health services must be accessible, acceptable, equitable, appropriate, and effective to be considered adolescent-friendly (9). Guidance exists to set up the scaffolding to support youth who, for a variety of reasons, may be reticent to access care on their own. These quality standards must be implemented across all aspects of health care delivery, including in the waiting room, with front desk staff, nurses, and medical assistants, in the exam room, in laboratory work, and in billing mechanisms, as well as in regard to institutional and national policies or regulations. In addition to these quality standards, the WHO has published the guidance for implementation as a part of its efforts to help improve adolescent health (10).

Accessible: In order for health services to be accessible, services must be affordable, and adolescents must be informed of their availability. If community members in the place where Azizah lives and works are aware of services and hours, they can direct her to appropriate care. The hours must be convenient for young people, especially those who work and support themselves.

Acceptable: Acceptability from youth is a crucial component. Once youth have accessed the health care system, it is critical to use strengths-based models to screen for concerns that may impact any aspect of their health and lives. Strengths-based models, which are discussed later in this chapter, help to identify and support the individual factors that will allow youth to feel empowered and successful (11). This, combined with trauma-informed models that address existing risk, helps to break down barriers that may exist because of cultural differences (12). Trauma-informed care takes into account the impact trauma can have on all aspects of someone's life, including their health and well-being, and requires that providers acquire a skill set to avoid retraumatizing patients, and to meet their specific needs.

TABLE 9.1   Suggestions to implement youth-friendly services in the health care setting

Tenets of youth-friendly services	Illustrative suggestions for local implementation of quality health care services within general practices
Accessible	Clinic décor, signs, and advertising reflective of all patients
Acceptable	Materials in varied languages that are brief so that they can be read in the clinic and not brought home
	Websites with information for patients to look up information on the phone
Equitable	Training of staff in youth-friendly principles, sensitivity to adolescent issues, and cultural humility
Appropriate and effective	Warm referrals available for psychiatry, gynaecology, or services that can provide support around interpersonal violence

Azizah must feel comfortable confiding the details of the sexual assault she experienced before leaving Bangladesh and trust that she will not be blamed or judged. The practitioner must implement the principles of trauma-informed care in practice. Individuals like Azizah, who have experienced trauma, may feel distress when there are invasive procedures (such as pelvic examinations), removal of clothing, physical touch, lack of privacy or confidentiality, or if they are asked embarrassing questions or asked to re-live the trauma (12). While a female provider may be preferable, a male provider who also implements these practices can help youth like Azizah feel comfortable. Measures include building rapport and trust over time, giving unhurried attention, explaining any and all procedures before beginning, giving the young person control over as many decisions as possible, validating their distress or reactions to the visit, encouraging questions about concerns, and placing a high priority on understanding their culture and values and how they may impact their responses and decisions (12).

Equitable: Patients must be treated with equal care and respect. A young person such as Azizah should be treated with the same care and respect as someone from Kolkata. This includes not restricting services, assuring that providers offer the same level of care, and that the support staffs are trained to do the same.

Appropriate and Effective: Services must reflect the needs of the population served. In the case of migrant young people, concerns such as mental health and sexual health must be addressed. However, before these can be addressed, the legal rights of these youth to access care are critical to understand. For example, Azizah has experienced the stress of being separated from family, and of the migration itself. The standard is that the health care providers are trained in evidence-based protocols, have the basic equipment to deliver services, and have the time and skills to work with young people.

The ideal of youth-friendly services can be difficult to achieve. Support of the local community, government, and humanitarian and developmental assistance programs is critical. Please refer to Table 9.1 for examples of suggestions to implement youth-friendly services.

SPECIFIC LEGAL AND HEALTH CONCERNS FOR MIGRANT YOUTH

Mental health concerns

Migrant adolescents are exposed to stressors during all stages of the migration journey and are particularly vulnerable to mental health issues, including anxiety and adjustment disorders (13). The lack of psychosocial support and inefficiencies in the migration processes generate further stress and contribute to the burden of mental health issues among migrants (14). Laws that ensure migrants' access to mental health services are needed to improve adolescent health. As of 2015, half of the WHO member states had a stand-alone law for mental health, yet 14% of member states indicate that the legislation is not acted upon and many existing laws are only partially implemented (15).

Mental health issues in adolescent migrants are exacerbated due to unacceptable housing conditions. Unaccompanied adolescents, especially young women, could benefit from separate accommodations to ensure their mental well-being and to limit the risk of gender-based violence. For example, in Ireland, migrants seeking asylum live in shared quarters for an indefinite amount of time, which increases their emotional and mental health issues (16). In 2015, Ireland had no national strategy to meet the unique mental health needs of migrants, and the Direct Provision programme limits asylum seekers' rights to access higher-level education, housing, and employment (16). Only 7 out of 21 EU member states studied provide housing to migrants seeking asylum or allow individually arranged housing without reservations (17). In addition, only 8 EU member states provide migrants with the same housing benefits as nationals, and only 14 member states prohibit housing discrimination on grounds of nationality (17).

While Azizah is fortunate to have housing, the crowded conditions and stress of living with people not known to her can negatively affect her mental health. This, in addition to processing her experience of sexual trauma, compounds her need for effective mental health services. Asking about her housing situation and providing resources can be helpful. While awaiting referral to mental health services, providing methods for managing stress demonstrates a commitment to Azizah's well-being.

Sexual and reproductive health concerns

Adolescents have among the highest rates of unmet need for sexual and reproductive health services (18). In particular, migrant girls face increased risk of sexually transmitted infections, exposure to HIV, sexual coercion, exploitation, violence, teenage pregnancy, and maternal mortality (2,19). This risk to their sexual health may be attributed to the conditions they fled from, the migration journey, or vulnerability upon arrival (2). Laws that limit adolescents' ability to access sexual and reproductive care, such as payment fees, are harmful to young women's health (20). In 2013, only 47 countries had laws that ensured the provision of free birth control (21). Many host countries have yet to implement systems that ensure migrant access to affordable health care. Some migrants arriving in the United States are automatically enrolled in Medicaid or are eligible for Refugee Cash Assistance and Refugee Medical Assistance; however, these provisions only operate in the short term (22).

Some countries also have laws that limit access to contraception by requiring parental or spousal consent, a medical prescription, or by limiting sexual and reproductive health services to married people (23). Similarly, parental or spousal involvement in minors' abortion access and HIV counselling and testing are significant barriers to care. Laws that require parental or spousal consent ignore the CRC's call for autonomous decision making and raise issues of patient confidentiality and privacy. In addition, these laws rely on the willingness of migrant adolescents' parents and spouses, who may be heavily influenced by customary and religious practices, to participate in the health-care-seeking process. Low acceptability of sexual and reproductive health services, whether for socioeconomic, political, or cultural reasons, can lead to the denial of medical procedures and the marginalization of adolescents who seek them, violating adolescents' rights to health and non-discrimination (10).

There are real concerns for Azizah's sexual health. In addition to pregnancy testing, and if positive, options for counselling and referrals to safe abortion or prenatal care, she must be screened for sexually transmitted infections and HIV. Regardless of the results of this testing, she will need to be engaged in ongoing sexual and reproductive health care. Education around her continued sexual health is also warranted.

LABOUR CONCERNS FOR MIGRANT YOUTH

Many adolescents migrate explicitly for labour, and working youth migrants are particularly vulnerable to occupational hazards and exploitation (2). Laws are needed to protect youth from hazardous work and work exploitation. In Latin America and the Caribbean, all countries have established minimum working age laws (24). However, some countries, such as Bolivia, allow children to work starting at the age of 10, which is below the international standard established by the International Labour Organization Convention No. 138 (24). In addition, migrant workers usually engage in hazardous work before the age of 18, and many low- and middle-income countries lack legislation that addresses child engagement with hazardous work or prohibits the involvement of children in illicit activities (25). Moreover, more than a third of the world's countries do not have laws prohibiting sexual harassment at work (26), a prevalent issue among adolescent working migrants (2). Consequently, adolescent migrants are exposed to more dangerous work and lower wages and are at a higher risk of work-related deaths in comparison to local children (27).

Work conditions may be hazardous or pose health risks. In finding work at a factory, Azizah is able to learn skills and earn money to send to her mother and sister. She also, however, may be exposed to occupational hazards as a part of her job.

ADDITIONAL CONCERNS SPECIFIC TO MIGRANT YOUTH EXPERIENCES

Migrant adolescents are also uniquely vulnerable to stressors during transit and upon arrival. Unaccompanied children are vulnerable to trafficking and sexual exploitation, and countries with non-entry policies may increase the risk of child trafficking (28). In addition, these young people encounter health barriers upon arrival, as 35 countries still impose travel restrictions for people with HIV (29). Once in a country, migrant youth often face fear of imprisonment or forced repatriation to their home country as well as significant language barriers (22) and discrimination in the health system (30,31), resulting in fewer young people seeking health and legal services. The United States, Australia, and some European countries, for example, continue to disregard migrant rights to *non-refoulement* and protection from incarceration upon illegal entry. Youth may need support with accessing additional services or education, and therefore consideration for other concerns must include safety, housing, and privacy.

STRENGTHS-BASED MODELS TO ENGAGE MIGRANT YOUTH

Underlying the health care and legal services, programs must be infused with an adolescent development lens and the principles of positive youth development. These frames view adolescent development from a strengths-based approach, encouraging efforts to engage and prepare youth rather than seek to prevent problems, with a focus on risk (32). Inputs that promote youth development and engagement (not specific to health care for migrant youth) include stable location, basic care and services, healthy relationships and connections with peers and adults, high expectations and standards for the engaged youth, role models, challenging experiences and opportunities to participate and contribute, and high-quality instruction and training (32). A strengths-based approach is widely accepted in the field of adolescent medicine as a best practice for engaging adolescents in care (11). This model emphasizes meaningful partnerships between adults and young people built on a respect for that young person's emerging sense of autonomy and identity (33).

Before migration, youth should be prepared for challenges they may encounter and be aware of their human rights. Ensuring that young people possess personal documentation and have copies with trusted adults in other locations is critical. As mentioned, youth travelling alone are at heightened danger for trafficking and exploitation. Lists and connections to safe spaces and programmes can impact safety. Examples of how to support youth who have migrated include encouragement of continued education and attainment of life skills. Community programmes and social networks can help young people navigate the milestones of migration, such as securing work and housing and connecting with other young people. The lack of dependable social networks should encourage development of alternative plans for resources or housing (2).

Rather than focussing on the negative experiences and vulnerabilities of youth, there can be the recognition of and support for resiliency. Resilience, the ability to overcome adversity, can help young people respond to, cope with, and recover from difficult situations, challenges, and setbacks (34). Resilient youth learn and employ healthy strategies that help improve their capacity to bounce back in a variety of contexts and in response to different stressors. Trusted adults and programmes can foster resilience and be an important resource for this paradigm shift. Building on the work of others in the field, Ginsburg's model of resilience is comprised of 7 Cs exhibited by resilient young people: competence, confidence, connection, character, contribution, coping, and control (34). This model is of particular utility for migrant youth.

In the clinical setting, a strengths-based model begins with engaging youth around their special skills or existing strengths. Rather than screen for a series of risks, the model encourages a deeper understanding of the young person's home environment, larger community (work or school), self-esteem, support network, coping mechanisms and concern for depression or mental health issues, experience with drugs and alcohol, sexual experience and risk, experiences of violence, and issues that threaten their safety in relationships or communities (35). By screening in these areas (often referred to as a psychosocial assessment; see Table 9.2, SSHADESS Screen), youth are given the chance to identify areas where they are in need of support and partner with adults who encourage successful navigation of the development.

If Azizah seeks care at a centre that provides youth-friendly services using a strengths-based model, she will be more likely to disclose her traumatic experience and be able to receive mental and reproductive health screening and services that can support her health and well-being. She can also be connected to other critically important legal and social services available in her community.

SUMMARY

Migration provides young people with great opportunity for economic empowerment, education, and improved security; however, it can also pose great risks to young people's safety and health. Youth development programmes and health care providers and systems

TABLE 9.2 Strengths-based psychosocial assessment (SSHADESS Screen)

Domains for a strengths-based psychosocial assessment	Sample questions for migrant adolescent clients seen in the health care setting
Strengths	How would you describe yourself? What are you most proud of?
School/work	What are you currently doing with your time? <ul><li>If work, what type of work are you doing?</li><li>If school, what school environment? Did you go to school in the past?<ul><li>How far along did you get?</li></ul></li></ul>What are your hopes for the future?
Home	Where and with whom do you live? Where does your family live? Do you have any family members here? Did you arrive in this country by choice? Who are you closest to at home? Can you talk to anyone you live with if you are stressed? Who do you share sleeping space with?
Activities	Since arriving here, are you able to engage in activities that you enjoyed in the past? What kind of things have you been able to do for fun? Have you made connections with anyone since arriving?
Drugs/substance use	Do you drink alcohol or use anything to get high? Have you gotten into trouble or had anything bad happen while you were using alcohol or drugs? Have you ever exchanged sex for drugs?
Emotions/depression	How do you feel about yourself? Are you mostly happy or sad? Have you ever thought about suicide? Have you ever tried to kill yourself? Who do you talk to when you are upset? Do you ever get so anxious that it interferes with your life or activities?
Sexuality	How would you describe your gender? How would you describe the people you are attracted to? If you have sex, do you have sex with females, males, or both? Are you having sex? <ul><li>Oral, vaginal, anal?</li></ul>Any history of molestation, rape, or abuse? Have you ever exchanged sex for money, drugs, or housing? Do you fear, hurt, or feel controlled by partner? When was your first sexual experience? How many partners have you had? Did you use condoms the last time you had sex? Are you on contraception? <ul><li>If no, are you interested in contraception?</li></ul>Have you had any pregnancies? <ul><li>What were the outcomes?</li></ul>

(Continued)

TABLE 9.2 (CONTINUED)   Strengths-based psychosocial assessment (SSHADESS Screen)

Domains for a strengths–based psychosocial assessment	Sample questions for migrant adolescent clients seen in the health care setting
Safety	Do you feel safe where you live? Do you feel safe travelling to and from home? Do you feel safe at work or school? Are you drinking alcohol or using drugs so much that you pass out or do something you regret? How often do you wear seatbelts or helmets? Have you been involved in any interpersonal violence? Do you carry a weapon? • If yes, for safety? Are you witnessing violence currently or have you in the past? Have you ever been arrested or imprisoned? Are you worried about your legal status in the country?

Source: Adapted from Ginsburg KR. In: Ginsburg KR, Kinsman SB, editors. *Reaching Teens: Strength-Based Communication Strategies to Build Resilience and Support Healthy Adolescent Development.* American Academy of Pediatrics; 2014.

can use strengths-based models to help young people build on their strengths, address health outcomes or concerns, and foster resiliency. Developmentally informed legal frameworks and accountability mechanisms that provide adolescent protection and autonomy are needed to allow adolescent migrants to reach their full potential, achieve their right to health, and build a sustainable future.

REFERENCES

1. Patton GC, Sawyer SM, Santelli JS et al. Our future: a Lancet commission on adolescent health and wellbeing. *Lancet.* 2016;387:2423–78.
2. Temin, M, Montgomery M. *Girls on the Move: Adolescent Girls and Migration in the Developing World.* New York, NY: Population Council; 2013.
3. Feldman SS, Elliott GR. *At the Threshold: The Developing Adolescent.* Cambridge, MA: Harvard University Press; 1990; 642.
4. UNFPA. *World Population Dashboard.* 2017.
5. Rogers CG, Kinsman SB. Adolescent development: stages, statues, and stereotypes. In: Ginsburg KR, Kinsman SB, editors. *Reaching Teens: Strength-Based Communication Strategies to Build Resilience and Support Healthy Adolescent Development.* American Academy of Pediatrics; 2014.
6. UNICEF. Uprooted: The growing crisis for refugee and migrant children. New York, NY: UNICEF Division of Data, Research and Policy. New York; 2016. 134 p.
7. United Nations Convention on the Rights of the Child. *United Nations [Internet].* 1989;25(December):1–5. Available from: http://www.unicef.org/rightsite/files/uncrcchilldfriendlylanguage.pdf
8. Hergenroeder AC, Benson PAS, Britto MT et al. Adolescent medicine: workforce trends and recommendations. *Arch Pediatr Adolesc Med.* 2010;164:1086–90.
9. World Health Organization. *Making Health Services Adolescent Friendly – Developing National Quality Standards for Adolescent Friendly Health Services.* World Health Organization [Internet]. 2012;3. Available from: http://www.who.int/iris/bitstream/10665/75217/1/9789241503594_eng.pdf?ua=1
10. World Health Organization. *Global Accelerated Action for the Health of Adolescents (AA-HA!).* *Guidance to Support Country Implementation.* Geneva: World Health Organization; 2017.

11. Ginsburg KR. The journey from risk-focused attention to strengths-based care. In: Ginsburg KR, Kinsman SB, editors. *Reaching Teens: Strength-Based Communication Strategies to Build Resilience and Support Healthy Adolescent Development*. American Academy of Pediatrics; 2014.

12. Bloom SL, Wise Z, Lively J, Almonte MO, Contreras S, Ginsburg KR. Trauma-informed practice: working with youth who have suffered adverse childhood (or adolescent) experiences. In: Ginsburg KR, Kinsman SB, editors. *Reaching Teens: Strength-Based Communication Strategies to Build Resilience and Support Healthy Adolescent Development*. American Academy of Pediatrics; 2014.

13. Kirmayer LJ, Narasiah L, Munoz M et al. Common mental health problems in immigrants and refugees: general approach in primary care. *CMAJ* 2011; 183.

14. Human Rights Watch. *EU/Greece; Asylum Seekers' Silent Mental Health Crisis*. Brussels; 2017.

15. World Health Organization. *Mental Health Atlas 2014*. WHO; 2014.

16. Department of Justice and Equality. *Working Group to Report to Government on Improvements to the Protection Process, including Direct Provision and Supports to Asylum Seekers*. Final Report. Ireland; 2015.

17. EWSI. *EWSI Analysis: Immigrant Housing In Europe*. 2016.

18. World Health Organization. *Unmet need for family planning*. Sexual and Reproductive Health. 2015.

19. Morris JL, Rushwan H. Adolescent sexual and reproductive health: the global challenges. *Int J Gynecol Obstet*. 2015;131:S40–2.

20. Woog V, Singh S, Browne A, Philbin J. *Adolescent Women's Need for and Use of Sexual and Reproductive Health Services in Developing Countries*. Guttmacher Inst [Internet]. 2015;(August). Available from: https://www.guttmacher.org/sites/default/files/report_pdf/adolescent-srhs-need-developing-countries.pdf

21. Finlay J, Canning D, Po JYT. Reproductive Health Laws Around the World. PDGA Working Paper No. 96. Cambridge, MA: Harvard University; 2013.

22. RHTAC. Access to Care. Refugee Health. 2011.

23. IPPF. *Qualitative research on legal barriers to young people's access to sexual and reproductive health services*. Inception Report. London; 2014.

24. UNICEF. Legal minimum ages and the realization of adolescents' rights. 2016.

25. Bureau of International Labor Affairs. *2016 Regional Outlook: Latin America and the Caribbean; Asia and the Pacific*. In: 2016. Findings of the Worst Forms of Child Labor. Washington, DC: ILAB; 2016.

26. UCLA. *Nearly 235 Million Women Worldwide Lack Legal Protections from Sexual Harassment at Work*. UCLA Newsroom; 2017.

27. ILO. *Migration and Child Labour: Essentials*. Geneva; 2011.

28. Gammeltoft-Hansen T, Tan NF. The end of the deterrence paradigm? Future directions for global refugee policy. *J Migr Hum Secur*. 2017;5(1):28.

29. UNAIDS. *Eliminating HIV-related travel restrictions*. 2014–2015 UBRAF Themat Report 2016;7.

30. Svenberg K, Skott C, Lepp M. Ambiguous expectations and reduced confidence: experience of Somali refugees encountering Swedish health care. *J Refug Stud*. 2011;24(4):690–705.

31. Tendayi A. Beyond prejudice: structural xenophobic discrimination against refugees. *Georg J Int Law*. 2014;45(3):323–589.

32. Pittman KJ, Irby M, Tolman J, Yohalem N, Ferber T. *Preventing Problems, Promoting Development, Encouraging Engagement: Competing Priorities or Separate Goals?* Washington, DC: Forum for Youth Investment; 2003.

33. Kreipe RE. Who's the expert? Terms of engagement in adolescent care. In: Ginsburg KR, Kinsman SB, editors. *Reaching Teens: Strength-Based Communication Strategies to Build Resilience and Support Healthy Adolescent Development*. American Academy of Pediatrics; 2014; 25–30.

34. Ginsburg KR. The 7 Cs Model of resilience. In: Ginsburg KR, Kinsman SB, editors. *Reaching Teens: Strength-Based Communication Strategies to Build Resilience and Support Healthy Adolescent Development*. American Academy of Pediatrics; 2014; 31–36.

35. Ginsburg KR. The SSHADESS Screen: A Strengths-Based Psychosocial Assessment. In: Ginsburg KR, Kinsman SB, editors. *Reaching Teens: Strength-Based Communication Strategies to Build Resilience and Support Healthy Adolescent Development*. American Academy of Pediatrics; 2014; 139–143.

CHAPTER 10

Health care for older and elderly migrants

Catherine A. O'Donnell

LEARNING OBJECTIVES

At the end of this chapter, the reader should be able to:

- Consider the needs of older and elderly migrants (hereafter referred to as 'older migrants') — in particular, those aged 60 and over
- Address the health care needs of such individuals
- Address the challenges facing health care providers and carers, as well as families, in meeting the needs of older migrant patients

---

INTRODUCTION

Migration is not only for the young. With over 65 million people displaced in the world today, migration affects people of all ages. Migration journeys can be forced on people by war, conflict, or natural disaster, or may be a conscious choice to seek work or education, or for family reunification. Whatever the reason, some of those migrating will be older people. In addition, those who migrated many years ago for work, family, or other reasons are now growing old in their country of resettlement. This means that health care, and primary health care in particular, needs to consider and address the needs of older migrant patients. For example, many settled migrants are now growing old and living with chronic diseases, dementia, and multimorbidity, as outlined in the following clinical vignette.

CLINICAL VIGNETTE

Mrs Chauhan moved to the UK from the Punjab region in Pakistan in 1966 to join her husband, who had found work in the UK. They had a family and she is now a grandmother. Her English language ability is good, but she is not fully fluent and has often relied on her children for more difficult issues, such as hospital and family doctor appointments. She is now 77 years old and has both diabetes and early-stage heart failure. In addition, she is showing early signs of dementia and, although she knows her immediate family, she is increasingly focussed on her early life in the Punjab region. She attends a day centre twice a week in her UK city of settlement, where she is one of several people who originally came from the Punjab region.

DEMOGRAPHICS OF OLDER MIGRANT POPULATIONS

Migrants — including older migrants — are not a homogeneous group. As well as gender and socioeconomic status, the influence of the migration trajectory must be acknowledged. Thus, individuals who moved to a new country for work, education, or family reunification may have very different needs and responses from those who have arrived seeking asylum. One framework which helps us to consider these issues is intersectionality, which draws attention to the ways in which multiple variables intersect and influence health use and outcomes (refer to Chapter 2).

In considering the needs of older migrants, the first difficulty is the lack of consensus on the age at which a migrant is considered 'older' (1). While some might consider the age of retirement to be an appropriate reference point, others suggest that the retirement age of 60 or 65 is too old. They suggest that migration trajectories and experiences, especially if difficult, and the resultant likelihood of physical and/or mental frailty, mean that 'older age' may be considered to start at 50 or 55 years of age (1).

The second difficulty is that obtaining accurate statistics in relation to age and migrant populations is not straightforward. This is in part related to the difficulty of collecting data on migrant status, but also due to different populations of older migrants, as described previously. For example, the United Nations High Commissioner for Refugees (UNHCR) estimates that of 10.9 million refugees, 3% are aged 60 and over, a population of approximately 327,000 people; four percent of the 29.3 million classified as being of concern (including asylum seekers and internally displaced persons) adds a further 1.17 million to that total (2). Many of those regarded as displaced or stateless will have lived in camps, often for many years, as is the case for Palestinian refugees in the Middle East. The Syrian conflict has led to a new population of older refugees. By the end of 2016, the UNHCR had registered 4.8 million Syrian refugees, many in the countries around Syria. Of these, 3.2% — around 154,000 people — were aged 60 and above.

Data from the 28 member countries of the European Union (EU) shows that while the age structure of non-EU nationals living in EU member states is significantly younger than that of EU nationals, there is nevertheless a substantial proportion of the population of non-EU nationals aged 60 and over (Figure 10.1). Many of these individuals migrated to their country of settlement in the 1960s and 1970s to find work as 'guest workers' or migrant workers. Others migrated from former colonies, as in the case of those coming from Caribbean countries to the UK. Later, EU nationals migrated within the EU and are now living in a different country from the one they were born in or are a citizen of; for example, Eastern Europeans now living and working in the countries of Western Europe.

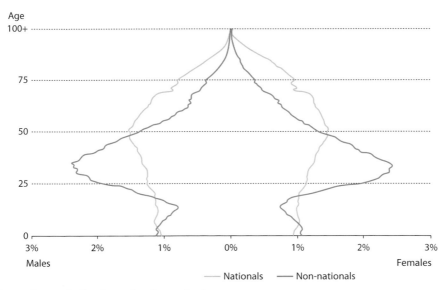

Source: Eurostat (online data code: migr_pop2ctz)

FIGURE 10.1   Age structure of EU nationals and non-EU nationals living in the 28 member states, 1 January 2016. (Eurostat. Migration and migrant population statistics. 2017. From http://ec.europa.eu/eurostat/statistics-explained/index.php/File:Age_structure_of_the_ national_and_non-national_populations,_EU-28,_1_January_2016_(%25).png#file.)

The third difficulty is that data on migrants within countries is often hard to find, due to a lack of data collection (3). This frequently means that using proxy measures, such as asylum applications, country of birth, or ethnicity, is often the only way to get an estimate of the number of older migrants living in a country. For example, in 2016 there were around 53,000 first-time asylum applications to the 28 member states of the EU, although only 1–2% of these were from people aged 65 and over. Analysis of Eurostat data found that the population of foreign-born persons aged 55 and over is increasing in the 20 European countries included in this analysis (4). Compared to country-level data from 2010, the rate of increase in this population in 2015 ranged from 2% in Cyprus to 74% in Luxembourg. The rate of increase in France, Germany, and the UK was 13%, 12%, and 24%, respectively, and the overall size of this population was just under 10 million people (4).

Analysis of the 2011 UK census data shows a similar picture. In England and Wales, 12% of the population born outside the UK were aged over 65 years, compared with 17% of the UK-born population — a population of 878,000 people (5). The three main nationalities represented were those born in India, Pakistan, and Ireland. A more detailed analysis focussed on language identified that of those aged 64 to 84, 17.5% (45,000 people) spoke Punjabi as their main language, with another 14% (37,000) speaking Gujarati. Proficiency in English decreased with age, especially among women, where only 40% of women aged 75 and over considered that they spoke English 'well' or 'very well' (5).

This growing population of older migrants, who moved for work and/or family reunification and are now growing old in their country of resettlement, is bringing new challenges to health care systems, the practitioners working in them, and to wider society (6). The growing population of older refugees and asylum seekers also has particular health needs. Biologically, such individuals may be facing the same challenges of chronic disease and multimorbidity as any other ageing population (refer to Chapter 18). However, there may also be particular issues, for example around language and communication, as well as cultural issues. A survey of older refugees in Europe conducted in 2002 identified poverty, language barriers, loneliness, and a lack of social networks as particular issues facing these populations (1,7).

HEALTH AND AGEING IN MIGRANT POPULATIONS

Several studies have examined mortality and healthy life expectancy among different groups of older migrants. Reus-Pons et al. explored mortality among migrants in Belgium, comparing them to non-migrants (8). They found that most migrant groups had a lower rate of mortality compared to non-migrants, although this pattern did not hold for all groups. For example, Turks and Eastern European men had higher rates of mortality, which they hypothesized was due to lower socioeconomic status. However, while there was some mortality advantage, the same group found that healthy life expectancy at age 50 was shorter for all migrant groups (9). This was true for men and women, and held true across several European countries (Belgium, the Netherlands, and England and Wales combined). The 'mortality paradox' has been reported for other migrant populations, most notably the Hispanic population in the United States, where mortality rates for foreign-born Hispanics aged 65 and over were closer to that of the settled White population despite the relatively lower socioeconomic status of the Hispanic population in general.

Cardiovascular disease, stroke, diabetes mellitus, some cancers, and arthritis have all been reported to be more prevalent in some migrant groups (10–13). Mental health conditions, including depression, anxiety, and schizophrenia, are known to be more prevalent among migrant groups compared to non-migrants, and especially among refugees and asylum seekers (14,15). Such increased risks remain in older migrant populations, especially among those who have experienced conflict and trauma. A survey of older refugees from Syria now living in Lebanon found a highly vulnerable population, with 60% reporting they had hypertension, 47% diabetes, and 30% heart disease (16). In addition to chronic disease, almost half had walking difficulties and one in four had eyesight problems. Many reported having anxiety or depression as well as feelings of loneliness or being scared.

The Survey of Health, Ageing and Retirement in Europe (SHARE) study with data from adults aged 50 and over in 11 European countries offers a unique opportunity to analyse health in a group of older migrants who moved to Europe from different settings, mainly to seek employment. The prevalence of depression was significantly higher in migrants compared to non-migrants, and was also higher for those living in Northern and Western Europe than in Southern Europe (17). Similar results were also reported in a review of the literature exploring the mental health of older migrants, which found evidence of a higher prevalence of depression in older refugees and asylum seekers, but also identified a lack of robust evidence in this area (18).

Although there is little work on the prevalence of dementia in migrant populations, the increase in dementia prevalence worldwide would suggest that, in time, older migrants will also be at risk of developing dementia (refer to Chapter 22). One UK-based study screened older (60 years and over) first-generation African-Caribbean migrants to the UK and compared them with the UK-born White population (19). They reported a higher prevalence of dementia in the African-Caribbean population compared to the White population (9.6% vs 6.9%).

This higher risk remained after adjusting for age and socioeconomic status. The sample was, however, relatively small (436 in total) and located in one area of London; such work needs to be replicated. A recent review of the international literature in relation to dementia in migrant and minority ethnic populations found that these groups were underrepresented in dementia research; there was, however, some evidence of an increased prevalence of dementia in non-Western migrant groups compared to the settled population (20).

The association between migrant status and chronic disease raises the issue of multimorbidity. Often defined as the presence of two or more coexisting chronic diseases, the prevalence increases sharply with age. This increase is exacerbated with increasing socioeconomic deprivation, at least until the oldest old (age 80 and above). However, there is little work looking at multimorbidity in migrant populations. A survey of health care use in one area in Switzerland found that approximately 40% of their asylum-seeking patients had multiple conditions, including chronic physical and mental health conditions (21). A study from Spain reported that the prevalence of multimorbidity was lower in people born outside Spain compared to the native-born population, although the prevalence of multimorbidity did increase with length of residency in Spain (22). Analysis of data from a Norwegian family practice found that multimorbidity varied by migrant group. Thus, compared to those moving for family reunification, multimorbidity was lower for labour migrants and those moving for education, but higher for refugees (23). This study also included patients aged 50 and over, and demonstrated the sharp rise in multimorbidity with age for all groups, except those migrating for education. However, this effect was also modified by length of stay, with the prevalence of multimorbidity doubling for all groups after 5-year stay in Norway. The SHARE study reported that relative to the native-born population, the risk for migrants of having two or more chronic diseases varied across countries: highest in Spain, Switzerland, and Italy, and lowest in Austria and France.

Related to this increase in chronic disease and multimorbidity is the increased risk of polypharmacy. Polypharmacy increases both with age and with multimorbidity (24). Increasing polypharmacy increases the chances of adverse drug reactions. Multimorbidity also leads to increased use of family practice and hospital appointments, leading to increased burden of care for both patients and carers – often described as 'treatment burden' (25). To date, however, there is little research considering the implications of multimorbidity, polypharmacy, or treatment burden in relation to older migrant patients. Clearly this area requires further investigation, given that such patients may experience other complications in relation to health care; in particular, entitlement and language and communication difficulties.

The SHARE dataset has also been used to explore health-related behaviour (26), self-reported well-being (27), and frailty (28). In general, migrants had poorer self-reported health and increased frailty compared to non-migrants, but there were complex patterns depending on region of origin and where in Europe migrants had settled. Of particular interest here was the finding that the gap in subjective well-being between older migrants and non-migrants was less in countries with more favourable policies on family reunification (27).

HEALTH POLICY ON ENTITLEMENT AND OLDER MIGRANTS

The finding that older migrants' subjective well-being is better in countries with more favourable policies on family reunification (27) raises the important role of policy and entitlement to health care. First, as discussed in Chapter 4, entitlement to health care for migrants varies depending on migrant status (29). For example, refugees and people in the process of claiming asylum often have full entitlement to access health care, whereas those whose asylum claim has been rejected or undocumented migrants have much more restrictive rights to health care (29). Entitlement of health care also depends on the health system itself, for example, whether access rights are based on citizenship via taxation or based on insurance. Entitlement to health care based on the ability to pay for insurance (social insurance or private insurance) may be problematic for older migrants, especially if access to social insurance is lost due to retirement.

Entitlement to access health care can also be gained or lost through policy change. For example, in the United States, changes to the eligibility rules for federal means-tested entitlements in 1996 saw older migrants lose their right to access federally funded health care (30). Older migrants were particular victims of this policy change, losing their rights to health care, and being portrayed in resulting congressional documents as 'non-contributing' members of society, a burden to US taxpayers and belonging to families who had the financial means to support their elderly relatives if they wished to. Such losses to entitlement can be reversed, however. State-level welfare reform and an improvement in Medicaid coverage improved health care coverage for some older migrants, especially those who were naturalized citizens (31). Concerted campaigns, first by migrant support organizations and activists, and later by some media outlets, highlighted the impact of lost entitlements to health and social care on elderly migrants, including incidences of suicide. This eventually led to a restoration of entitlements (30). However, a related issue is the way in which depictions of being a 'non-contributing' or 'undeserving' member of society may impact how older migrants access and use health care services.

ACCESS TO, AND USE OF, HEALTH CARE INCLUDING PRIMARY CARE

While there is a substantial body of literature looking at health care access by migrant groups, fewer studies have explicitly examined health care use and access by older migrants. Work using the SHARE database found that, compared to non-migrants, migrants used more health services, including visits to family doctors/general practitioners (GPs) and hospital stays (32). This varied by country and by the variable examined. In general, however, migrants accessed family doctors more than non-migrants, except in Austria, Italy, and Spain. Controlling for health care needs and some sociodemographic variables led to some changes: the reduced use of GPs remained in Austria and Spain, disappeared in Italy, and emerged in Germany. Usage also appeared greater for newer migrants, compared to long-stay migrants, at least for hospital-based care. Visits to family doctors were also higher in countries where the GP did not act as a gatekeeper to hospital care. However, when Diaz et al. examined the factors associated with frequent attendance at general practice in Norway, they found that older migrants attended less frequently than older Norwegians (33).

Some studies focussed on access to services for older migrants have also identified these issues. Ahaddour et al., in a review of literature on health and social care services for elderly Moroccan and Turkish migrants in Belgium, found that such services were largely inaccessible due to language, cultural, financial, and religious barriers. A lack of knowledge of such services and assumptions on the part of both older migrants and service providers that families would provide such care were further barriers (34). A lack of health literacy was also reported by Gracie et al. in the United States, where poverty and a lack of English language skills, health care insurance, and social support intersected to reduce access to health and social care (35). These issues, along with a lack of knowledge of health and social care services, were reported as key barriers to accessing health and social care for black and minority ethnic (BME) seniors in Vancouver (36). Similarly, a lack of knowledge of services was identified in a series of focus groups conducted with older people from the BME community in England, including migrants from the Somali, Polish, and Central European communities (37). This suggests that these barriers to access appropriate health and social care services may be universal across countries and health care systems. This should also help to identify and facilitate service redesign to address these barriers.

Much has been written about the barriers and facilitators to migrants' access and use of health care services, including primary care, with a number of international reviews of the evidence published (38,39). However, none explicitly considered the issues facing older migrants (refer to Chapter 6).

MEETING THE NEEDS OF OLDER MIGRANTS

A range of service approaches have been suggested to meet the needs of older migrants. The provision of appropriate and accessible interpreter services is an obvious starting point and is discussed in Chapter 20. However, in addition to this, there is the need to consider the accessibility of services, the cultural sensitivity of services, and approaches to address social isolation and loneliness, as well as health conditions. In this section, several examples of services designed to address the needs of older migrant populations are described. This is by no means an exhaustive list, but merely serves to outline some examples of good practice and to consider, more generally, some approaches that might be worth developing.

To date, much of the attention in developing services for older migrants in the UK has focussed on well-established BME communities, including those who came to work and older family members who came to join spouses and children. However, with the steady, albeit small, increase in older asylum seekers (as described earlier), entitlement to health and social care will become more of an issue than it is currently.

A lack of information and knowledge about services available for older migrants is often cited as a barrier to accessing care (36,37). This finding is replicated across countries and across different groups of migrants. Therefore, approaches to support information sharing and increase health literacy have been considered. In Australia, older Italian and Greek migrants were asked about their use of information and communication technology (ICT) to access health information. Unsurprisingly, this group did not use ICT to any great extent and were reluctant to do so (40). Instead, they were more likely to use local newspapers, radios, television, friends and family, and service providers, including doctors for information. They also used information from their country of origin, as well as their country of settlement (Australia). This preference for printed sources of information and a reliance on social networks and family members for information also surfaced in a review conducted in the United States (35) and interviews with older refugees in London. This suggests that interventions and services that use existing social networks, such as religious groups, social clubs, or lunch clubs, might offer solutions to caring for older migrants.

Another model of care provision is the home health care or home-based primary care model for older migrants being developed in the United States (41,42). These models provide primary care and/or community-based services directly to a patient's home, including supporting self-management for chronic diseases, supporting mental health needs, and providing medicine management. Pilot studies in the United States reported improvements in patient outcomes, including diabetic outcome measures and blood pressure (43), pain and anxiety levels, and medication management (42). A literature review of home-based primary care found that there was little evidence of best practice in the provision of this model, for example which health care professional was best placed to provide home visits (44). Building on the literature review by Febles et al., the team developed a conceptual model of care (41), which suggests that inputs include linguistic communication, cultural safety, and the interprofessional team; outcomes include improvements in health outcomes, quality of life, and health care professionals' collaboration.

Another approach which could be adapted to improve health literacy and access to appropriate services for older migrants is the use of community navigators or health advisors (45). While these models have not targeted older migrants, the approach of providing peer support and information to migrants to help them to self-care and access services in a more appropriate manner could be a viable approach in the care of older migrants. A scoping review of the community navigator model found substantial improvements in health outcomes such as diabetic control, improvements in diet and physical activity, and reductions in missed appointments for screening programmes (45).

Two clinical areas that are of particular importance in relation to older migrants are end-of-life care and care of dementia patients (refer to Chapter 22). End-of-life care has received little attention to date. Badger et al. conducted a review of end-of-life care in UK residential care homes; they found little work to guide care workers in the care of older patients from minority ethnic groups (46). A scoping review in the UK, supported by Marie Curie Cancer Care, suggested that minority ethnic groups were less likely to access palliative or end-of-life care; however, while acknowledging the role of migration in increasing the diversity of the UK population, there was no consideration of the impact of migration journey or type of migrant on the use of end-of-life care by migrants (47).

Migration has been considered more clearly in relation to dementia care, with the increasing prevalence of dementia amongst migrant groups identified (19,20,48,49). Thus, primary care will be required to meet the needs of patients such as Mrs Chauhan, described in the clinical vignette, and those described in Chapter 22. Weisman and colleagues reviewed some approaches to caring for migrant patients with dementia, in particular bicultural effectiveness training, an approach which focusses on teaching families to communicate both with the family member with dementia and with each other (48). Recognizing the importance of interpersonal relationships, cultural influences, and intergenerational hierarchies, this approach was viewed as one worth pursuing in the care of migrants with dementia. Individuals with dementia tend to lose recent memories first, so it may be beneficial to develop and tailor services to address the individuals' needs. When caring for older South Asian dementia patients it also recommended that services need to be culturally tailored to client groups, for example, by employing staff with similar cultural backgrounds (50). Other issues identified in this review were a limited understanding of the signs and symptoms of dementia, a lack of awareness of services, stigma in relation to mental health conditions, and culturally preferred coping strategies. Migration experiences were also identified as important for understanding people's experiences of services and of caring. Therefore, services need to consider early life experiences, the impact of their migrant journey, and acculturation in the host journey.

SUMMARY

Primary care practitioners are caring for increasingly ageing and diverse patient populations. Migrants are not a homogenous group, and this is particularly true of older migrants; some may have lived for many years in the country of settlement; others may be newer arrivals. Some migrants will have chosen to move; others will have been forced to flee. Primary care practitioners may not be aware of all of these complex interplays when dealing with older migrant patients. However, being aware of the wider social and structural environments in which people are living may give practitioners a greater insight into both the illnesses being presented to them and the way in which patients do, or do not, respond to health and medication advice. Considering the migration trajectory of a patient may therefore be valuable in working with that patient to decide on the best course of action and to facilitate shared decision making in the consultation.

REFERENCES

1. Connelly N, Forsythe LA, Njike G, Rudiger A. *Older Refugees in the UK: A Literature Review*. London: Age Concern, Refugee Council; 2006.
2. UNHCR. *Statistical Yearbook 2015*. Geneva; 2017.
3. Rechel B, Mladovsky P, Devillé W. Monitoring migrant health in Europe: a narrative review of data collection practices. *Health Policy*. 2012;105(1):10–6.
4. Ciobanu RO, Fokkema T, Nedelcu M. Ageing as a migrant: vulnerabilities, agency and policy implications. *J Ethn Migr Stud*. 2017;43(2):164–81.
5. Office for National Statistics. 2011 Census: detailed characteristics for England and Wales, March 2011. 2013.
6. Zubair M, Norris M. Perspectives on ageing, later life and ethnicity: ageing research in ethnic minority contexts. *Ageing Soc*. 2015;35(5):897–916.
7. Knapp A, Kremla M. Older refugees in Europe: survey results and key approaches. London: ECRE; 2002.
8. Reus-Pons M, Vandenheede H, Janssen F, Kibele EUB. Differences in mortality between groups of older migrants and older non-migrants in Belgium, 2001-09. *Eur J Public Health*. 2016;26(6):992–1000.
9. Reus-Pons M, Kibele EUB, Janssen F. Differences in healthy life expectancy between older migrants and non-migrants in three European countries over time. *Int J Public Health*. 2017;62(5):531–40.
10. Arnold M, Razum O, Coebergh J-W. Cancer risk diversity in non-western migrants to Europe: an overview of the literature. *Eur J Cancer*. 2010;46(14):2647–59.
11. Dassanayake J, Gurrin L, Payne WR, Sundararajan V, Dharmage SC. Cardiovascular disease risk in immigrants: what is the evidence and where are the gaps? *Asia Pac J Public Health*. 2011;23(6):882–95.
12. Yun K, Fuentes-Afflick E, Desai MM. Prevalence of chronic disease and insurance coverage among refugees in the United States. *J Immigr Minor Health*. 2012;14(6):933–40.
13. Vandenheede H, Deboosere P, Stirbu I et al. Migrant mortality from diabetes mellitus across Europe: the importance of socio-economic change. *Eur J Epidemiol*. 2012;27(2):109–17.
14. Levecque K, Lodewyckx I, Vranken J. Depression and generalised anxiety in the general population in Belgium: a comparison between native and immigrant groups. *J Affect Disord*. 2007;97(1):229–39.
15. Hollander A-C, Dal H, Lewis G, Magnusson C, Kirkbride JB, Dalman C. Refugee migration and risk of schizophrenia and other non-affective psychoses: cohort study of 1.3 million people in Sweden. *BMJ*. 2016;352:i1030.
16. Strong J, Varady C, Chahda N, Doocy S, Burnham G. Health status and health needs of older refugees from Syria in Lebanon. *Conflict Health*. 2015;9:12.
17. Aichberger MC, Schouler-Ocak M, Mundt A et al. Depression in middle-aged and older first generation migrants in Europe: results from the Survey of Health, Ageing and Retirement in Europe (SHARE). *Eur Psychiatry*. 2010;25(8):468–75.
18. Virgincar A, Doherty S, Siriwardhana C. The impact of forced migration on the mental health of the elderly: a scoping review. *Int Psychogeriatr*. 2016;28(6):889–96.
19. Adelman S, Blanchard M, Rait G, Leavey G, Livingston G. Prevalence of dementia in African–Caribbean compared with UK-born White older people: two-stage cross-sectional study. *Br J Psychiatry*. 2011;199(2):119–25.
20. Kumar BN, Spilker RS, Price R, Qureshi S, Diaz E, Ruud MIA. *Dementia, Ethnic Minorities and Migrants. A Review of the Literature*. Oslo: Norwegian Centre for Migration and Minority Health; 2017. Contract No.: NAKMI Report No 2.

21. Pfortmueller CA, Stotz M, Lindner G, Müller T, Rodondi N, Exadaktylos AK. Multimorbidity in adult asylums seekers: a first overview. *PLOS ONE*. 2013;8(12):e82671.
22. Gimeno-Feliu LA, Calderón-Larrañaga A, Díaz E et al. Multimorbidity and immigrant status: associations with area of origin and length of residence in host country. *Fam Pract*. 2017;34(6):662–6.
23. Diaz E, Kumar BN, Gimeno-Feliu L-A, Calderón-Larrañaga A, Poblador-Pou B, Prados-Torres A. Multimorbidity among registered immigrants in Norway: the role of reason for migration and length of stay. *Trop Med Int Health*. 2015;20(12):1805–14.
24. Roberts ER, Green D, Kadam UT. Chronic condition comorbidity and multidrug therapy in general practice populations: a cross-sectional linkage study. *BMJ Open*. 2014;4(7).
25. Mair FS, May CR. Thinking about the burden of treatment. *BMJ*. 2014;349:g6680.
26. Arsenijevic J, Groot W. Lifestyle differences between older migrants and non-migrants in 14 European countries using propensity score matching method. *Int J Public Health*. 2018;63(3):337–47.
27. Sand G, Gruber S. Differences in subjective well-being between older migrants and natives in Europe. *J Immigr Minor Health*. 2018;20(1):83–90.
28. Brothers TD, Theou O, Rockwood K. Frailty and migration in middle-aged and older Europeans. *Arch Gerontol Geriatr*. 2014;58(1):63–8.
29. O'Donnell CA, Burns N, Mair FS et al. Reducing the health care burden for marginalised migrants: The potential role for primary care in Europe. *Health Policy*. 2016;120(5)495–508.
30. Yoo GJ. Constructing deservingness: federal welfare reform, supplemental security income, and elderly immigrants. *J Aging Soc Policy*. 2001;13(4):17–34.
31. Nam Y. Welfare reform and older immigrant adults' Medicaid and health insurance coverage: changes caused by chilling effects of welfare reform, protective citizenship, or distinct effects of labor market condition by citizenship? *J Aging Health*. 2012;24(4):616–40.
32. Solé-Auró A, Guillén M, Crimmins EM. Health care usage among immigrants and native-born elderly populations in eleven European countries: results from SHARE. *Eur J Health Econ*. 2012;13(6):741–54.
33. Diaz E, Gimeno-Feliu L-A, Calderón-Larrañaga A, Prados-Torres A. Frequent attenders in general practice and immigrant status in Norway: a nationwide cross-sectional study. *Scand J Prim Health Care*. 2014;32(4):232–40.
34. Ahaddour C, den Branden S, Broeckaert B. Institutional elderly care services and Moroccan and Turkish migrants in Belgium: a literature review. *J Immigr Minor Health*. 2016;18(5):1216–27.
35. Gracie B, Moon SS, Basham R. Inadequate health literacy among elderly immigrants: characteristics, contributing, and service utilization factors. *J Hum Behav Soc Environ*. 2012;22(7):875–95.
36. Koehn S. Negotiating candidacy: ethnic minority seniors' access to care. *Ageing Soc*. 2009;29:585–608.
37. Manthorpe J, Iliffe S, Moriarty J et al. 'We are not blaming anyone, but if we don't know about amenities, we cannot seek them out': black and minority older people's views on the quality of local health and personal social services in England. *Ageing Soc*. 2009;29:93–113.
38. Scheppers E, van Dongen E, Dekker J, Geertzen J, Dekker J. Potential barriers to the use of health services among ethnic minorities: a review. *Fam Pract*. 2006;23(3):325–48.
39. Gil-González D, Carrasco-Portiño M, Vives-Cases C, Agudelo-Suárez AA, Castejón Bolea R, Ronda-Pérez E. Is health a right for all? An umbrella review of the barriers to health care access faced by migrants. *Ethn Health*. 2015;20(5):523–41.
40. Goodall K, Ward P, Newman L. Use of information and communication technology to provide health information: what do older migrants know, and what do they need to know? *Qual Prim Care*. 2010;18(1):27–32.
41. Nies MA, Febles C, Fanning K, Tavernier SS. A conceptual model for home based primary care of older refugees. *J Immigr Minor Health*. 2018;20(2):485–91.
42. Miner SM, Liebel D, Wilde MH, Carroll JK, Zicari E, Chalupa S. Meeting the needs of older adult refugee populations with home health services. *J Transcult Nurs*. 2017;28(2):128–36.
43. Nguyen DL, DeJesus RS. Home health care may improve diabetic outcomes among non-English speaking patients in primary care practice: a pilot study. *J Immigr Minor Health*. 2011;13(5):967–9.
44. Febles C, Nies MA, Fanning K, Tavernier SS. Challenges and strategies in providing home based primary care for refugees in the US. *J Immigr Minor Health*. 2017;19(6):1498–505.

45. Shommu NS, Ahmed S, Rumana N, Barron GRS, McBrien KA, Turin TC. What is the scope of improving immigrant and ethnic minority healthcare using community navigators: a systematic scoping review. *Int J Equity Health*. 2016;15(1):6.
46. Badger F, Pumphrey R, Clarke L et al. The role of ethnicity in end-of-life care in care homes for older people in the UK: a literature review. *Divers Equal Health Care*. 2009;6:1–7.
47. Calanzani N, Koffman J, Higginson IJ. Palliative and end of life care for Black, Asian and Minority Ethnic groups in the UK: demographic profile and the current state of palliative and end of life care provision. London: King's College, Cicely Saunders Institute; June 2013.
48. Weisman A, Feldman G, Gruman C, Rosenberg R, Chamorro R, Belozersky I. Improving mental health services for Latino and Asian immigrant elders. *Prof Psychol Res Pr*. 2005;36(6):642–8.
49. Truswell D. Black, minority ethnic and refugee (BMER) communities and the National Dementia Strategy: the London experience. *Divers Equal Health Care*. 2011;8:113–9.
50. Giebel CM, Zubair M, Jolley D et al. South Asian older adults with memory impairment: improving assessment and access to dementia care. *Int J Geriatr Psychiatry*. 2015;30(4):345–56.

CHAPTER 11

Family and group as a unit of care

Bridget Kiely and Berit Viken

LEARNING OBJECTIVES

At the end of this chapter, the reader should be able to:

- Develop an awareness of different definitions of family, family structures, and roles within families between cultures
- Understand some of the specific challenges facing families who migrate
- Gain insight into how both of the above impact families' health and well-being and can create challenges both within the clinical consultation and for preventative health and health promotion
- Get an introduction to some techniques and tools for overcoming these challenges

---

INTRODUCTION

The influence of the family on health and the importance of the family unit in society are well recognized (1). Increasingly, it is recognized that a life-course perspective and a greater focus on culturally appropriate health promotion are necessary in promoting migrant health (2). An important challenge for health practitioners is to identify how family members create or select health-related conditions and processes in a given set of constraints and opportunities provided by the home environment and the general social context (3). Family norms in host countries often differ from those in the migrant families' country of origin (4). Indeed, societies in general can differ significantly in their tendency towards an individual or collective focus (5). This can create challenges for health practitioners and families alike. The process and pace of acculturation along with changing roles within the family structure can create tension among migrant families, and is important for health practitioners to have an awareness of this (6).

Settings-based health promotion is consistent with an ecological view on health. Bronfenbrenner (7) proposed an ecological theory of development that has been relevant to the design of ecological models applied in health promotion. In this framework, behaviour is viewed as both being affected by, and affecting, multiple levels of influence, described as the micro-, meso-, exo-, and macrosystem levels. The microsystem refers to face-to-face influences in a specific setting, for example, the home or the clinical practice. The mesosystem is the system of microsystems and pertains to the interrelations among the various settings in which the individual and family are involved. The exosystem refers to forces within the larger social system in which the individual is embedded. Finally, the macrosystem refers to the overarching institutional patterns of the culture or subculture that influence both the microsystem and the mesosystem (7). Green et al. contend that the settings approach sees health as dependent on the interaction between individuals and subsystems of the ecosystem, and the settings approach therefore offers the potential for shaping these elements to maximize health gains. It shifts the goal away from specific behaviour change towards creating the conditions that are supportive of health and well-being (8).

In this chapter we review the challenges faced by migrant families and how this affects their health and their ability to access health care service, in particular preventive and health promotion services. We discuss the challenges that health practitioners may face in caring for such families and offer some practical approaches to overcome these and promote health within the family unit.

CLINICAL VIGNETTE

Mohamed Al Tahir's family from Somalia, consisting of wife Nour (40 years old) and children Bashar (male, 12 years old), Fatima (female, 10 years old), Omar (male, 8 years old), Nawras (male, 5 years old), and Ahmad (male, 3 years old), arrived 1 week ago to a European country to join their husband and father Mohamed. Mohamed is 42 years old and arrived 1 year earlier. He had been renting a single room in the city after finding work as a night porter. The family is initially housed in hotel accommodations in an isolated part of the country due to pressures on the homeless services near where Mohamed had been living. At their first assessment things are slightly chaotic, but everyone is well. The family members are very happy to have arrived in a country where they can safely stay. Mohamed has given up his job in the city to be close to his family and smokes heavily. Nour is a housewife. Both parents are overweight, with BMIs of 29. Only the two eldest children have been to school. The children are given catchup vaccinations and the family is screened for infectious disease as per local guidance.

THE FAMILY AS A CONTEXT FOR HEALTH

'Family is the natural and fundamental group unit of society and is entitled to protection by society and the State' according to Article 16 of the Universal Declaration of Human Rights (9). The United Nations High Commissioner for Refugees (UNHCR) explicitly recognizes the importance of the family and advocates for family reunification in the context of involuntary migration, stating that 'The refugee family is essential to the successful integration of resettled refugees' (1). There is no internationally agreed upon definition of family, but a flexible approach is advocated for by UNHCR, especially to take into account looser definitions of family to include extended family that are more expansive than the Western concept of the nuclear family. Broadly, family can be considered as any group of two or more people connected through marriage or blood lineage who live together and/or are economically or emotionally dependant on each other. The family context can be presented as a dynamic social system encompassing a set of multidirectional influences stemming from the interplay of different home settings and family processes: environmental, social, developmental, and cognitive (3).

Migrant families tend to be from cultures with a more collectivist view and a broader definition of family, and health promotion materials or approaches that are more individualistic are less likely to be successful (10). The need for a life-course approach in order to promote the health of migrant families is becoming more recognized (2) (Chapter 7). Included in the life-course approach are family members of all ages, including elderly migrants. Research from Norway shows that the most important issue when growing old in a new homeland as an ethnic minority migrant is to be surrounded by one's family (11).

The medical sociologist Antonovsky saw stressors as a normal part of life that could be both positive and negative. In his Salutogenic Model of Health, he focusses on the strengths of individuals and their successful adjustment to life stressors (12) (Chapter 5). Antonovsky proposed that the human response to psychosocial stressors is based on the mobilization of generalized resistance resources, and the ability to use these resources is dependent on one's sense of coherence. Sense of coherence is a global orientation that all persons have a pervasive, enduring though dynamic feeling of confidence that the stimuli deriving from one's internal and external environments are structured and predictable (comprehensible), resources are available to meet the demands (manageable), and the demands are meaningful challenges worthy of overcoming (meaningful). Such orientation enables individuals to effectively cope with a wide variety of stressors and promote healthy well-being. According to Antonovsky, the concept of sense of coherence can be applied at an individual as well as a family level. Family sense of coherence refers to the family's global belief that the environment is comprehensible (structured, predictable, and explicable), manageable (resources are available to meet demands), and meaningful (demands are challenges worthy of investment) (13).

Any phenomenon can be characterized by the degree to which it creates these three important experiences: consistency, load balance, and participation in decision making. Antonovsky's understanding was not focussing on stressors alone, nor focussing on resources alone, but focussing on their combined effect to create life experiences that are characterized by consistency, load balance, and participation in decision making. Such experiences are conducive to a high sense of coherence, and therefore move a person towards health (13,14).

STRESSORS FOR THE MIGRANT FAMILY

The previous vignette sets the scene for some of the challenges facing many migrant families after a short 'honeymoon' period after reunification. This family will probably be struggling to cope with the stresses of reunification, social isolation and loss of wider family supports, loss of traditional roles, differing paces of acculturation for the members of the family with consequent mental and physical health effects, and lack of access to appropriate interpretation services. When young men migrate first and reunify with their families, later significant stress can be caused due to differing expectations about socioeconomic status. Often with family reunification the same level of support for integration for refugees and asylum seekers is not available. Studies have shown that reunification is a particular time of stress for families and can indeed lead to family breakups (10,15).

Migrants who come from a more collectively oriented society, like the Al Tahir family, with a wider definition of family, are accustomed to getting the majority of their social support from family and not the state (16). Individualistic societies have loose ties that often only relate an individual to his/her immediate family. They emphasize the 'I' versus the 'we'. Its counterpart, collectivism, describes a society in which tightly integrated relationships tie extended families and others into in-groups (5). When this wider network is disrupted, members of collectivist societies instead turn to the nuclear family for support (6). The family may not be able to offer the support in its reduced state, or children have to provide support to parents. Emotional problems may never make it to the consultation room as there may be a preference for emotional problems to be discussed and managed within the family, with very few expectations of the state to provide support (17,18). As a consequence, psychological problems that are the cause of, or are contributing to, symptoms may not be apparent in consultations unless specifically asked about, leading to unsuccessful attempts to treat individuals and clinical problems when a more holistic family focus is needed.

Changing roles within families are another source of stress. Men who lose their role as breadwinner and patriarch suffer from loss of identity in the new environment, leading to self-esteem and mental health issues (4,6). As we see in our clinical vignette, the family was homeless on arrival and the father, who had previously settled, had to leave his job, reducing his capacity to support the family and his sense of self-worth as a provider. Parental stress can impact children already coping with their individual stress of migrating and reduce their supports. Enuresis, poor sleep, behavioural issues, low self-esteem, and avoiding interaction with other children have been reported in children undergoing acculturation (19). While many children have had traumatic experiences in their countries of origin, the stress they experience on arrival in the host country has been found to be the greatest predictor of psychological problems in the future (20).

The process of acculturation is discussed in depth in Chapter 2, but briefly, it is a complex social and psychological process which implies cultural learning and behavioural adaptation to a non-native country (21). Different family members adapt at different rates. For older members, cultural heritage can become the only form of identity left. They can be resistant to adapting and actively prevent younger members from participating in activities that are perceived to not be aligned with their cultural identity (22). Younger family members adapt more quickly through more exposure such as school, sports, and entertainment. In certain cases, eager to overcome discrimination, living in socially disadvantaged areas and coping with previous and ongoing trauma due to family stresses, young adults from migrant backgrounds are at risk of delinquency (4). This can cause stress within the family and parents can feel that their children are abandoning their cultural heritage. This feeling of abandonment can lead to depression (15) as well as to conflict within families, as seen in the clinical vignette that follows. Families who have migrated have had a significant erosion of their resources, both material and emotional, and parents are left less able to provide a protective shield for their children. Often they have lost standing within the community and within the family due to changing roles and loss of breadwinner status, undermining their perceived parental control. Parents are often not familiar with the new culture that their children have to navigate, such as social media, and find it difficult to support their children. Authoritarian parenting styles allow for very little discussion between parents and their children, and this can hinder family discussions around adapting to a new culture (22).

THE ROLE OF THE FAMILY IN MENTAL HEALTH

Families have often a role to play in contributing to stress and mental health problems, and the lack of normal family supports can exacerbate stressful situations, as seen in the following vignette. Two of the most significant impacts on mental health are the loss of the extended family social network and worry about family members left behind (15). Family members left behind are often grandparents who provide crucial support to parents. Parents in turn worry about the health of the grandparents, who often do not have access to services. In some cases, families may have no way of knowing about the well-being of other family members and this can lead to prolonged grief reactions. As we will soon see in the vignette, shortly after arrival Nour is worried and is constantly thinking about her mother. The reason may be that she does not know anything about her mother's condition, but it could also be that she has received bad news from home. Many migrants maintain close links with their family members in their country of origin through the Internet. The identity and social practices of migrants transcend national borders, and migrants retain lasting ties with their country of origin (23).

CHALLENGES IN CLINICAL PRACTICE

A FIRST FOLLOW-UP

After 2 months, the staff at the homeless accommodation centre ask you to see Nour again. They have witnessed her shouting at the children and crying. You see her with an interpreter as she still has only a few words of English. She is feeling depressed, has poor sleep, and cannot stop thinking about her mother, who has stayed behind in Somalia. Her husband has been very irritable lately and the children are hard to manage without the support of her extended family. She denies any domestic violence or having hit the children. Mohamed has actually come to the consultation and is pacing outside the room; at Nour's request you invite him in. He is also finding the situation difficult, especially as he has had to quit smoking due to the increased cost of cigarettes. He complains that there is no help for Nour with the children and she has not been able to attend English classes run by a local charity.

The most frequently cited challenges of working with migrants in general are related to language and communication, managing multiple family members attending interviews and promoting health in a group perceived to have other priorities (24). There is also the often-unidentified challenge of cultural differences. While clinicians might quickly identify the migrant families' culture as different, they might find it more difficult to understand that their own culture is unique and strange compared to others (25).

Language and communication

Language is one of the most significant barriers in migrant families accessing health care services, including health promotion (Chapter 20). If the professional practitioner and the family members do not understand each other, it is the practitioner's obligation to advocate for the rights of the family members to understand information that is being given. For various reasons, including funding, availability, and administrative, professional interpreting services are frequently not available at the time of consultation. Family members with better host language skills often attend to translate for their relatives. Indeed, family members often attend even if they are not translating, in particular, husbands and mothers-in-law, as this would have been culturally acceptable in their country of origin. Women in particular report difficulties with this type of model, inventing illnesses to discuss rather than discussing certain issues in front of family members or not actually wanting the specific family member to be present at all in the case of antenatal care and mothers-in-law (26). There is also the concern about information not being fully translated, or indeed censored, with one review of interpreting services in an obstetrics unit noting that husbands intervened even with the presence of professional interpreters (27).

Using children as interpreters also further inverts the parental role and can assign inappropriate responsibilities to children and cause them stress. Interpreting in a consultation expects them to have a significant vocabulary in a second language and often puts a burden on them outside the consultation room, with responsibilities for reminding parents or grandparents about medication or helping them to navigate transport systems and hospital appointments. Practitioners often find it difficult to ask questions of a personal nature or to discuss issues such as contraception or mental health while using children as interpreters (24,27).

To avoid these and other possible problems, it is imperative for the family's access to and effective use of the health care services that interpreting services are available until the family members reach adequate language proficiency, despite the time it takes. While interpreting services can be costly and time consuming, having a professional interpreter is widely recognized as best practice (24). If personal interpreters are not available, telephone interpretation services, while not ideal, remove the need for inappropriate translation by a child. Indeed, in Norway it is now forbidden to use children as interpreters outside emergency situations. It is important for clinicians to be familiar with the local arrangements for funding and accessing interpreters, and to advocate for them if they are not available. It may also be necessary to advocate with family members to allow professional interpreter services to be used, explaining the importance of independence, proficiency with medical terminology, and privacy for the patient. Families may have concerns about confidentiality or that the interpreter may be from a rival tribe or group, and it is important to understand and address these concerns. If a family has not requested an interpreter in advance and it has not been possible to obtain one on short notice, even over the phone, it is important to discuss with them for future visits and to note on the patient record to book an interpreter in advance. Having a professional interpreter also facilitates a private consultation, giving the patient the opportunity to discuss personal issues. Continuity of interpreters can help to build trust with both the clinician and the patient (18). Dedicated clinic times for migrant families can make it easier to engage interpreters, although this should not restrict access at other times if more urgent reviews are required.

Managing multiple family members

Clinicians often struggle with multiple family members being present in a consultation. While there may be different attitudes to privacy within families across cultures, there is a distinct clash here with the importance of autonomy and confidentiality. Often clinicians can find themselves discussing an individual's health in front of and often with a brother, husband, or cousin. Due to the hierarchical nature of some family structures, this would not seem abnormal; indeed, it would be necessary for there to be this interpretation of what is best for their family member and to implement any management plan as they deemed fit. However, there is a balance to be struck between respecting an individual's privacy and involving the family in a holistic solution. As mentioned earlier, individuals may invent illnesses to avoid discussing private issues in front of their family (26). Clinicians need to be alert to the risk of casually denying the right to access health by failing to ask a family member to wait outside, at least for the initial part of the consultation. However, family members can be a useful source of collateral information and in supporting their loved one with a management plan, as we saw in our clinical vignette when Mohamed was able to add further context to the family's situation, and their input should be sought at an appropriate time (28).

Promoting health in a group perceived to have other priorities

From a health promotion perspective, participation and user involvement are important to enable people to improve their health. If the family was viewed as a functional unit, Mohamed could have been included in the consultation from the start. The health practitioner could, for example, focus on the sense of coherence of the wife and husband. How do they understand the situation, how do they manage, and what is meaningful for them? In the consultation, the practitioner should be open-minded and could use questions, for example, from solution-focussed therapy (29), such as looking for previous solutions, inviting the client to do more of what is working, scaling questions, or coping questions – for example: 'How have you managed to carry on?'

A settings approach in health promotion

The settings approach has been attributed to the Ottawa Charter's (30) assertion that: 'Health is created and lived by people within the settings of their everyday life; where they learn, work, play and love'. The settings approach involves a shift from individual behavioural approaches towards considering the contributions of major settings to health. Not only do settings impact directly on health and well-being, but individual choices about health and health behaviour are taken in the settings encountered in day-to-day life – the home, community, workplace, and school (WHO, 1999 in [8]). Since the settings approach sees health as dependent on the interaction between individuals and the subsystems of the ecosystem, it offers the potential for shaping these elements to maximize health gains and creating the conditions that are supportive of health and well-being (8).

VIGNETTE, FOLLOW-UP

With the family's agreement, you speak with the accommodation centre management and arrange a meeting with the language teachers, the schoolteachers, the local crèche, and mental health services. Resources are found for some childcare for the younger children so Nour can go to English classes. The schoolteachers volunteer to set up some afterschool sports for the children, and the centre management sets up a games room. The local mental health team is starting some group sessions on stress management. You encourage Nour to attend the group sessions, and prescribe some nicotine replacement therapy for Mohamed.

The health practitioner here is taking into consideration the context of the family and their general resistance resources. By mediating between different microsystem services such as the accommodation centre, the school, the crèche, and mental health services she will strengthen the mesosystem of the family. Utilizing the resources in their environment in this way can help to empower the family.

Community participatory approach

A practical method for working with health promotion in the community is the Participatory Learning and Action as described by Pretty et al. (31) (Chapter 24). In these participatory methods, they make use of, for example, play and nonverbal techniques to get people involved and active in shaping their own circumstances. Prost et al. (32) did a systematic review of women's groups practicing participatory learning and action and concluded that they are a cost-effective strategy to improve maternal and neonatal survival in low-resource settings (32). Encouraging Nour to take part in a women's group with a varied set of methods could therefore be a good health promotion strategy.

THE SECOND FOLLOW-UP

A couple of months later you see Nour again for another follow-up. Things had initially improved, but the family has subsequently moved to social housing and so Nour is no longer attending the group. She is accompanied by her daughter, Fatima, who interprets for her, as interpreting resources are no longer provided. She complains of generalized pain and fatigue. You note she has gained weight. At your enquiry, Nour tells you her husband is less irritable and now only smokes the occasional cigarette, but he is very bored. She is very worried about her eldest son who is out with his friends from football a lot and often misses prayer. Mohamed and the son frequently fight about this. Nour feels very isolated and has no one to talk to.

Taking a holistic view of the family, you make some enquiries about services available locally to support recently arrived refugee families and make contact with the resettlement worker, the local school, and local volunteer group. This follows the health promotion strategy of mediating between different professionals and groups in society.

PRIORITY SETTING FOR MIGRANT FAMILIES

Clinicians often perceive that migrant families prioritize socioeconomic needs above health (24), and may well be correct. In turn, unemployment leads to low mood, inactivity, inadequate funds to access healthy food options, and increased rates of smoking and alcohol use (33), and thus over time reverses the healthy migrant effect (15). We saw this with Mohamed in the clinical vignette. Migrant families are often very present-oriented due to the precariousness of their situations and the pressure to ensure basic needs of food and shelter are met (34). Health promotion in this context can be very difficult, as a potential future benefit for a current cost or effort is not sufficient to warrant the investment. Clinicians may have to concede that there is a logic to prioritizing socioeconomic concerns over health to a degree, as socioeconomic status is such a strong upstream determinant of health, but as these are often beyond the individuals' or families' control they manifest in the consulting room either as depression, psychosomatic symptoms, or the impact of chronic stress and restricted lifestyle options on cardiovascular disease. Attitudes to food and body shape vary across cultures. 'You've got fat!' is a surprising compliment in West Africa, where larger body size is seen as a sign of health and prosperity and thinness as a sign of poverty and ill health. Families may struggle to access foods that they are familiar with and be limited in what they can afford, especially in relation to fresh fruits and vegetables (22,35,36). This does not mean that it is impossible to promote health, but an understanding of where people are at in their journey as well as their cultural norms will help to inform the best approach.

CLINICAL VIGNETTE, FOLLOW-UP

At your next review with Nour, you enquire how she would feel about reattending group support and also having a family consultation. With her agreement and with support from an in-person interpreter, you meet with the family and spend an hour reviewing their challenges, exploring attitudes towards cooking, meal times, exercise, and discussing family communication. Equipped with a better understanding of how the family functions, you can begin setting goals with the family around exercise, healthy eating, and improved communication to help reduce family stress. You also have the opportunity to build rapport and suggest to the family that they could share their goals with their resettlement worker who can link them with local sports clubs and activities.

SUMMING UP

Understanding the social and cultural contexts of the migrant family is paramount to understanding their needs and capacity to implement change or manage a particular treatment plan. Clinicians can often feel inhibited from making these enquiries due to time constraints, language barriers, and a feeling that it is not their role. Indeed, in research into migrants' perceptions about being asked about social issues, some migrant families did not feel it is the clinician's role, but were not upset, and many were glad that they were asked about their journey and social circumstances (37). Many best-practice guidelines for migrant health recommend an assessment by a multidisciplinary team in order to fully put the family in context in terms of their structure, socioeconomic status previously and now, their cultural heritage, problem-solving skills, and capacity for change (38). Such an assessment is valuable to clinicians, although in reality they are often a luxury rather than the norm. Simple awareness of the different cultural norms, in particular around family, will help a clinician tailor approaches and information in a more understandable way and allow a shift from the very individual-focussed approach typical in Western health care models.

It is hoped that reading this chapter will have gone some way towards creating an awareness of different family structures and roles, and give clinicians more confidence in navigating the balance between individual privacy and an inclusive approach that recognizes the importance of family for many migrants.

The degree to which any of the suggested approaches can be adopted will depend on local resources, but having an awareness of the importance of family and the specific needs of the migrant family allows clinicians to adopt, or advocate for, an approach that has a life-course perspective and follows the principles of equity, disease prevention, and health promotion.

CONCLUDING THOUGHTS

This chapter has reviewed some of the challenges facing migrant families, the stress of migration, changing roles, the differing pace of acculturation within the family in a new culture, different attitudes towards family and the role of family, and language barriers to accessing health and how they manifest in the family unit. The clinician dealing with migrant families needs to be aware of these cultural differences and stressors the family is facing in order to put their health in context, avoid common pitfalls in providing health care for migrant families, and provide health care that not only addresses immediate health needs but takes a preventive perspective and promotes health.

While there are many challenges facing families and clinicians caring for them, they are not insurmountable. It is worth bearing in mind the recommendations of the Commission on Social Determinants of Health of the World Health Organization, 'investment in the early years provides one of the greatest potentials to reduce health inequities within a generation…that mothers and children need a continuum of care from pre-pregnancy, through pregnancy and childbirth, to the early days and years of life'. The Commission accordingly calls for health care systems to be based on principles of equity, disease prevention, and health promotion' (33).

The impact of migration on families is significant, and the road to acculturation is one fraught with the risks of losing the healthy migrant effect due to stress, poor socioeconomic circumstances, and lack of culturally and linguistically appropriate support for families to access services, including health promotion services. Supporting migrant families takes time, a different approach, and working with other agencies, but it is ultimately very rewarding.

REFERENCES

1. UNHCR. Annual Tripartite Consultations on Resettlement [Internet]. 2008 [cited 2017 Oct 15]. Available from: http://www.unhcr.org/3b30baa04.pdf
2. Familife. Familife project | NEWS [Internet]. 2016 [cited 2017 Oct 22]. Available from: https://www.familifeproject.com/news
3. Soubhi H, Potvin L. Homes and families as health promotion settings. In: *Settings for Health Promotion: Linking Theory and Practice* [Internet]. Thousand Oaks, CA: SAGE Publications; [cited 2018 Jul 6]: 44–85. Available from: http://sk.sagepub.com/books/settings-for-health-promotion/n2.xml
4. Betancourt TS, Abdi S, Ito BS, Lilienthal GM, Agalab N, Ellis H. We left one war and came to another: resource loss, acculturative stress, and caregiver-child relationships in Somali refugee families. *Cultur Divers Ethnic Minor Psychol* [Internet]. NIH Public Access; 2015 Jan [cited 2017 Nov 10];21(1):114–25. Available from: http://www.ncbi.nlm.nih.gov/pubmed/25090142
5. Hofstede G. *Culture's Consequences: Comparing Values, Behaviors, Institutions and Organizations Across Nations* [Internet]. 2002 [cited 2017 Oct 22]. Available from: https://books.google.ie/books?hl=en&lr=&id=9HE-DQAAQBAJ&oi=fnd&pg=PP1&ots=lKteuRv1NM&sig=Tmip0sTl6d4beUSF1eNAdnL8q0g&redir_esc=y#v=onepage&q&f=false
6. Samarasinghe K, Arvidsson B. 'It is a different war to fight here in Sweden' – the impact of involuntary migration on the health of refugee families in transition. *Scand J Caring Sci* [Internet]. Blackwell Science; 2002 September 1 [cited 2017 Oct 15];16(3):292–301. Available from: http://doi.wiley.com/10.1046/j.1471-6712.2002.00089.x
7. Bronfenbrenner U. Toward an experimental ecology of human development. *Am Psychol* [Internet]. 1977 [cited 2018 Jul 6];32(7):513–31. Available from: http://content.apa.org/journals/amp/32/7/513
8. Green J, Tones K, Cross R, Woodall J. *Health Promotion, Planning and Strategies.* Thousand Oaks, CA: SAGE Publications; 2015.
9. United Nations. The Universal Declaration of Human Rights. 1948 [cited 2015 Jun 14]; Available from: http://www.un.org/en/documents/udhr/index.shtml#a25
10. Samarasinghe K, Fridlund B, Arvidsson B. Primary health care nurses' promotion of involuntary migrant families' health. *Int Nurs Rev* [Internet]. 2010 June [cited 2017 Oct 22];57(2):224–31. Available from: http://www.ncbi.nlm.nih.gov/pubmed/20579158
11. Thyli B, Hedelin B, Athlin E. Experiences of health and care when growing old in Norway – From the perspective of elderly immigrants with minority ethnic backgrounds. *Clin Nurs Stud* [Internet]. 2014 May 26 [cited 2018 Jul 6];2(3):52. Available from: http://www.sciedupress.com/journal/index.php/cns/article/view/3724
12. Antonovsky A. *Health, Stress and Coping.* 1979 San Francisco: Josey-Bass.
13. Antonovsky A, Sourani T. Family sense of coherence and family adaptation. *J Marriage Fam.* 1988;(50):79–92.

14. Vinje HF, Langeland E, Bull T. Aaron Antonovsky's Development of Salutogenesis, 1979 to 1994. In: Mittelmark MB, Sagy S, Eriksson M et al., editors. *The Handbook of Salutogenesis* [Internet]. Springer; 2017 [cited 2018 Jul 6]. Available from: https://link.springer.com/content/pdf/10.1007%2F978-3-319-04600-6.pdf

15. Carballo M, Divino JJ, Zeric D. Migration and health in the European Union. *Trop Med Int Heal* [Internet]. Blackwell Publishing; 1998 December 1 [cited 2017 Oct 22];3(12):936–44. Available from: http://doi.wiley.com/10.1046/j.1365-3156.1998.00337.x

16. Bordone V, de Valk HAG. Intergenerational support among migrant families in Europe. *Eur J Ageing* [Internet]. Springer Netherlands; 2016 September 4 [cited 2017 Oct 22];13(3):259–70. Available from: http://link.springer.com/10.1007/s10433-016-0363-6

17. Gonçalves M, Moleiro C. The family-school-primary care triangle and the access to mental health care among migrant and ethnic minorities. *J Immigr Minor Heal* [Internet]. Springer US; 2012 August 27 [cited 2017 Oct 21];14(4):682–90. Available from: http://link.springer.com/10.1007/s10903-011-9527-9

18. Riggs E, Davis E, Gibbs L et al. Accessing maternal and child health services in Melbourne, Australia: reflections from refugee families and service providers. *BMC Health Serv Res* [Internet]. BioMed Central; 2012 May 15 [cited 2017 Nov 10];12:117. Available from: http://www.ncbi.nlm.nih.gov/pubmed/22587587

19. Samarasinghe KL. A conceptual model facilitating the transition of involuntary migrant families. *ISRN Nurs* [Internet]. 2011 [cited 2017 Nov 10];2011:824209. Available from: http://www.hindawi.com/journals/isrn/2011/824209/

20. Measham T, Guzder J, Rousseau C, Pacione L, Blais-Mcpherson M, Nadeau L. Refugee children and their families: supporting psychological well-being and positive adaptation following migration. *Curr Probl Pediatr Adolesc Health Care* [Internet]. Mosby; 2014 August 1 [cited 2017 Nov 11];44(7):208–15. Available from: http://www.sciencedirect.com/science/article/pii/S1538544214000303?_rdoc=1&_fmt=high&_origin=gateway&_docanchor=&md5=b8429449ccfc9c30159a5f9aeaa92ffb

21. Berry JW. Stress perspective on acculturisation. In: *The Cambridge Handbook of Acculturation Psychology*. Cambridge: Cambridge University Press; 2006: 43–57.

22. Halliday JA, Green J, Mellor D, Mutowo MP, de Courten M, Renzaho AMN. Developing programs for African families, by African families. *Fam Community Health* [Internet]. 2014 [cited 2017 Oct 22]; 37(1):60–73. Available from: http://content.wkhealth.com/linkback/openurl?sid=WKPTLP:landingpage&an=00003727-201401000-00008

23. Levitt P. *The Transnational Villagers*. Berkeley: University of California Press; 2001.

24. Priebe S, Sandhu S, Dias S et al. Good practice in health care for migrants: views and experiences of care professionals in 16 European countries. *BMC Public Health* [Internet]. BioMed Central; 2011 December 25 [cited 2017 Oct 15];11(1):187. Available from: http://bmcpublichealth.biomedcentral.com/articles/10.1186/1471-2458-11-187

25. Abma TA, Heijsman A. Crossing cultures: health promotion for senior migrants in the Netherlands. *Health Promot Int* [Internet]. 2015 September [cited 2017 Oct 22];30(3):460–72. Available from: http://www.ncbi.nlm.nih.gov/pubmed/24001443

26. Barron DS, Holterman C, Shipster P, Batson S, Alam M. Seen but not heard – ethnic minorities' views of primary health care interpreting provision: a focus group study. *Prim Health Care Res Dev* [Internet]. Cambridge University Press; 2010 April 28 [cited 2017 Oct 21];11(02):132. Available from: http://www.journals.cambridge.org/abstract_S1463423609990399

27. Yelland J, Riggs E, Szwarc J et al. Compromised communication: a qualitative study exploring Afghan families and health professionals' experience of interpreting support in Australian maternity care. *BMJ Qual Saf* [Internet]. 2016 April [cited 2017 Oct 22];25(4):e1–1. Available from: http://www.ncbi.nlm.nih.gov/pubmed/26089208

28. Kirmayer LJ, Narasiah L, Munoz M et al. Common mental health problems in immigrants and refugees: general approach in primary care. *CMAJ* [Internet]. Canadian Medical Association; 2011 September 6 [cited 2017 Nov 10];183(12):E959–67. Available from: http://www.ncbi.nlm.nih.gov/pubmed/20603342

29. Institute for Solution Focused Therapy. What is solution-focused therapy?–Institute for Solution-Focused Therapy [Internet]. [cited 2018 Jul 6]. Available from: https://solutionfocused.net/what-is-solution-focused-therapy/

30. WHO 1986. The Ottawa Charter for Health Promotion. http://www.who.int/healthpromotion/ conferences/previous/ottawa/en/

31. Pretty JN, Guijt I, Thompson J, Scoones I. A trainer's guide for participatory learning and action [Internet]. Sustainable Agriculture Programme, International Institute for Environment and Development; 1995 [cited 2018 Jul 6]. 267 p. Available from: https://books.google.ie/books?hl=en&lr=&id=uu-BPsudVog C&oi=fnd&pg=PP14&dq=participatory+learning+and+action+pretty+et+al&ots=j1RUZqx9Mi&si g=rW-3yZO3l-FC2ouh_enKL-TD_L4&redir_esc=y#v=onepage&q=participatory learning and action pretty et al&f=false

32. Prost A, Colbourn T, Seward N et al. Women's groups practising participatory learning and action to improve maternal and newborn health in low-resource settings: a systematic review and meta-analysis. *Lancet* [Internet]. 2013 May 18 [cited 2018 Jul 6];381(9879):1736–46. Available from: http:// www.ncbi.nlm.nih.gov/pubmed/23683640

33. CSDH. Closing the gap in a generation: health equity through action on the social determinants of health. [Internet]. Geneva; 2008 [cited 2017 Nov 10];246. Available from: http://apps.who.int/iris/ bitstream/10665/43943/1/9789241563703_eng.pdf

34. Bechtel G, Davidhizar R, Spurlock WR. Migrant farm workers and their families: cultural patterns and delivery of care in the United States. *Int J Nurs Pract* [Internet]. Blackwell Science Pty; 2000 December 1 [cited 2017 Oct 15];6(6):300–6. Available from: http://doi.wiley.com/10.1046/j.1440-172x.2000.00221.x

35. Gibbs L, Waters E, Christian B et al. Teeth tales: a community-based child oral health promotion trial with migrant families in Australia. *BMJ Open* [Internet]. BMJ Publishing Group; 2015 June 11 [cited 2017 Oct 21];5(6):e007321. Available from: http://www.ncbi.nlm.nih.gov/pubmed/26068509

36. Connor A, Rainer LP, Simcox JB, Thomisee K. Increasing the delivery of health care services to migrant farm worker families through a community partnership model. *Public Health Nurs* [Internet]. Blackwell Publishing; 2007 July 1 [cited 2017 Nov 10];24(4):355–60. Available from: http://doi.wiley. com/10.1111/j.1525-1446.2007.00644.x

37. Yelland J, Riggs E, Wahidi S et al. How do Australian maternity and early childhood health services identify and respond to the settlement experience and social context of refugee background families? *BMC Pregnancy Childbirth* [Internet]. 2014 December 6 [cited 2017 Nov 10];14(1):348. Available from: http://www.ncbi.nlm.nih.gov/pubmed/25284336

38. Faculty of Public Health. Migrant Health-The Health of Asylum Seekers, Refugees and Relocated Individuals. Royal College of Physicians of Ireland; 2016.

III

Health challenges
at the clinic

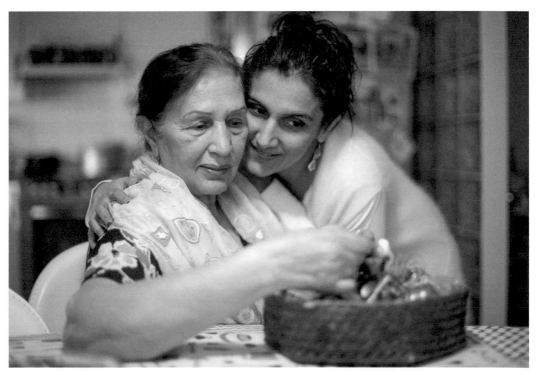

Photo credit: Iffit Querishi/NAKMI.

CHAPTER 12

Health challenges at the clinic

Maria van den Muijsenbergh

LEARNING OBJECTIVES

This section addresses some of the health challenges at the clinic when meeting patients with migrant backgrounds. Specifically, this chapter will make the reader aware of:

- The complexity of several dimensions that might be present in consultations with migrants
- The need for person-centred, culturally sensitive, integrated care

---

SEVERAL LAYERS OF COMPLEXITY

General practitioners often encounter challenges at the clinic when taking care of migrants. These challenges include very different dimensions, such as:

a. Communication: Dealing with language differences, limited health literacy, and low literacy, and sometimes with cultural differences in presentation of symptoms, illness beliefs, and health care expectations
b. Differences in prevalence and treatment due to genetic differences and country of origin
c. Complex and often difficult-to-resolve psychosocial problems related to migration, especially in refugees, further complicated by perceived discrimination and social exclusion

The case of Mariam presents a typical example of a combination of these challenges.

CLINICAL VIGNETTE

Mariam is your last patient today. She is 22 years old and originally from Sierra Leone. Your practice assistant Anne arranged for her your last time slot, as she already assumed you would need a lot more time than the usual 10 minutes. Mariam had not made an appointment by telephone but came this morning to your practice and pleaded with your practice assistant for an urgent appointment. At least, that is what Anne understood. Mariam spoke very little English but pointed to her belly, said 'Baby' and 'Problem' and 'Doctor, now please'.

As instructed by you, Anne took her aside to a separate room to try to get some more information. Mariam showed an old health insurance card, from which the assistant took her name and date of birth (01-01-1996) and her place of birth (Kabala — the assistant Googled it, and found it is a city in the northern part of Sierra Leone). It became also clear that Krio is Mariam's mother tongue. Asked about her address, it turned out to be the shelter for undocumented homeless women familiar to you.

Anne checked the blood pressure (150/90), pulse (104/minute), and urine (protein +, no sign of infection) and asked the GP trainee to have a quick look at the belly of Mariam to exclude urgent pathology. The trainee examined her and concluded, judging by the size of her belly, Mariam had to be some 4 months pregnant, and there were no signs of appendicitis, HELPP syndrome, or any other acute morbidity. Anne then scheduled the appointment with you for this afternoon. She put it in Mariam's telephone and wrote it down in English.

A bit to your surprise, Mariam was already in the waiting room (later you found out that she had spent the whole day in the neighbourhood of your practice, afraid of not being able to find it again in time). You arranged for a telephone interpreter in Krio and started your conversation with Mariam. As you are used to doing with new patients, you wanted to get some biographical background. However, Mariam did not look at you, gave very short and often vague answers to questions about her life and especially about her country of origin, length of stay in, and journey to the Netherlands. You are just told that she was rejected in her asylum application and she now lives in the shelter home. You felt there was a reason for this reluctance and changed to more factual questions about her reason for the encounter. Now Mariam looked more interested and told you she is pregnant with her first baby and she wants to keep it. She says she does not know who the father is and if you try to ask a bit more about how and when she got pregnant, she does not reply. She tells you she had heard that if it is a girl there is a chance she may stay in the country (because of the risk of female genital mutilation [FGM] in Sierra Leone). So, she wants to know if it is a girl. And she wants to know if everything is all right with the pregnancy. She had a pain in her belly last week. She stopped eating carrots, as she understood that would harm the baby, and started to drink a potion that she got from a compatriot that should help to get a healthy girl.

After half an hour you wrap up the consultation, although you still have many questions. You reassure Mariam that she will get all the help she needs, and you make a new appointment for 2 days hence — as by then you will have found out to whom to refer her, etc. Mariam leaves the consultation room with some sort of a smile and a much brighter face than when she entered.

You now try to list all the different issues you heard and want to address now or later:

1. Immediate attention will need to be given to the somatic aspects related to her pregnancy: Did Mariam herself undergo FGM? Has she been infected with HIV or hepatitis? What does she know about pregnancy — did she take folic acid? What is the potion she taking, and could that cause harm? Does she have anaemia — maybe a hemoglobinopathy? Does she have any parasitic infection? A blood pressure of 150/90 is high for a pregnant young girl; does she suffer from hypertension, and if so, what does this mean in migrants with an African background? Is there real proteinuria or was it just contamination? Why does she have a pain in her belly?
2. You worry about her migration history and her vague account of the father: did she suffer from sexual violence, or has she perhaps been forced into prostitution? Does she suffer from PTSD or depression, as she seemed so 'dull'? Is she all on her own to raise the child? Should you inform the child protection board?
3. You also worry about her access to health care: What midwife or gynaecologist would be willing to help her, given her undocumented (and thus uninsured) status; will she be able to get maternity assistance after birth; would she have money to buy all necessary things, and to pay for public transport to visit the hospital or midwifery practice? Will she be able to make an appointment? Should you make the appointments for her?
4. In general, you worry about her financial means and a place to stay for her, now and after the birth of her child. Would there be any social security or other help to obtain for her? What are the rules concerning pregnant migrants, and is there a possibility to get them into an asylum-seeking centre?

You give a deep sigh; so many different issues, so many things you do not know — but at least you have the feeling you can do something for her.

COMMUNICATION

The challenges in communication related to language barriers, health literacy, and cultural differences have been described in detail in Section I. Cultural differences and taboo typically play a role in consultations related to mental health problems (Chapter 17) and reproductive health (Chapter 13), two of the themes that are further considered in this section. The presentation of disease, particularly the expression of pain, is another challenge often pointed out in communication with some migrant groups (1), that is dealt with in Chapter 15. However, also for consultations dealing with other clinical problems, the juxtaposition of all the layers of complexity described previously often means that the GP has to put more time and effort into understanding the patient and their problem, to provide understandable information, negotiate the way forward, and check what the patient is able to further deal with regarding the commonly agreed solution of the health problem.

DIFFERENCES IN PREVALENCE OF DISEASE

Although migrants and the majority population present the same diseases and risk factors, prevalence varies among groups. Mental health problems, cardiovascular disease, overweight, diabetes mellitus, some infectious diseases (hepatitis B/C, HIV, tuberculosis, parasitic infections), and reproductive health problems are generally more prevalent among refugees and other groups of migrants, especially among those originating from South Asia, Africa, and the Caribbean, than among the host populations (2–4). Some diseases with a genetic origin like hemoglobinopathies and hypovitaminosis D occur more often in migrant populations in high-income countries than in the host population, or ask for a different approach, like hypertension in people of West African descent. Besides, migrants from some countries suffer from culturally determined health problems like FGM. On the other hand, some diseases like cancer are generally less prevalent among migrants, although with differences among groups (Chapter 16). This section covers some of these clinical areas of knowledge without attempting to give detailed information for each disease or risk factor for each migrant group. It is not possible for the GP to have detailed knowledge on prevalence for all diseases for each migrant group at a given point in time, but some general knowledge and attention to these issues can be useful to keep in mind when meeting migrant patients. For detailed information, the interested reader is invited to go to the references included in the chapters.

COMPLEX PSYCHOSOCIAL CONTEXT

In addition to the challenges directly related to the migration history of the person, the lack of social support and finances further limit the self-management skills of some groups of migrants (5). Also, many migrants have to deal with adverse psychosocial circumstances (poverty, discrimination, poor housing, grief about their loss of family or friends and social position, etc.) that can negatively affect their health due to chronic stress and can hinder effective management of their diseases (6,7). Furthermore, prevention of chronic diseases might need a special approach for some migrant groups, as described in Chapter 14. In consequence, the care of migrants in the clinic often requires a more active engagement of the doctor or practice nurse if we are to give equitable health care to these patients.

THE NEED FOR PERSON-CENTRED, CULTURALLY SENSITIVE INTEGRATED CARE

The specific socioeconomic and cultural context of migrants like Mariam, in combination with different morbidity patterns and challenges in communication, ask even more than in other patients for a person-centred approach tailored to their medical as well as psychosocial needs, in a culturally sensitive way in person-centred care (8), as discussed in Chapter 3. To be able to deliver such care, health care professionals need cultural competencies (Chapter 20). In addition to a shift from disease/problem-oriented care to care aiming at the goals the patient himself has set (9), special care must be paid to the social and spiritual dimensions and the integration of health and social well-being. In this, it can be important to target not only the individual and his family, but also the community, as discussed in Chapter 24. Some interventions to improve healthy lifestyle, for instance, are most effective if supported by health policies targeting the whole community or neighbourhood. This kind of person-centred care, integrated in a broad population-oriented approach within a strong primary care system, has proven to contribute to the diminishing of health disparities of vulnerable social groups like migrants (10).

For health professionals in daily practice this means that he/she:*

1. Has knowledge of and acknowledges social and cultural differences between patients.

---

* Adapted from: J. De Maeseneer et al., *Primary healthcare as a strategy for achieving equitable care.* A literature review commissioned by the Health Systems Knowledge Network. 2007.

2. Asks for life and health priorities of persons attended and respects these whenever possible (e.g. when confronted with conflicting treatments in cases of multimorbidity person-centeredness), and involves patients in decision making.

3. Is available and accessible for all people, in physical, financial, and cultural respects. This means, among other things, that the practice organization and the communication in consultations are adapted to the language and literacy level of the patient.

4. Strives for personal continuity of care. Seeing as much as possible the same doctor or nurse increases satisfaction, trust, and confidence and improves communication with a patient (11).

5. Knows of the specific social determinants of health (education, income, migration background, living circumstances) and the influence on health in his patients (community orientation).

6. Collaborates with other disciplines in the field of social well-being and public health, in prevention and care (integrated care).

CONCLUSION

Together, these challenges can be very demanding, as GPs need more time than they usually have available, require the organization and use of (expensive) interpreter services, and need to improve their cultural competence and specific knowledge about groups they might not see often. Furthermore, as with other vulnerable patients, the GP can sometimes feel overwhelmed by the amount of problems they cannot solve. On the other hand, as GP you can mean so much to these patients if you treat them in the typical person-centred way that is characteristic for good GP care. Last but not least, the main ingredient of good health care for migrants is something all health professionals should be able to provide — a smiling face, a welcoming gesture, and sufficient time, compassion, and respect.

REFERENCES

1. Hjörleifsson S, Hammer E, Díaz E. General practitioners' strategies in consultations with immigrants in Norway — practice-based shared reflections among participants in focus groups. *Fam Pract* 2018;35:216–21.

2. Hadgkiss EJ, Renzaho AM. The physical health status, service utilisation and barriers to accessing care for asylum seekers residing in the community: a systematic review of the literature. *Aust Health Rev.* 2014;38:142–59.

3. Agyemang C, Addo J, Bhopal R et al. Cardiovascular diseases, diabetes and established risk factors among populations of sub-Saharan African descent in Europe: a literature review. *Global Health.* 2009;5:7.

4. Wit MAS, Tuinebreijer WC, Dekker J et al. Depressive and anxiety disorders in different ethnic groups. *Soc Psychiatry Psychiatr Epidemiol.* 2008;43(11):905–12.

5. O'Donnell CA, Burns N, Mair F et al. Reducing the health care burden for marginalised migrants: the potential role for primary care in Europe. *Health Policy.* 2016;1:1.

6. Schulz AJ, House JS, Israel BA et al. Relational pathways between socioeconomic position and cardiovascular risk in a multi-ethnic urban sample: complexities and their implications for improving health in economically disadvantaged populations. *J Epidemiol Community Health.* 2008;62:638–46.

7. Agyemang C, Goosen S, Anujo K, Ogedegbe G. Relationship between post-traumatic stress disorder and diabetes among 105,180 asylum seekers in the Netherlands. *Eur J Public Health.* 2012;22(5):658–62.

8. Saha S, Beach MC, Cooper LA. Patient centeredness, cultural competence, and healthcare quality. *J Natl Med Assoc.* 2009;100(11):1275–85.

9. De Maeseneer J, van Weel C, Daeren L et al. From 'patient' to 'person' to 'people': the need for integrated, people-centered healthcare. *Int J Pers Cent Med*. 2012;2(3):601–14.

10. De Maeseneer J, Willems S, De Sutter A, Van de Geuchte I, Billings M. Primary healthcare as a strategy for achieving equitable care: a literature review commissioned by the Health Systems Knowledge Network. 2007.

11. Razavi MF, Falk L, Wilhelmsson S. Experiences of the Swedish healthcare system: an interview study with refugees in need of long-term health care. *Scand J Public Health*. 2011;39:319–25.

CHAPTER 13

Gynaecology and obstetrics

Berit Austveg and Kathy Ainul Møen

LEARNING OBJECTIVES

In this chapter, the reader will learn about:

- Specific aspects regarding sexual and reproductive health among migrant women that challenge the mutual understanding between the patient and the GP
- The most commonly presented reproductive health issues among migrant women
- Relevant topics, such as antenatal care, which is crucial to reducing the risk for adverse outcomes of pregnancy and could improve reproductive health among migrant women

---

INTRODUCTION

More than 40 million female migrants, nearly 11% of the female population, lived in Europe in 2017 (1). Most of these women have migrated from Africa, Latin America, and Asia, and the proportion of non-Europeans continues to increase (2). Migrant women are heterogeneous and therefore there will be large variations in the socioeconomic backgrounds in addition to ethnic differences, and the GP must give this due consideration. Moreover, many female migrants are employed in the informal economy, particularly as caretakers, private nurses, or domestic helpers, and this will have consequences in terms of their social position and access to resources, including access to health care (3). Women migrant workers face significant vulnerabilities to health risks that stem from their gender, their migration status, their employment and living conditions, and workplace contexts (4).

Women's reasons for migration can vary, and their rights in the new country often depend on the cause of migration. This is discussed in detail in Chapter 4. All European countries have ratified important human rights conventions that the governments are obliged to follow. For sensitive issues like the ones dealt with in obstetrics and gynaecology, and especially for irregular migrants who are almost stripped of rights, dual and conflicting roles can become disturbing for the GP. On the positive side, having a long-term relationship with patients representing different cultures, and who often have complex and interesting medical conditions, can be very rewarding and inspiring. Assisting patients in deeply human issues like aspirations to having a fulfilling sexual life and forming a family in situations that otherwise can be stressful is a fascinating task for a GP.

Reproductive rights are part of human rights. They imply the right of the individual to decide when to have children, and to have the means to regulate their fertility. Over the past few years, migration has been debated globally, and anti-migration sentiments are quite common. GPs are part of society and thus also influenced by societal sentiments and pressures. Therefore, the need to listen carefully to the woman and assist her in achieving her reproductive goals cannot be overemphasized.

Finally, as mentioned earlier, as migrants are heterogeneous, the sexual and reproductive health, traditions, and rights will differ among groups. This chapter deals primarily with migrant women in Europe, mainly from Asia, Africa, Latin America, and East Europe, and with women who have only been in the host country for a relatively short period. However, several themes covered could also be applicable to other migrants in different settings.

CLINICAL VIGNETTE 1

A female patient from Kenya was sent to a GP in Norway by 'free health help for irregular migrants' by the Red Cross. She told the GP that she had been vomiting for days and couldn't eat or drink because of nausea. Initial laboratory results showed that she was pregnant and dehydrated. The patient wouldn't tell how she got pregnant or about her living conditions. She was admitted to hospital for further treatment. Some days after, the GP was contacted by the police for a meeting. The GP learned from the police officer that the patient was a victim of human trafficking and had been forced into prostitution.

CLINICAL VIGNETTE 2

A female Pakistani patient, recently migrated to Europe and a mother of four children, had an appointment with the GP for contraception. After some discussion, she decided for an IUD. Three months later she came back to the GP and asked the GP to remove the IUD. She claimed that she had gotten air in her shoulders as an unwanted side effect of the IUD. The GP explained that anatomically it was impossible to have air in the shoulders; there was simply no space for air. The GP palpated the patient's shoulders, found some tenderness, and referred her for physiotherapy.

Some weeks later, the patient came back because of another complaint. The GP asked if she had seen a physiotherapist for her shoulders, and the patient told that she had not. Then the GP asked about the IUD, and if the trouble was still there. The patient looked away and mumbled that the IUD had 'fallen out'.

A few weeks later, the GP was invited to a language class for migrant women to provide health education. Some of the women asked the doctor whether it was dangerous to remove an IUD by themselves. The GP responded that a doctor or midwife should remove it, but the women insisted in their question and claimed that health care providers had not always complied the women's wish to remove the IUD and told the women that they 'had enough children already'. Reluctantly, the GP said that what health staff would do, would be to pull the threads of the IUD under visual control, but in principle it was the same thing if a woman could find the threads in her vagina and pulled. The GP felt embarrassed when she realized that the women have experienced not being listened to by their health care providers and wondered if that was the situation with the patient she had seen a short while ago.

CLINICAL VIGNETTE 3

A pregnant woman from a country that practices female genital mutilation (FGM) came for antenatal care. The woman asked her GP if the GP could perform FGM after the child was born if the child was a girl. The GP asked the woman to come back with her husband for a discussion. The GP anticipated that the man would be in favour of the procedure. When they both came, the GP explained that it would be illegal to perform FGM, and it was also harmful to the health. To her surprise, the husband agreed with her and said that FGM would cause damage. The pregnant woman, however, got upset and hurt, saying that it implied that her husband meant that she was 'damaged'.

CLINICAL VIGNETTE 4

Two Muslim women visited a GP for antenatal care during Ramadan. The first woman was pale and weak, and the GP saw that she was anaemic. The GP asked if she was fasting, and she said yes, 'my religion demands it'. The second patient looked sound and healthy and had no anaemia. When she was asked about whether she was fasting, she said, 'Of course not, my religion says that pregnant women should not fast'.

The previous vignettes describe some of the cases that GPs might come across. Many high-income countries also experience that trafficking of women and girls for prostitution and forced labour is one of the growing areas of concern (5). These women are often promised better living conditions, attractive jobs, and education by those who are responsible for trafficking. Migrant sex workers can either be women who have migrated for that purpose, or persons who have come in a dire economic and social situation where they see themselves forced to prostitution, as seen in Clinical Vignette 1. Debt because of the travel cost can be one reason; demands for sending money to the home country can be another. Migrants may in general not have full rights to health services, and for persons who reside illegally in the host country, the combination of high risk for health problems and lack of rights can be detrimental.

VARIATION IN SEXUAL AND REPRODUCTIVE RISKS AND PATTERNS

Migrant women in Europe differ in their reproductive health and disease patterns as compared to the majority populations. It has been shown that some groups have lower access to use of contraceptives, higher risks of unwanted pregnancies and abortion, lower use of antenatal care, and higher risk for adverse pregnancy outcomes (6,7).

Europe has had an increase in migration, and many of the migrants are still relatively young compared to the general population. Very little is known about long-term effects of the higher risks that women in reproductive age are facing, so there is little knowledge about gynaecological problems among elderly migrant women. Acculturation in terms of reproductive health seems to differ among offspring of migrants: some adopt the majority patterns relatively quickly, whereas other groups follow traditions for a longer time (8).

Migrant sex workers face the same health hazards as other sex workers. In addition, they could be more stigmatized than their majority counterparts, and more exposed to violence and to sexually transmitted infections (9,10). When migrants are in an irregular situation and outside the ordinary health care system, with no health insurance, their vulnerability can be extreme. To the extent that they are cared for at all, it is often thanks to charities and voluntary health workers.

CULTURAL AND SOCIOECONOMIC DIFFERENCES

Cultural differences are real and important. All the same, 'culture' can be used as a convenient box in which to put what is not immediately understood, and what requires some extra effort. It is indeed a huge topic and can only be touched upon here (see also Chapters 4 and 5). There are cultural differences in how we see health and illness, how to get a good life, how to deal with ill health, and whom to consult and how. Sexuality and sexual health are heavily loaded with cultural attitudes. Cultural awareness can be a good guide to know what to be looking for, and for asking relevant questions. However, cultural knowledge and cultural awareness alone cannot give all the answers. The clinician must also relate to the individual's needs.

Clinical examination and diagnosis are often based on perceptions related to the cause for the presenting complaints. The perceptions regarding these causes can vary between cultures. In countries where religions still play an important role in people's daily lives, God or fate can more frequently be thought of as causes for health problems. One example of the importance of this discrepancy in understanding health and disease is genetic counselling in families that have an increased risk for having a child with a hereditary disease. Explaining percentages of risks for having a child that can live or not, that can have a debilitating condition or not, is difficult enough in a conversation between persons from the same culture. If the migrant woman says that 'it is up to God' or to 'fate', it requires compassion and a great amount of understanding from health care providers to secure good communication. Also, explanations that are based on natural causes can be a challenge for the GP.

When the patient and the physician do not share the same views on the reason for a complaint, giving a mini-lecture on human anatomy or physiology may not be the best approach. In Clinical Vignette 2, about the IUD, it would have been better to ask the patient to describe what she felt in her shoulders, to see if they could have found a common ground, a description of the problem that they both could agree on. Based on their common understanding they might find a solution to it. Then the GP could explore whether the woman was uncomfortable with the IUD for some reason since she felt the IUD was the cause of her trouble. Negative health care experiences among migrants are an important concern; inadequate exchange of information, perceived differences in expectations between patients and care providers about medical procedures, and feeling of rejection from optimal care because care providers were prejudiced or discriminate have been reported by migrants (11). In some traditional medicine schools, humoral theories play a central role in the origin of complaints, and air in the body is a reasonable explanation for a variety of complaints. These complaints include what in Western medicine is discomfort of muscular or other origin.

Consultations in the GP's office are asymmetrical situations where one person is seeking help and the other is supposed to give the help. The potential for learning increases as the concerns of the patient become clearer. To give the patient the best possible assistance for their complaints, it is essential to negotiate common ground.

Socioeconomic differences between patients and health care providers have a substantial impact on the communication and on the quality of the health care that is provided. The social status of migrants reflects complex patterns. Their socioeconomic status in the host country often changes for the worse, with little recognition of previous education or wealth. These changes in socioeconomic status likely affect women and men in different ways, and this influences the rapport between the parties in the consultation room. Social differences may be exacerbated when sensitive issues are at stake.

FEARS AND EXPECTATIONS

The epidemiological picture in the countries of origin might give guidance to health practitioners in Europe dealing with recently arrived migrants. Particularly for those who are relatively new in the host country, it also reflects the migrants' own experience of what are serious conditions and what are not, what to seek help for, and what to fear. This can have an impact on their health behaviour. Because maternal mortality is high in many countries migrants come from, they may have experienced pregnancy-related deaths among family members, friends, and neighbours. When migrants are settling in their new country and are told that there is a complication in a pregnancy, it can give rise to more anxiety than the GP is used to. Unsafe abortions are common in countries with strict abortion legislation and poor health services, so the decision to terminate a pregnancy can cause fear of serious health effects. They may be used to substandard cancer treatment, so being told that they have irregular cervix cells can also cause greater alarm than for non-migrant patients. It is important for the GP to have knowledge about how to handle such anxiety.

The coverage of health insurance in a European country might be better than what the migrant women were used to from their home countries, and reproductive health care is often well covered. Hospital care in particular could amount to catastrophic expenses in many countries from which migrants originate, including from complications in pregnancies. It is important to explain the rights and the financial implications of the use of services in these situations. While patients might express relief and gratitude for their rights, they may also have difficulties navigating in health services, and the GP is well placed to assist them in this task.

SPECIFIC CLINICAL ISSUES AND DILEMMAS

The roles and responsibilities of GPs in relation to gynaecological complaints and pregnancies vary across Europe. The following explores the most common issues that GPs are dealing with, as well as issues that are specific to migrant women.

Choice of contraceptives

There is a general trend that migrant women in Europe less often use contraceptives than non migrant women (6). Migrants may have myths and misconceptions about specific contraceptives. They may have heard rumours that IUDs can cause infertility, or that contraceptive pills cause cancer, for example. They may also have experience of coercive use of provider-controlled methods such as IUDs, injections, and sterilization, or that contraceptives are not provided for unmarried women (12).

Some contraceptive methods cause changes in bleeding patterns. There are culturally based views on the importance of an appropriate amount of bleeding during menstruation. Anaemia is more prevalent among some migrant women, and for them, increased bleeding can be harmful. Decreased bleeding can lead to a feeling of dirt accumulating in the body, leading to a variety of discomforts. Increased bleeding can also lead to anxiety. Some women can express excessive fatigue for a relatively small increase in bleeding, based on cultural views of the blood's effects in the body. It is important for the GP to talk about these issues when choosing the optimal contraceptive method with the woman.

Spontaneous abortion, miscarriage, and infertility

Fertility varies greatly between the migrants' countries of origin and is closely linked to cultural values related to gender roles and ideals. It is a general tendency that fertility changes with migration (13). Over a relatively short period of time, the migrants adapt their fertility, which becomes closer, if not always equal, to that of the host country. It is surprising how quickly such important changes are made, taking into consideration how fundamental fertility is for the life projection of the individuals.

While substantial differences in fertility exist among migrants, there is a tendency that it is higher than in the host population, specifically for the first years in the host country (13). The loss of a wanted pregnancy can be difficult to cope with for a variety of reasons. Having a baby in an insecure situation can create a sense of meaning and optimism for the future, and may be wanted by the woman even under circumstances that would seem suboptimal for others. Furthermore, reproductive decisions and aspirations may be more of a collective effort than what is common in a European culture, and family members and in-laws in the home country can be involved.

Infertility also has important cultural bearings. Again, individual differences may far outweigh the cultural ones, but knowing a bit about cultural views on importance of having offspring can help in posing the right questions. In some cultures, arranged marriages are the norm, and collective views decide the timing and number of children a couple is expected to have, with less emphasis on the wishes of the individual.

The process of investigation and treatment for infertility can take a long time and be costly. Good planning is important to avoid frustration for both the patient and the physician, and it is important to be aware of plans for travels and absences.

Termination of pregnancy

Rates of termination of pregnancies vary greatly across the globe. It is highest in Vietnam and in Eastern European countries, while the countries with the lowest rates are in Europe (14). Migrants generally have higher rates than the non-migrant population. This could reflect the continuation of practices from the country of origin, but it might also reflect insufficient accessibility of contraceptive services, and thus a failure of health services.

While abortion legislation is liberal in most European countries, it is strict in many of the migrants' countries of origin. Strict abortion laws do not lead to lower rates of abortions, but to unsafe abortions and related mortality and morbidity (14). When a need for termination of a pregnancy arises, it may cause distress in women based on knowledge from her country of origin of the detriment that abortions can lead to. While there are religious arguments for supporting women's choices and trusting their abilities to make moral and ethical decisions, many religious leaders condemn abortion. Religious convictions can lead to stigma and condemnation from others and invoke feelings of shame. For these reasons, migrant women who wish to terminate their pregnancy may need some extra care to prepare them, with a thorough explanation of the procedure and its effects. They may also need follow-up and support after the procedure.

Antenatal care

GPs responsible for antenatal care should consider if special efforts are needed to guide the patient safely through the pregnancy and help in planning delivery in the best possible way. Possible risks for certain groups of patients should be considered, while also making sure that all the routines for antenatal check-ups are being followed and that the woman understands what is going to happen where, and who to contact in case of doubts or emergencies.

There are some conditions that occur more frequently during pregnancy among migrant women. Migrant women of Asian and African decent in Norway have statistically higher risk of adverse pregnancy outcome, operative vaginal delivery, emergency caesarean sections, and some other complications than the native population (7). As mentioned previously, anaemia is more prevalent among migrant women than in the host population. Nutritional deficiencies are the most common reasons (iron, folic acid, and vitamin B_{12}), but infrequently seen conditions like thalassemia and sickle cell anaemia may be present. Chronic infections and infestations, such as hepatitis, HIV, hookworm, and malaria may also be present, but it is important not to forget common causes, and avoid being overwhelmed with exoticisms. Gestational diabetes in pregnancy has been shown to be many times more frequent among South Asian migrants in Europe and other high-income countries compared to other groups (15). Thus, several conditions and risk factors might occur more often in pregnant migrant women, and if untreated lead to complications and adverse pregnancy outcomes. Migrant women with special risk factors should be followed carefully. A good strategy can be for the GP to have close cooperation with a specialist while maintaining continuous contact with the patient.

Preparing for delivery is an important part of antenatal care. Since onset and development of delivery are unpredictable events, logistics planning, including planning for the assistance of a translator, needs to be considered carefully. It is important to give information on what will happen, both in the case of a normal delivery and if complications should arise. A fine balance needs to be drawn between giving the right amount of knowledge and avoiding creating unnecessary fear and overload of information.

Postnatal care

As mentioned previously, delivery complications are more common in certain migrant groups. The GP should be aware of any such complication and assist the woman in coming to terms with what has happened to her and her baby. There are important cultural differences in the appropriate way of treating a woman during her delivery, and for behaviour for a woman who has just given birth. To what extent women want to uphold such traditions varies greatly. Some women want special forms of massage during the puerperium; they want to avoid certain types of food and be sure they get other types of food. Some are reluctant to take showers and prefer steam instead, and some believe that being exposed to fresh air right after birth is harmful. Women who are used to less high-tech deliveries than what is common in European countries may feel assured and feel taken well care of. But the women may also miss traditional practices and worry that their health or that of their baby may be in jeopardy.

It may be wise to include the husband or partner and members of the extended family in the support of a woman during the puerperium, especially when there have been complications. Friends can also give practical and emotional support. However, care should be taken that the women's needs are at the centre.

Cervical cancer screening and treatment

Cervical cancer is one of the few preventable cancers if detected early. It is the third most common cancer and the fourth most frequent cause of cancer deaths in women worldwide (16). However, cervical cancer prevalence and mortality are not evenly distributed. More than 85% of the cases and deaths occur in low-income and middle-income countries (17). Cervix cancer is slightly more common in some migrant groups, especially women from East, West, and Central Africa and Melanesia (18).

Migrant women have lower participation in cervical cancer screening. There are several barriers for cervical cancer screening, including poor knowledge about the disease, language barriers, fear of pain and procedural discomfort and fear of bad news, lack of perceived necessity, sociocultural barriers such as stigma attached to the disease, poor health literacy, and economic constraints. There are also system-related barriers, such as lack of trust in the health system and access to female physicians (19).

Strategies like information letters about the disease and screening in women's native language; educating women about the benefits of the test and their right to have a translator under consultation; raising awareness through schools, religious gatherings, or health clinics; information given by GPs; and initiating a recall system in the native language could increase attendance. In addition, future possibilities like HPV home testing would also promote migrant women taking the test.

However, culture and individual need should be understood by the GPs when they meet migrant women. For some women, being a virgin until marriage is important and they are afraid of taking the test because they feel the procedure would endanger their virginity. Cervical cancer screening might not be relevant when the woman has never had any form of sexual encounter. On the other side, there is evidence that the GPs often take for granted that migrant women from low-income countries will not be interested in taking the test, and do not even bother to invite to the procedure. Therefore, the GP should get to know the patient's cultural and religious background when it comes to sensitive issues like cervical cancer screening by talking to the women rather than relying on prejudices.

Female genital mutilation

FMG is a tradition practiced primarily in sub-Saharan Africa. The various forms of FGM cause different medical problems. Infibulation, with a partial closure of the vaginal orifice, causes the most complications, especially in relation to menstrual pain, sexual intercourse, and pregnancies. Other forms of FGM can also cause problems because of scar tissue and cysts, and because of the trauma that they inflict.

Preventing new cases of FGM is a priority in European countries, and most of the countries have a ban on the practice. It is harmful and a violation of basic human rights.

While clear standpoints against the practice can be important for prevention, they can cause stigma for girls and women who are living with the mutilation. Those who want medical help for their problems can be ambivalent about receiving treatment. As a minority in the host country, they can feel that their identity is threatened in the first place and living with FGM can be part of their identity. Even though no religion mandates FGM, it is often believed that it does. This reinforces the belief that it is necessary. Infibulation is often, wrongly, seen as a proof of virginity. Requesting an opening intervention before marriage can therefore be frowned upon, and the woman can fear for her reputation if it becomes known that she is requesting, or getting, treatment. We have good experience with giving the woman a medical statement saying the treatment was necessary for her to show to protect her reputation.

Experience has shown that health staff may be more reluctant to talk about FGM than women who are living with the consequences. When GPs are reluctant to bring up the issue and are uncomfortable discussing it, it can be a serious barrier to good treatment (20). If, on the other hand, the GP has acquired knowledge about the issue on beforehand, and shows an open mind, the women who are affected are normally eager to discuss their symptoms and their wish for help. When examining a woman with FGM, extra care should be given so that she feels she is in control of the process at all times. She may need counselling beforehand, which may be given by a person she knows and trusts, such as a GP. When women are asked about what they remember about having gone through the procedure of FGM, almost all say that they remember the pain (21). Pain is also often the main problem in the long run. Because of previous trauma, and because many of the nerve endings have been cut, many women who live with FGM are extra sensitive to pain and may experience even the slightest touch as painful. An examination should start with just looking, and only when she is ready, palpation and exploration should be performed.

The treatment can sometimes be very simple, but at other times more complicated. Cysts and infections may arise. De-infibulation, which is an opening of the closed orifice, should be considered for all women to improve their quality of life, and it is necessary for a vaginal delivery. There are good reasons for being de-infibulated before pregnancy, and it makes monitoring of the pregnancy much easier. If it is to be done during pregnancy, the second trimester is preferred. At the latest, it should be done during delivery. It should always be the woman herself deciding the timing of the de-infibulation, based on information, and if needed, counselling. De-infibulation during the first trimester should be avoided to prevent a perceived association between de-infibulation and a spontaneous abortion, if that should occur. The surgical intervention should be done by a specialist, but the GP can play an important role in diagnosing, motivating for treatment, informing, and supporting women during their process. It is important that the GP becomes familiarized with the issue.

Menopausal challenges

Previous literature shows that culture shapes the experience of menopause (22). However, the symptom experience of migrant women during menopausal transition should be understood within the context of their migration transition. Studies show that migrant women less often report vasomotor symptoms like hot flushes than non-migrant women, and are more likely to report physical symptoms such as skeletal and muscular pain than vasomotor symptoms (23) and psychological symptoms like depression more often than women from host countries (24).

Many migrant women are sceptical about hormone treatment for their symptoms and prefer self-management. Moreover, migrant women often describe this in terms of convenience and protection against unplanned pregnancies. Traditional medicines and change of dietary and lifestyles are often used as self-management. The GP should understand migrant women's own perceptions of menopause, becoming familiar with the cultural and psychosocial influences of menopause, and then empower them to make decisions regarding management. This will help improve the care of perimenopausal and menopausal women. As for all other non-migrant women, health care providers should be cautious not to medicalize the symptoms, but to show respect for women's views of normality of the menopausal transition.

Expression of pain

The physical examination can be a challenge. Anxiety can increase sensitivity to pain. If the woman is uncertain that she has been understood, or if she fears that she is being discriminated against, she can express it as physical pain. Previous traumas can also make the patient extra sensitive. Refugees in particular have frequently experienced sexual abuse and assaults, and may therefore need extra care. Finally, there are cultural differences in how pain is expressed, and in what ways pain should be expressed by a mature and sensible person (25). When a patient expresses pain stronger than expected, it should never be ignored and seen as 'low threshold of pain', or 'their culture' but rather as a way of communication or a pathology that we did not count on. Pain is always subjective; it is the behaviour that can be experienced by others, and it is the GP's task to try to make sense of the patient's pain behaviour.

Virginity

In some traditional cultures, preserving virginity until marriage is seen as vital. The belief that there is a hymen that should be intact in unmarried girls can be strong. Depending on the degree of acculturation, young girls might fear that a gynaecological examination can damage the hymen, which can be a barrier to seeking necessary medical help. It is important that the GP is aware of this and discusses with the patient how she can still be examined without endangering virginity.

Where virginity is a requirement for entering marriage, women who are going to be married may request hymen repair if they have had sexual intercourse or otherwise fear that the hymen has been broken. It is our experience from our clinical work that sometimes the mere explanation of the fact that the hymen has different forms and sometimes is absent all-together, is enough to relieve this anxiety. In societies that put a great emphasis on the hymen, and occasionally on a blood-stained sheet after the wedding night to 'prove' virginity, women have ways of dealing with it. The mother, aunt, or another trusted woman can be a good ally and help in difficult situations. Surgical intervention to 'restore' the hymen is therefore generally contraindicated and should be avoided (26).

ROLE OF THE GP

Gender of the GP and of the interpreter

In taking the history, cultural issues can come up, as explained previously. It is also common that the gender of the health care provider can play a role. When there is need for an interpreter, the gender of the interpreter can also be an issue. A sensible policy could be to try to allocate a female physician and translator to women with a strong wish for that. Nevertheless, different European countries have different policies when it comes to abiding by patients' gender preferences for their service provider. In some countries, there are laws that regard it discrimination to require a specific sex. In all cases, effort should be made to build a good relationship with the patient and show respect for her wishes, explaining why they can or cannot be met in cases where it is not possible.

Not infrequently, women who say that they don't want to be examined by a male physician can accept one if that male physician is sympathetic towards them and uses the necessary time to create an alliance with the woman and her involved relatives. However, accepting a male interpreter might be more difficult, and if there is a problem accepting the interpreter, some may find it easier to have a translator by phone, who does not see the patient and who does not need to know her identity. When there are no other alternatives, the translator is placed out of sight of the patient in the consultation room, as it is better to have a translator than no translator.

There are ideological discussions about the role of an interpreter. Some schools insist that only pure, word-by-word translation is accepted, while others favour translators who are also cultural mediators. Whichever model is used, it is important to keep in mind that a gynaecological history may be particularly sensitive. Therefore, extra effort may be needed to make sure that the patient's views and concerns are well understood.

Khan et al. mention barriers that Pakistani migrants faced in Germany, where they state that coordination between the family doctor and specialists about the patient's illness was also a barrier (27). When a GP refers a migrant patient to a specialist, it may be necessary to give more information than usual to the specialist, including on socioeconomic and legal concerns. In referring, it is also important to mention the need for an interpreter, and what language it should be. GPs could experience inadequate help given to migrant patients by specialists because of linguistic barriers, and at the same time, specialists could feel that the referrals from GPs are not adequate to understand the patient's problem. Thus, good communication between the GP and the specialist is important to give the migrant patient optimal health care.

General practice is based on continuity and coordination. The GP can have the privilege of knowing the patient for a long time and be aware of the conditions that the patient is living under. A migrant patient may require more follow-up after having been seen by a specialist than non-migrants do. The GP should therefore consider offering a consultation after a referral to explain the outcome and clarify any misunderstandings that may arise.

SUMMARY

Providing sexual and reproductive health services to migrant women can be a very rewarding task for a GP. It touches upon existential aspects that are fundamentally important for all persons, and especially for persons who have been uprooted and relocated. However, it can also pose challenges. The right to affordable health care can be a challenge, especially for women without legal residence in the host country. Migrant women can face higher risk for many conditions related to gynaecology and obstetrics, and for lower quality of health care.

The GP's understanding of cultural aspects of the migrant patient is particularly relevant for understanding the views and behaviours related to sexuality and reproduction. Knowledge of cultural concerns can help the GP pose more relevant questions. However, only the patient can provide the information that is specific for her. In cases when a consultation is required, there is a need for a closer cooperation than usual between the GP and the specialist. Moreover, the GP should secure continuation and coordination of often long-lasting themes, such as reproductive health.

ACKNOWLEDGEMENT

We would like to express our very great appreciation to Dr Birgitta Essén for her valuable and constructive suggestions of the manuscript.

REFERENCES

1. United Nations. Trends in International Migrant Stock: the 2017 revision. Available from: http://www.un.org/en/development/desa/population/migration/data/estimates2/docs/MigrationStockDocumentation_2017.pdf (accessed December 2017).
2. Migration Policy Institute. Between Integration and Exclusion: Migrant Women in European Labor Markets. Available from: https://www.migrationpolicy.org/article/between-integration-and-exclusion-migrant-women-european-labor-markets (accessed March 2011).
3. Anthias F, Kontos M, Morokvasic-Müller M. *Paradoxes of Integration: Female Migrants in Europe.* Springer Netherlands: Springer; 2013.
4. Hennebry JW, Keegan; Walton-Roberts, Margaret. *Women working worldwide: a situational analysis of women migrant workers.* United Nations Entity for Gender Equality and the Empowerment of Women (UN Women); 2017. Report No.: 978-1-63214-056-2.
5. Kok G. Trafficking of women for the purpose of sexual exploitation in Europe. *Biomed Health Sci Res.* 2014;**2**.
6. Omland G, Ruths S, Díaz E. Use of hormonal contraceptives among immigrant and native women in Norway: data from the Norwegian Prescription Database. *BJOG.* 2014;121(10):1221–8.
7. Bakken KS, Skjeldal OH, Stray-Pedersen B. Higher risk for adverse obstetric outcomes among immigrants of African and Asian descent: a comparison study at a low-risk maternity hospital in Norway. *Birth.* 2015;42(2):132–40.
8. Pailhé A. The convergence of second-generation immigrants' fertility patterns in France: the role of sociocultural distance between parents' and host country. *Demogr Res.* 2017;36(45):1361–98.
9. Keygnaert I, Vettenburg N, Temmerman M. Hidden violence is silent rape: sexual and gender-based violence in refugees, asylum seekers and undocumented migrants in Belgium and the Netherlands. *Cult Health Sex.* 2012;14(5).
10. Platt L, Grenfell P, Fletcher A et al. Systematic review examining differences in HIV, sexually transmitted infections and health-related harms between migrant and non-migrant female sex workers. *Sex Transm Infect.* 2013;89(4):311.
11. Suurmond J, Uiters E, de Bruijne M, Stronks K, Essink-Bot M-L. Negative health care experiences of immigrant patients: a qualitative study. *BMC Health Serv Res.* 2011;11(1):10.
12. Sedgh G, Hussain R. Reasons for contraceptive non-use among women having unmet need for contraception in developing countries. *Stud Fam Plann.* 2014;45(2):151–69.
13. Tønnessen M. Fertility rates and other demographics among immigrants and children of immigrants born in Norway Oslo, Norway: Statistics Norway; 2014. Available from: https://www.ssb.no/en/forskning/demografi-og-levekaar/fruktbarhet-og-familiedemografi/fertility-rates-and-other-demographics-among-immigrants-and-children-of-immigrants-born-in-norway.
14. World Health Organization. *Safe Abortion: Technical and Policy Guidance for Health Systems.* 2nd ed. Geneva: WHO; 2012.
15. Anand SS, Gupta M, Teo KK et al. Causes and consequences of gestational diabetes in South Asians living in Canada: results from a prospective cohort study. *CMAJ Open.* 2017;5(3):E604.
16. Jemal A, Bray F, Center MM, Ferlay J, Ward E, Forman D. Global cancer statistics. *CA Cancer J Clin.* 2011;61(2):69–90.

17. Ferlay J, Steliarova-Foucher E, Lortet-Tieulent J et al. Cancer incidence and mortality patterns in Europe: estimates for 40 countries in 2012. *Eur J Cancer.* 2013;49(6):1374–403.
18. Ferlay J, Soerjomataram I, Dikshit R et al. Cancer incidence and mortality worldwide: sources, methods and major patterns in GLOBOCAN 2012. *Int J Cancer.* 2015;136(5):E359–E86.
19. Gele AA, Qureshi SA, Kour P, Kumar B, Diaz E. Barriers and facilitators to cervical cancer screening among Pakistani and Somali immigrant women in Oslo: a qualitative study. *Int J Womens Health.* 2017;9:487–96.
20. WHO. *WHO guidelines on the management of health complications from female genital mutilation.* Geneva: World Health Organization; 2016.
21. Johansen RE. Pain as a counterpoint to culture: toward an analysis of pain associated with infibulation among Somali immigrants in Norway. *Med Anthropol Q.* 2002;16(3):312–40.
22. Stanzel KA, Hammarberg K, Fisher J. *Experiences of Menopause, Self-Management Strategies for Menopausal Symptoms and Perceptions of Health Care among Immigrant Women: A Systematic Review.* Taylor & Francis Group; 2018; p. 101–10.
23. Hafiz I, Liu J, Eden J. A quantitative analysis of the menopause experience of Indian women living in Sydney. *Aust N Z J Obstet Gynaecol.* 2007;47(4):329–34.
24. Blumstein T, Benyamini Y, Hourvitz A, Boyko V, Lerner-Geva L. Cultural/ethnic differences in the prevalence of depressive symptoms among middle-aged women in Israel: the Women's Health at Midlife Study. *Menopause.* 2012;19(12):1309–21.
25. Helman CG. *Culture, Health and Illness.* 5th ed. London: Hodder Arnold; 2007.
26. Wild V, Poulin H, McDougall CW, Stockl A, Biller-Andorno N. Hymen reconstruction as pragmatic empowerment? Results of a qualitative study from Tunisia. *Soc Sci Med.* 2015;147:54–61.
27. Khan N, Saboor H, Qayyum Z, Khan I, Habib Z, Waheed H. Barriers to accessing the German health-care system for Pakistani immigrants in Berlin, Germany: a qualitative exploratory study. *Lancet.* 2013;382:18.

CHAPTER 14

Chronic disease prevention and management: An understated priority

Nicole Nitti

LEARNING OBJECTIVES

At the end of this chapter, the reader should be able to:

- Demonstrate the importance of addressing chronic diseases and their risk factors in migrant populations
- Understand unique challenges faced by migrants and special considerations for their care
- Identify best practices in chronic disease management that relate to migrant populations

---

INTRODUCTION

Before I began working with migrants and refugees in Toronto, I excitedly began reading up on tropical medicine and communicable diseases. I even bought a communicable disease handbook for my desk. Months later, that book was gathering dust and my appointment slots were filled with people struggling with their diabetes and hypertension or other chronic diseases. Many of them had inadequate understanding of their conditions and how their long-term health may be affected. I began to realize that if we really wanted to improve the health of our clients, we needed a new approach.

CHRONIC DISEASE IS IMPORTANT TO MIGRANT HEALTH

Chronic diseases are the number one cause of death worldwide with heart disease, cancer, respiratory illnesses, and diabetes contributing to 70% of deaths related to chronic disease (1) and affecting quality of life of more and more people and communities. Once thought to be a concern felt mainly by the developed world, the World Health Organization data indicate that the countries most affected are low- and moderate-income countries such as India and countries in the Middle East and Africa, and that developing countries have the fastest rising prevalence. Since most chronic disease is largely related to modifiable risk factors, with 80% of heart disease, stroke, and diabetes being preventable (2), action should become a priority.

Many of the migrants seen in health clinics come from countries with the highest rates of diabetes and hypertension. Even in refugee populations previously thought to have low risk of chronic disease, a higher prevalence of chronic diseases and their complications have been observed (3). A Canadian study looked at diabetes prevalence in Ontario residents and found that overall there was a higher prevalence in newcomers than long-term residents. Those of South and Southeast Asian descent, refugees, elderly women, and those living in the lowest income quintile were at highest risk (4).

Traditionally, migrant health guidelines have emphasized infectious disease, malnutrition, and mental health, which are common, often highly symptomatic, and create imminent risk to the individual and the people around them. However, there is significant risk in overlooking chronic diseases and their risk factors. The 'healthy migrant effect' (refer to Chapter 2) is strongly related to development of chronic diseases. Primary health care plays a huge role in reducing this through meticulous identification and developing effective chronic disease prevention and management strategies.

UNIQUE CHALLENGES FACED BY MIGRANTS AND SPECIAL CONSIDERATIONS FOR THEIR CARE

Chronic disease places a large burden on the people living with it and their families. Extending far beyond managing medication regimens and maintaining a healthy diet, the activities involved in managing conditions like diabetes have a layered effect on daily life including productivity, energy, leisure time, mental health, and for the populations being discussed here, the ability to thrive in a new country.

Sociodemographic factors

Health care is 25% of health and well-being, with the social environment being the most important (5).

CASE STUDY

Jane is a 42-year-old woman from the Caribbean living in Toronto for 10 years. She is a single mother on social assistance working towards her diploma in nursing. She has insulin-dependent type 2 diabetes with obesity and hypertension and struggles with prioritizing her health care needs as there simply isn't enough time to make all the appointments, find time to exercise, and cook nutritious meals. She often feels guilty that she can't manage her health better and lies awake worrying about being around for her son as he gets older.

Rates of chronic diseases and their risk factors are higher in populations of lower socioeconomic status. Regrettably, migrants are more likely than long-term residents to live in poverty and be underemployed, putting them at risk of poor health outcomes. Precarious employment and food insecurity (poor access to culturally acceptable food) makes following through with treatment recommendations next to impossible. Without medication coverage, prescriptions are useless. In addition to financial cost, there are many hidden costs for people living with chronic disease. Time, energy, and emotional capacity are all implicated. An effective care plan explores and incorporates the individual's specific pressure points and needs.

When patients cannot manage all the expectations of their physician, they are often considered to be 'noncompliant' and labelled as 'difficult'. Sometimes providers bring an agenda that is unreasonable, and 'noncompliance' has nothing to do with the patient's motivation to follow recommendations. Damaging to the patient-provider relationship, this erodes an already fragile confidence in their ability to be successful. It pays to listen.

Language and cultural considerations

A language barrier creates major obstacles for migrants trying to manage a chronic disease. Impeded communication with providers, untranslated education materials, and difficulty participating in groups removes the tools and supports patients need. It cannot be overemphasized how important it is for providers to employ professional interpretation (reference Chapter 20). Attempting to explain the complexities of medication and monitoring regimens to someone with limited proficiency in the language being spoken is neither effective nor safe. Although frequently practiced as an acceptable alternative, using family, friends, or untrained individuals who speak the same language as the patient is problematic and often leads to poorly communicated messages, and impinges on privacy and autonomy. Professional interpretation is available worldwide at affordable rates, and either over the phone or in person should be the standard (6).

Approaches to health and illness differ from culture to culture and affect people's behaviours and methods to maintaining wellness. Different explanatory models of illness can be traditional, biomedical, or a mixture of both, and has developed over generations. To ensure that patients are comfortable with treatments prescribed and understand why a behaviour is harmful, it is imperative to ask patients about their understanding of the illness and how it should be treated.

CASE STUDY

Reza is a 50-year-old man with hypertension who presents with a headache. In his home country of Iraq, he used to get 'injections' from his doctor for his headaches and is requesting the same treatment. He is also prescribed hydrochlorothiazide 25 mg to reduce his blood pressure, which he takes whenever he feels it is high. His blood pressure is 160/100 in the office. He wants a referral to a specialist.

The concept of chronicity in illness can be particularly challenging. Taking medications when one feels perfectly well may be counterintuitive to some, and remission of symptoms may be considered a reason for discontinuing treatment (7). Some may not understand the incurability of the chronic condition (8) or simply believe it is their destiny (9). Again, seeking to understand the patient's perspective by encouraging open discussion provides an opportunity to incorporate long-held beliefs and traditions into evidence-based recommendations. This is supported by providing translated and culturally adapted patient education materials and self-management tools. Some patients may have had little or no exposure to basic education, making many of the conventional methods insufficient.

'Health care culture' varies across countries and impacts expectations of health care providers and systems. In particular, patients may not understand primary health care systems, as health care systems are still in early stages of development of many parts of the world. Their previous care may have been fragmented and profit driven, leading to increased medicalization and over-investigation that lacks an evidence-based approach. Patients like Reza can become upset when they don't receive the treatment they expect, and feel that they are not receiving the best care. Sometimes it can take multiple visits, patiently explaining the reasoning behind a decision while gently but firmly resisting unwarranted investigations or treatments to gain acceptance and trust.

Patients need to feel safe, cared for, and respected in order to develop a trusting and productive relationship with their primary care provider and the team. Migrants already feel out of place and disconnected and have likely experienced discrimination in the community, including health care settings, making them wary of staff and services. Careful attention needs to be paid to the patient's experience from the minute they walk in the door. The physical space, interactions with all staff, and communications all contribute to building a strong rapport. Clinic policies need to include clear language around inclusiveness, anti-oppression, and anti-discrimination, and expectations of staff. Regular staff training in cultural competency (refer to Chapter 5) and behaviour modelling by leadership is essential.

COMORBIDITY – MENTAL ILLNESS

A valuable advantage primary care has is the breadth of expertise across the spectrum of health conditions. This allows for screening, diagnosing, and treatment of chronic conditions that commonly concur, such as mental illness (refer to Chapter 17).

CASE STUDY

Mohammed is a 45-year-old man from Ethiopia who arrives in Canada as an asylum seeker after years of imprisonment and torture. He has a diagnosis of depression and complex post-traumatic stress disorder (PTSD) as well as uncontrolled hypertension and type 2 diabetes. He is separated from his family and has few contacts close to him. He is a smoker and has blood pressure readings of 160/95 and 155/92; his HbA1c is 8.5%. He comes to clinic inconsistently and sometimes is lost to follow-up for months at a time.

Migrant populations are known to be at risk of mental health conditions which are linked to an increase in both incidence and poor outcomes of diabetes and heart disease (10). Identifying mental illness with the help of appropriate screening tools allows for concurrent treatment of mood disorders and/or anxiety, which gives patients a better chance of success. Both counselling and medical management with SSRI/SNRIs are helpful. When antipsychotics are indicated, a metabolically neutral choice is best practice.

The experience of violence, persecution, and torture on any individual's level of function is complex and devious. For many, it undermines the ability to have faith in one's self and trust in others, making it difficult to consistently manage their illness. PTSD is known to be a chronic stress reaction with prolonged elevations of stress hormones such as catecholamines, which are also linked to physiologic changes. There is a potential causal link between PTSD and the development of heart disease (11). Although many patients with PTSD can be managed within primary care with medications and counselling, some will benefit from more intensive treatments, such as exposure therapy, that require both specialist expertise and patient readiness.

IMPACT OF POOR ACCESS TO HEALTH CARE

Dr Tedros Adhanom Ghebreyesus, WHO Director-General, stated on Human Rights Day on 10 December 2017: 'The enjoyment of the highest attainable standard of health is one of the fundamental rights of every human being without distinction of race, religion, political belief, economic or social condition'. Despite that, anyone working in health care knows this has not been actualized. Many vulnerable migrant groups, especially refugees (3) and undocumented people, do not have access to care. Further, when health care is available it is often limited to infectious disease and emergency services, while the ongoing needs of maintaining control of chronic disease are not met.

CASE STUDY

Rui is a 30-year-old man, previously well, who presents to a non-insured clinic feeling very unwell with a history of weight loss, polyuria, and weakness. He is tachycardic with a blood pressure of 100/60, and a finger prick glucose test reveals severe hyperglycaemia. He and his wife are undocumented migrants from Portugal and live with their two young children. They have no coverage for health services outside the clinic. His work in construction (roofing) supports the family.

Precarious migration status and lack of health insurance often create crisis situations due to fear of cost or deportation as a result of seeking care. Providers often feel restrained in their recommendations because they are concerned about the individual's ability to pay. Patients are sometimes forced to make difficult decisions and compromises in regard to their health, and providers need to have frank discussions about the consequences both of treatment and non-treatment in order for them to make an informed decision. If a condition is life threatening, that needs to be made clear. In these situations, a 'health first and worry about the rest later' direction needs to be stressed (refer to Chapter 6). In non-emergent cases, care planning becomes a balance between what is recommended and what is doable. Thinking outside the box and finding creative solutions using all resources available can be surprisingly effective. Even when the solution is imperfect, the positive effect of compassion and understanding cannot be underestimated.

Refugees are at risk of poor access due to disruption of systems in their home country and long periods in transition countries with absent or limited access to health care. This can also be a turbulent time fraught with loss, discrimination, and disorder, making accessing care difficult even when available. Other migrant groups might also be at risk both in the country of origin and in the country of destination for a number of reasons. Without proper monitoring and support, chronic diseases such as diabetes and hypertension are likely to be undetected or poorly controlled with early onset of complications. Assessing this is an important part of initial assessments.

ASSESSMENT OF NEW ARRIVALS

CASE STUDY

Asef is a 60-year-old woman originally from Syria and has been living in Lebanon for the last 3 years. She is staying in a refugee shelter where she presents to the drop-in clinic held there for a prescription renewal. She has hypertension treated with 10 mg of amlodipine, which was initially prescribed in Syria. While in Lebanon she purchased her medication through an unlicensed pharmacy and did not see a physician as she felt she would be mistreated. Her blood pressure is 102/55 and blood work shows an HbA1c of 10%.

Newcomers are faced with many challenges and changes. Their first health assessment is a chance to gain a full understanding of their health status and needs as well as introducing them to the health system. If the patient is experiencing symptoms, the first step is to determine the need for urgent investigations and referrals. Once stability is established, a comprehensive history, physical, and evidence-based screening investigations can take place. Incorporating appropriate screening for cardiovascular disease and diabetes and risk factors, such as obesity and smoking status, into initial visit protocols will help avoid missed opportunities for improved health outcomes in the long term.

Obtaining the medical history can be painstaking, with confusing timelines and medical records that are incomplete and not translated. The medications patients bring with them may be inadequate, unnecessary, or unexplained. A careful history of the course of illness including onset, investigations done, different doctors seen, and hospitalizations, is needed to piece together the story and lay down a stronger foundation on which to make clinical decisions. It is also an opportunity to inquire about access to care before leaving and along their journey. Gaps in care indicate the need for a low threshold for suspicion of unidentified complications and comorbidities. Medication adjustment and deprescribing often needs to be considered.

For patients with chronic disease arriving from tuberculosis (TB)-endemic countries, screening for latent TB is especially important as they are at higher risk of reactivation due to both recent migration and the presence of chronic disease (12).

CASE STUDY

Nicolette is a 62-year-old refugee from Burundi. She has known diabetes and takes 20 units of NPH daily. Her BP is 145/90. Her lab results are as follows: HbA1c 7.5%, LDL 3.7, eGFR 65. Rather than continuing with insulin, it was decided to trial a combination of metformin, sitagliptin, and canagliflozin as well as starting a statin and ACE inhibitor. She was referred to the diabetes nurse and supported with self-monitoring, diet, and exercise. Three months later her HbA1c was 7.1%, her BP and LDL to target, she had lost 3 kg, and was very happy not to be on insulin.

For migrants coming from low and middle income countries countries it is not uncommon to present with outdated and inappropriate treatments. These need to be carefully replaced with more appropriate and evidence-based regimens. What happens first, in what order, and how quickly is dependent on clinical urgency and ability of the provider to follow up. Of course, the patient needs to be a central part of this process with a clear understanding of what is changing and why. They must be allowed to express concerns and set the pace of change, and unless there is a safety issue, have the choice of no change. Astute clinical skills and collaboration with other providers and caregivers will support decision making.

The initial few assessments should prioritize stabilization of uncontrolled illness, identifying patient concerns and follow-up needs, collecting and compiling reports and results that can be forwarded to continuing providers, and supporting the patient to understand next steps. When patients move on to another provider, results and a summary of care provided will ensure continuity of care and reduce duplication of testing. Facilitating connection to ongoing primary care is an essential role of the transitional provider.

Newcomers are most likely unfamiliar with navigating health and social systems. Facilitating resources like case managers, settlement workers, or volunteer groups are sometimes needed when family support is not available.

APPROACH TO CARE

Chronic disease management differs from episodic care in that most of the work is done outside the office appointment with the onus on the patient to follow through. It is a long-term endeavour intermingled with many aspects of daily life and is affected greatly by life circumstances. Approach to care for anyone must take into consideration all of the individual's medical, social, and psychological needs and avoid being disease specific. Treatment targets must be individualized and incorporate patient goals and preferences. For migrant populations, understanding the unique challenges they face can help identify strategies that would be most helpful. The cornerstone to doing this well is an effective patient-provider relationship based on trust and respect, supported by an interprofessional team.

Traditional office-based practice is not well set up for effective chronic disease management, as appointment times are short and can easily be dominated by urgent concerns, pushing mundane activities of monitoring and managing conditions such as diabetes to the side. This is what Dr Ed Wagner, of the MacColl Center for Healthcare Innovation at the Kaiser Permanente Washington Health Research Institute, referred to when he described the 'tyranny of the acute' (13). In the 1990s, he spearheaded the development of the Chronic Care Model, which promotes high-quality health and community systems with well-developed organizations and tools to create productive interactions between an informed provider and an engaged patient leading to better health outcomes. This model has been adapted by several countries including Canada, the UK, Holland, Spain, and Russia (14) as an improved approach to chronic disease management. The graphic developed for use in Canada is shown in Figure 14.1. Each of the elements in this model can be adapted to meet the needs of migrant populations (see also Tables 14.1 and 14.2 for details).

Supporting self-management is the Chronic Care Model attributed most linked to achieving success with chronic disease management (16). Unlike traditional patient education techniques, self-management teaches problem-solving skills targeted to the individual and fosters self-efficacy — the belief in one's ability to make behaviour change. In a qualitative evaluation of self-management attitudes amongst Vietnamese, African American, Caucasian,

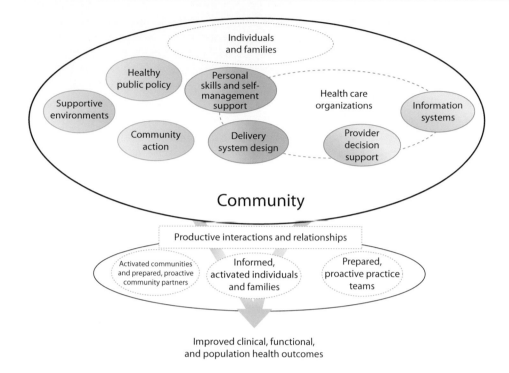

FIGURE 14.1 The expanded Chronic Care Model.

and Latino patients with chronic disease, Shaw et al. found that low health literacy and cultural beliefs serve as barriers to effective self-care regimes (7).

Models of self-management education, such as the Stanford model and the Expert Patient programme, use both peers and professionals to empower patients and give them the skills they need to manage their health. These models can be adapted to migrant populations successfully and have been shown to make a difference in both behaviour and health outcomes (17).

CASE STUDY

Maria is a 55-year-old woman from Colombia who has been living with diabetes for the last 10 years. Recently, it has been more difficult to maintain her sugar levels and Maria became disheartened. She joined a 6-week self-management group run by a Spanish-speaking community health worker. By the end of the programme, she had learned much more about how foods affect her sugar levels and that if she went for a walk after dinner, she could prevent her typical evening high levels. She buddied with another woman in her neighbourhood to help motivate her. Maria lost 5 kg and was able to lower her HbA1c.

Peer support is frequently cited in the literature as an effective way to build self-management skills. Peers are people of the same culture with or without the diseases and can be paired with health professionals, such as nurses, to bring united and relevant messages and support about living with chronic disease. Peer-led support groups have been shown to be very effective in creating behaviour change as well as some impact on clinical outcomes such as lowering HbA1c (18).

Behaviour change associated with living with chronic disease often takes multiple encounters before the patient is willing and able to adopt them. Expecting an individual to change something that brings them pleasure or stress relief is likely to be met with resistance even when they know it is harmful (think of a personal example…). Rather than chastizing or using scare tactics, exploring their personal challenges with making changes will reduce frustration on both sides, strengthen the relationship, and allow for practical problem solving. Motivational interviewing is a goal-oriented and patient-centred counselling technique that encourages behaviour change through resolving ambivalence. It is a skill set that is easily learned by a wide range of professionals, and works cross-culturally (18).

TABLE 14.1   Elements of the Chronic Care Model with examples

CCM element	Examples
Delivery system design: delivery of effective, efficient clinical care and self-management support	• Team-based care – team composition should be based on patient need and should include mental health support, settlement workers, or culturally specific community health workers. Diversity of staff will enrich the team. • Language support with professional interpreters. • Ensuring appointments are available when people need them. • Exploring access strategies that do not require the patient to come in. • Develop a continuing quality improvement approach. • Include patient's representative of the practice population in the practice design. • Outreach and access strategies to bring care to those most in need.
Decision support: promote clinical care that is consistent with scientific evidence and patient preference	• Clinical guidelines embedded into electronic health record. • Initial visit screening templates. • Comparative tables of medications and their costs. • Opportunities for inter-professional care conferences.
Clinical information systems: organize patient and population data to facilitate efficient and effective care	• Collecting and reviewing data to understand the practice population, e.g. levels of insurance, ethnocentric info, migration status, prevalence of chronic diseases. • Electronic health records that facilitate communication between team members. • Repositories of community resource information.
Self-management support: empower and prepare patients to manage their health and health care	• Culturally adapted tools and education. • Peer-led programmes. • Self-management support training such as motivational interviewing for providers and teams.
The community: mobilize community resources to meet needs of patients	• Cultural and faith-based organizations. • Mental health case management. • Community based self-management programmes. • Physical activity and cooking groups. • Social supports such as food banks and language classes.

Source: Chronic Care Model - Model Elements. n.d. Retrieved from Improving Chronic Illness Care: http://www.improvingchroniccare.org/index.php?p=Model_Elements&s=18 (15)

TABLE 14.2 Macro, meso, and micro examples of prevention activities

Level of interaction	Examples
On the patient level (micro)	• Consistent screening for risk factors • Repeated non-judgmental messaging around importance and benefits of change • Linking behaviour change to symptom improvement and overall well-being • Offering referrals and support with behaviour change
On a practice level (meso)	• Collecting data on risk factors in the practice population • Culturally appropriate health promotion materials in waiting rooms and other frequented places • Developing culturally/language appropriate group programmes that meet the need of the practice population, such as walking groups, cooking classes, and smoking cessation programmes
On a systems level (macro)	• Advocating for cultural adaptation of health promotion programmes • Community based research demonstrating effectiveness of prevention programmes in migrant populations • Working with cultural groups to develop meaningful messaging

EMPHASIZING PREVENTION

CASE STUDY

Rohinder is a 35-year-old man from India complaining of low back pain. He says he is otherwise completely healthy and is only looking for something for pain. He has a BMI of 35 and is a smoker.

In primary health care, there is immeasurable potential to reduce the swelling tide of chronic disease. By reducing modifiable risk factors, the vast majority of conditions such as diabetes, heart disease, and COPD can be prevented. Unfortunately, prevention programmes and services tend to be underemphasized and underfunded. Considering that unhealthy habits and modifiable risk factors such as smoking and obesity increase the longer newcomers live in North America (19), it is clear that there needs to be a shift towards putting more energy and resources to upstream initiatives. It can be helpful to approach prevention from a macro-, meso-, and microperspective.

CONCLUSION

Chronic disease prevention and management is as vital to the health of migrants as it is to the native-born population. This means shifting the approach to care and adapting tools and services to meet the needs of the individuals and the communities they live in. The importance of an effective patient-provider relationship has been strongly emphasized throughout this chapter, as it is essential in supporting people with the ongoing management of their health. When working with migrants, building this relationship means taking time to understand their perspective on health, current and previous life circumstances, and how these factors affect their well-being and what they most need from the provider and the team.

It is important to realize the inequity many migrants face in managing their illness. Considering that migrants are over-represented in low-income and underemployed populations and struggle with many of the social determinants of health, there needs to be cross-sectoral partnership and advocacy, and with intentional effort to provide access to culturally appropriate, person-centred team-based primary health care, the inequities experienced can be significantly reduced.

REFERENCES

1. WHO. Noncommunicable Diseases. Retrieved from http://www.who.int/news-room/factsheets/detail/noncommunicable-diseases 2018, June 1.
2. WHO. Global Health Observatory Data. Noncommunicable diseases (NCD). 2018. Retrieved from http://www.who.int/gho/ncd/en/
3. Amra HA. Noncommunicable disease among urban refugees and asylum-seekers in developing countries: a neglected health care need. *Global Health*. 2014;10:24.
4. Creatore MI, Moineddin R et al. Age- and sex-related prevalence of diabetes mellitus among immigrants to Ontario, Canada. *CMAJ*. 2010;182(8):781–9.
5. Keon WJ. *A Healthy, Productive Canada: A Determinant of Health Approach*. Ottawa: The Standing Senate Committee on Social Affairs, Science and Technology Final Report of Senate Subcommittee on Population Health; 2009.
6. Shakya YB. *Addressing Racialised Disparities in Access to Health Care and Quality of Care: A Literature Review*. Toronto: Access Alliance Multicultural Health and Community Services, The Wellesley Institute; 2007.
7. Shaw SJ. The role of culture in health literacy and chronic disease screening and management. *J Immigr Minor Health*. 2009;11(6):460–7.
8. Heerman WJ, Wills MJ. Adopting models of chronic care to provide effective diabetes care for refugees. *Clin Diabetes*. 2011;29(3):90–5.
9. Changani KP. Hypertension beliefs and practice among South Asian immigrants: a focus group study. *J Immigr Refug Stud*. 2011;9:98–103.
10. Chapman DP, Perry GS, Strine TW. The vital link between chronic disease and depressive disorders. *Prev Chronic Dis*. 2005;2(1):A14.
11. Kubzansky LD, Koenen KC. Is post-traumatic stress disorder related to development of heart disease? *Future Cardiol*. 2007;3(2):153–6.
12. Centers for Disease Control and Prevention. *Latent Tuberculosis Infection: A Guide for Primary Health Care Providers*. Global Tuberculosis Institute, National Center for HIV Viral Hepatitis STD and TB Prevention. New Jersey Medical School, Rutgers, The State University of New Jersey; 2013.
13. Bodenheimer T, Wagner EH, Grumbach K. Improving primary care for patients with chronic illness: the Chronic Care Model, Part 2. *JAMA*. 2002;288(15):1909–14.
14. Improving Chronic Illness Care. Retrieved from http://www.improvingchroniccare.org/index.php?p=About_US&s=6
15. Chronic Care Model - Model Elements. n.d. Retrieved from Improving Chronic Illness Care: http://www.improvingchroniccare.org/index.php?p=Model_Elements&s=18
16. Chen RAA. *Chronic Disease Self-Management Support Strategies for Ethnic Minorities: A Systematic Review*. Toronto; 2017.
17. Babamoto KS, Sey KA et al. Improving diabetes care and health measures among Hispanics using community health workers: results from a randomized controlled trial. *Health Educ Behav*. 2009;6(1):113–26.
18. Hettema J, Steele J, Miller WR. Motivational interviewing. *Annu Rev Clin Psychol*. 2005;1:91–111.
19. Koya, DL, Egede LE. Association between length of residence and cardiovascular disease risk factors among an ethnically diverse group of United States Immigrants. *J Gen Intern Med*. 2007;22(6):841–6.

CHAPTER 15

Understanding unexplained and complex symptoms and diseases

Morten Sodemann

LEARNING OBJECTIVES

In this chapter the reader will learn:

- The benefits of obtaining a full clinical history and that core concepts of body, mind, disease, and health are not universal and therefore require to be decoded
- To improve the understanding of health care professionals when meeting a patient with complex symptoms and diseases
- Examples of important symptoms and disease groups that are easily misdiagnosed, overlooked, or ignored
- Tools to discuss and assess health complaints that are awkward or strange

---

CLINICAL VIGNETTE

A 46-year-old woman from a country in West Africa is referred to a medical emergency ward with 4 years of muscle stiffness, as well as universal and rapid onset of muscle fatigue even with light exercise. She also describes bilateral pain in the thigh muscles, shoulders, and upper arms. The patient's mother and two siblings have similar symptoms. The patient arrived in Denmark through family reunification to the spouse (who came earlier as a political refugee) in 2009. She has given birth to five children, of whom three are in Denmark. The oldest of her children is now 41 years old, the second-oldest is 38 years old, and the youngest is 18 years old.

She also suffers from obesity, type 2 diabetes, and hypertension and is on treatment with insulin injections, two types of antidiabetic tablet medicines, an antihypertensive drug, and a cholesterol-lowering drug.

For a number of years, her family doctor has tried to motivate the patient to lose weight, but without success. The patient states that muscle fatigue prevents her from walking more than 4–5 minutes and attempting to use a training centre had to be abandoned for the same reason. The patient has been seen several times at the emergency ward with similar symptoms. Specialist doctors in rheumatology have assessed the patient and suggested that the patient should stop taking the cholesterol-reducing drug, as this is the most likely cause for the patient's symptoms. This has not helped, and the family physician has given up further clinical investigations and suggests that the patient has 'ethnic pains' and premenopausal symptoms.

The patient does not speak very much Danish. She speaks a language for which there are only one or two interpreters in Denmark, so her own doctor has tried without interpreter or through her husband, who has limited English proficiency. The 18-year-old son, who goes to high school, has occasionally served as an interpreter and driver, but he has exams and is unable to interpret. The patient is illiterate and has difficulty understanding clinical findings, investigations, and treatment.

CULTURE AND HEALTH

Over 200 culture-related syndromes, also referred to as ethnic psychoses or atypical culture-bound reactive syndromes, have been documented (1). Distinguishing between essentially very rare culture-bound syndromes and frequently misunderstood patient symptoms is a challenge to any medical doctor. Culture-specific diagnoses cover a dissimilar group of illnesses whose syndrome constellations are unique to certain cultural groups (2). While general medical conditions which localize to certain geographic regions or genetic groups have been historically included with the culture-specific diagnoses, the term is now primarily used to refer to mental health conditions. As early as the eighteenth century, scientists were identifying differences in illnesses based on the geographic origin of the sufferer. In 1733, George Cheyne, a Scottish physician practicing in England, wrote of disorders which he felt were more common amongst the English in *The English Malady* (3). He attributed these disorders of low spirit, nervous distempers, melancholy, and hypochondria to the cultural factors of poor diet, 'manner of living', and geographic factors including weather. By the late nineteenth century, the now famous Malaysian-specific disorders of *amok* and *latah* were identified by W. Gilmore Ellis (3). For a full list of culture-bound syndromes, see Smith (3). For a number of reasons, doctors tend to overinterpret unusual presentations of normal diseases as cultural expressions, rare tropical diseases, medically unexplained symptoms, or a functional disorder.

DECISION MAKING IN THE CONSULTATION

Doctors usually apply epidemiological evidence in individual contexts but fail to incorporate information about the individual into the clinical decision-making process and thereby enhance the marginalization of migrants in doctor-patient interviews. It has also been shown that the doctor's differential diagnostic considerations are highly influenced by the doctor's perception of the patient's migrant background. Furthermore, physicians feel more sure about their diagnosis when the patient has a higher education. A study of doctors' decision-making processes showed that the more diagnostic or treatment options doctors face, the more uncertain they become and the more likely they are to choose not to treat or to choose the simplest treatment or a secure 'conservative' diagnosis.

The combined influence of language barriers and cognitive biases is a disadvantage to migrant patients who lack the communicative strength to challenge the clinical and psychosocial generalizations that they experience. The result is that symptoms are misdiagnosed or ignored, and remain 'unexplained' from the patient's point of view. Migrant patients can easily end up with a 'culture bound' chronic non-malignant pain syndrome mixed with medically unexplained symptoms that are interpreted with stigmatizing and counterproductive terms such as 'cultural expressions' or 'ethnic pain'. Medical staff may tend to construct typical illnesses that are presumably typical in migrants, such as *morbus Bosphorus* (the infamous 'Mamma mia syndrome'), *ganzkörperschmerz* (pain all over the whole body), or g*astarbeiter ulkus* (migrant workers' ulcus; referring to the higher incidence of ulcers in migrant workers) (4). The well-attested emergence of stereotypes concerning migrants' health that developed from the 1970s onwards lead to a widespread stigmatization of migrants' illness, a perception that has complicated clinical decision making by prematurely assigning meaningless labels to complex expressions of bodily distress and trauma (5,6). The reference to the patient's 'foreign,' 'exotic,' 'unfamiliar' culture hides the fact that an unbiased treatment of a specific patient might not be the intention of health care workers or is regarded to be too difficult — intercultural problems might easily turn out to be problems of hierarchies or social difference.

DIFFERENCES IN PRESENTATION OF DISEASE, DIAGNOSTIC PROCEDURES, AND TREATMENTS

The relationship between migrant background and health is usually attributed to three explanations: (i) a biological explanation (differences in genetics, differences in infections), (ii) a psychological explanation (adaptation, integration, stress, trauma, minority status, residence, language acquisition), and (iii) an environmental explanation (social networking, socioeconomic status, linguistic exposure) (Chapter 2). However, informal and structural barriers in access to health care for migrant patients and inequality in treatment to these patients compared to majority patients apparently play an equal role in unfavourable health outcomes for migrants in most societies (Chapter 6). Furthermore, there are virtually no available studies to explain why the quality of hospital treatment is so much lower for migrant patients, and there is not even a basis for finding out what the possible barriers include (7).

Expressions of somatization vary widely between ethnic groups, partly because of different ways of expressing illness and symptoms, but social and educational factors also play a role (8,9). Physical symptoms are frequent in primary care among some migrant groups, especially among trauma survivors, including those who have experienced sexual abuse (10,11). These symptoms continue or even get worse during the course of medical investigations — the sometimes ambiguous results, provoking even more blood tests, endoscopies, and CT scans, leading the patient into a slippery slope involving serial medical and surgical procedures and frustrating random attempts at diagnosis and care often ending in a multi-drug challenge with financial implications. In such cases, the symptoms may be considered fulminant, provoking patient anxiety and physician stress. Patients' symptoms often become milder or disappear when the focus of the clinical process is shifted from invasive procedures to patient education and support for coping with their bodily experiences.

Patients may have difficulty talking about certain subjects if the doctor does not bring them up or make it clear that it is permissible to talk about other subjects, and doctors often do not know the unwritten rules or silent messages from nonverbal signs, as they normally would when it comes to majority patients. Sexual abuse history or other trauma such as war, torture, or disasters have often been overlooked during the acute phase, and as long as the patient is not aware of the link between psychological trauma or physical abuse and subsequent bodily sensations, the vicious circle will continue. Atypical depression, severe anxiety disorders, or some personality disorders and atypical schizophrenia are often not considered, but can present in the same way. Somatic investigation may evoke these past traumas. Clinical management should consider a shift away from continuing clinical investigations to adaptation, normalization, and cognitive training (12).

It is a self-understanding among doctors, and an expectation of the patients, that doctors evaluate patients objectively and without prejudice, using biomedical observations from the physical exam combined with blood tests and other paraclinical investigations to diagnose and set up a treatment plan. Unfortunately, a large number of studies indicate that this is not the case (13,14). Van Ryn has published a review of studies documenting discrimination and/ or treatment choices that lack medical foundation: osteoporosis treatment and prevention, smoking cessation, alcohol overuse, mammography, breastfeeding, pain management, referral to dialysis, cardiac surgery, renal transplantation, and psychiatric treatment (15). Others have confirmed that physician uncertainty in diagnostic processes, choice of clinical investigations, and treatment were more frequent in migrant patients (16,17). Patients with language barriers get more blood samples and other tests ordered than majority patients, resulting in longer hospital stays (Chapter 6). Differences are diagnosis dependent, so that patients with language barriers who present abdominal pain trigger a CT scan of the stomach three times more frequently than language proficient patients with abdominal pain, while there was no difference in frequencies of chest pain (18).

Some studies indicate that migrants often struggle to understand the meaning of medical encounters, and while some patients are comforted by the idea of a connection between body and mind, others become even more anxious when presented with the idea that their physical body sensations may stem from poor mental health, trauma, isolation, depression, or grief (19) (Chapter 2).

Even in the case of common chronic diseases that are strictly regulated by guidelines and evidence, such as cardiovascular illness and diabetes, management and outcome seem to vary both by country of origin and by recipient country (20–23). Some migrant groups have higher mortality rates from diabetes and cardiovascular illness but also higher mortality from certain cancers and infectious diseases (24–27). Social determinants seem to play a strong role in these differences, but availability of data across countries and migrant groups is lacking in many countries (24,28).

THE GREAT MIMIC: POST-TRAUMATIC STRESS SYNDROME

Post-traumatic stress syndrome (PTSD) is often overlooked or misdiagnosed in medical and psychiatric care, where comorbidity of PTSD and other psychiatric diagnoses is particularly frequent (29) (Chapter 17). The combination of life threat and traumatic loss may be particularly undermining to the psychological well-being of refugees, and consequent comorbidity of PTSD and depression may be associated with longer-term psychosocial dysfunction (30,31).

PTSD can be expressed as universal neurogenic pains (6), and some of these patients are likely to misdiagnosed as somatization and therefore not offered relevant treatment.

On the other hand, pain can wrongfully be ascribed to diagnosed PTSD, thereby overlooking cancer, cardiovascular disease, or rheumatic illnesses. Clinicians should screen all torture survivors for depression as well as for generalized anxiety and PTSD. Torture survivors rarely suffer from factitious diseases or somatization disorders. However, their somatic symptoms are usually culture-specific expressions of emotional distress; for example, an underlying depression (32). A large Canadian population study with almost 37,000 people showed that a PTSD diagnosis (corrected for socioeconomic factors, other mental illnesses) was significantly correlated with increased risk of cardiovascular disease, pulmonary disease, chronic pain conditions, gastrointestinal diseases, and cancer. The PTSD diagnosis was also associated with suicide risk, physical and mental disability, and low quality of life (33). Misdiagnosed or overlooked PTSD comorbidity seems to be a frequent experience among migrant patients, especially refugees.

Worldwide deaths from occupational injuries have fallen, but at the same time have increased among migrants (34). Occupational hazards are often not reported because of lack of knowledge or symptoms are discarded as 'cultural expressions' of job fatigue. These occupational cases have frequently been misdiagnosed as somatization. There seems to be a link between PTSD and risk of occupational diseases or accidents in a vicious circle, where PTSD patients suffering from dissociation or flashbacks are more prone to accidental exposures that lead to long-term sick leaves and loss of job.

CONSEQUENCES OF THE PRACTITIONER'S CROSS-CULTURAL CLINICAL SKILLS AND COMPETENCIES FOR THE PATIENT

Physicians find it difficult to distinguish patient's somatic complaints from social needs, and indicate this as a reason for experiencing difficult contact with a patient. The patient's illness concepts and ideas about healthy living might be difficult to grasp for the doctor because of cultural and language barriers. Doctors often complain that migrant patients compromise communication because they, from a physician point of view, present their symptoms in an excessive or exaggerated manner. A Dutch analysis of migrant differences in patient safety found that all reported patient safety breaches involving patients with language barriers were due to administrative and professional failure: (i) inappropriate response to obvious barriers (language) and obvious risk factors (country of origin, trauma, genetics); (ii) misunderstandings between patient and therapist due to obvious differences in disease experience, information level, and expectations for treatment; and (iii) inappropriate treatment due to the therapist's biased perception of patient needs and behaviour and stereotypical notions of patient response patterns (35).

The consequence of low-quality bilingual clinical communication is that patients do not understand the diagnostic or treatment plan and are unable to follow it (Chapter 20). Patients with language barriers often have inadequate understanding of their diagnosis, the medication they receive, what the treatment plan is, and whether there is need for follow-up checks at the hospital (36). In a study of patient uptake of information after a medical consultation at the emergency medical department in a hospital, 61% of the migrant patients were unable to recall or explain the diagnosis, treatment, or plan for follow-up — this was a problem for 41% of majority patients (36).

If it is not taken into account, language barriers affect the doctor's way of recording sickness history and make it difficult to have a coherent story that makes sense for medical purposes and often ends with many gaps in the information that can lead to erroneous diagnoses. Diseases whose diagnosis may be difficult due to the fact that many organs are or can be involved and develop over many years are diagnosed very rarely among migrants (37). These disease entities risk being stereotyped, as the previously described unexplained diffuse culturally bound symptoms and syndromes. Table 15.1 presents some examples of common blind spots in communication involving patients with language barriers.

In a study from The Migrant Health Clinic at Odense University Hospital, nearly a third of the referred patients had social, economic, or mental problems of central importance

TABLE 15.1 Selected examples of common blind spots in communication involving patients with language barriers

Patient factor	Medical consequence and/or background
Learning the rules and playing the game: Adopting doctor's social codes and acquiring health professional's language. Afraid of the doctor and afraid to stress or annoy the doctor. Only offers the physician information on a need-to-know basis. Patients will go very far to avoid (what is perceived as) humiliation. Assumptions about the doctor's ability to understand health complaints. Respects, but does not trust the doctor.	Only present one symptom and just ask one question. No interaction, no response, no information – or only 'neutral' information exchange out of fear that the doctor will not understand the problem or situation – better to be silent than exhibit vulnerability, as the doctor (maybe) may trivialize concerns, which feels humiliating. Hesitates to take up difficult sensitive issues. Patient willing to change and model their story, omit information, highlight 'favourable', and suppress 'dangerous' information, etc. Accept an unwanted clinical exam or treatment. In many cultures respect for doctors is taken for granted but trust only if they really help – no help, no trust, which can be confusing for some doctors who mistake the respect for patient acceptance of their plan and skills. No spontaneous information given. Holds back important clinical information.
Illness symptoms and disease concepts. Concepts of illness are coded and rooted in maternal language and perceived in a different social context and mindset.	Has difficulty explaining symptoms to the doctor and might completely avoid mentioning it to the doctor (hot/warm syndromes, Koro syndrome, Jinn, etc.). Bilingual patients often need interpreters to help when they obtain an illness because concepts of illness are rooted and formed in childhood in the maternal language. Conversation too simple with low content in second language. Important details are omitted or missed. Clinical history lacks detail.
Shame, fear, stigma, and taboo. Shameful about his/her second language skills. Shameful to ask for an interpreter. Shame about the health problem and does not dare mention it to the doctor (or stigma related). Shame about poverty/financial situation. Believes that it is not acceptable to have detailed knowledge of body parts, their functions and excretions. Mental illness is a handicap or a taboo. Fears stigma and social isolation.	Simple health complaints or serious warning signs are not mentioned (incontinence, blood in urine, diarrhoea, weight loss, coughing [TB stigma]). Socioeconomic reasons for compliance issues are overlooked (cannot afford medication). Talk about organs such 'kidneys', 'liver', or 'gallbladder' does not make sense. Patient is uncomfortable discussing diseases arising in kidneys, urine, bladder, and reproductive organs. Will not mention or discuss mental health issues, does not want psychiatric evaluation or medication.

to their symptoms or disorders, compliance failure, or an unexplained chronic condition. Every fourth patient had an overlooked significant health condition, while every fifth had a condition that was misjudged or misinterpreted (38). Besides the fact that language barriers, low health literacy, and simple lack of knowledge constitute the core of impaired access to quality hospital care, several unexpected issues of clinical importance emerged.

Over 65% of the patients referred suffered from chronic PTSD and 75% had not previously been diagnosed with the condition. The effect of PTSD on several cognitive functions including sleep, memory, and ability to concentrate, understand and combine information seems to impair language acquisition, empowerment, and compliance to such an extent that it explains most of the compliance issues these patients experience when they contract a chronic disease like diabetes, HIV, or hypertension. PTSD and the related conditions impair compliance and health literacy during the entire process from healthy to sick by delaying seeking help, introducing doctor delay because of misinterpretation of symptoms, cancelled investigations (blood tests, colonoscopies, MR scans, and x-rays) because they remind patients of previous trauma, refusal of life-saving treatment because of fear of side effects, and lack of follow-up because of lack of knowledge of its value. These effects are boosted by overall anxiety, mistrust in the health care system, and insecurity about their residence status in the country. Finally, these patients are characterized by loneliness and very small social networks that offer little support in the case of illness. Increasing compliance and improving care for these patients require new competencies that include collaboration with other specialties and tailor-made patient information and follow-up.

The clinical vignette presented at the beginning of this chapter is a good example of the complexity in communication, diagnosis, and treatment in the encounter between migrants and the health care system.

On examination the female patient in the clinical vignette in the beginning of this chapter had obvious difficulties mobilizing from a chair, and a physical examination showed clear signs of quadriceps muscle atrophy. The patient was referred to a dietician with an interpreter but in spite of this she didn't lose weight. It turned out that the patient eats at night because she suffers from sleeplessness due to nightmares, and food gives her peace of mind and relieves her anxiety. She was subjected to severe psychological trauma in her home country, information she had never shared with her husband, and she had subsequently developed symptoms of PTSD. She was referred to a treatment centre for trauma and torture survivors and put on relevant supportive medical treatment.

The patient was referred to rheumatological for reassessment because blood tests indicated decay of muscle fibres. A muscle biopsy showed signs of polymyositis, which is a good explanation for her significant muscle fatigue, and the patient was put on relevant medical treatment.

Finally, the patient and her husband were asked to explain the observation that some of her children were 'too old' for her age – she would have been 4 years old when she had her first child. The husband admitted that he did not know his wife's birthday so he just put a random date and birth year on the application for family reunification. The patient investigated the matter in her home country and discovered that she was actually 67 years old – and therefore entitled to old age pension, a fact that may also have contributed to her physical function level.

Sparse and inadequate cultural competences among health care workers have been documented in virtually all European countries (39). It is well-founded that patients who have experienced discrimination based on their migrant origin or distrust the health care system more often fail hospital appointments, more often choose to stop medical treatment or clinical investigations, and wait longer to collect their prescription medicine (40,41).

Diseases that vary in intensity or present with several different symptoms such as asthma, rheumatoid arthritis, or inflammatory bowel disease, are underreported among migrants. Hemoglobinopathies are often overlooked because they are considered to be rare, but in fact they are frequent among migrants in Europe: a Dutch study found 16% positive among pregnant migrant women (42,43). Furthermore, foci with particularly high prevalence among migrants have been detected in London, Copenhagen, Paris, Brussels, and Madrid (44). Undetected heterozygotic thalassemias with low-grade anaemia and hepatitis B carrier status can be expressed as fatigue, and universal low-grade pains just as pronounced vitamin D deficiency.

Other not so prevalent diseases like systemic lupus erythematosus are also underdiagnosed among some groups of migrants (45). Familial Mediterranean fever (hereditary polyserositis) is frequently a challenge to clinicians unfamiliar with the hereditary syndrome. The fever syndrome has been shown to be as frequent among migrants as in their home countries, with a prevalence of 173/100,000 among Turkish migrants and 124/100,000 among Lebanese migrants living in Sweden (46). It is commonly mistaken for 'cultural pain expression', juvenile rheumatic arthritis, somatization, atypical depression, polyarthritis, low chest pain, appendicitis, acute cholecystitis, dissecting aortic aneurysm, or rheumatic fever (47). The syndrome most often presents during childhood but if overlooked it can be a frequent cause of multiple emergency hospitalizations and anxiety.

A clear but unintended spinoff of the increasing specialization in hospital care is that migrant patients seem to end up as a group of patients in no-man's land — they are too complex and time-consuming for the general practitioner and they are often too complex, with more than one chronic disease, and time-consuming for a highly specialized hospital department. This is a general tendency seen among a growing number of marginalized vulnerable patients with low school education and low socioeconomic status, but the effect is boosted by language problems and low health literacy leading to increasing inequity in hospital care among ethnic minorities.

SOME PRACTICAL TOOLS

The clinical problems encountered when meeting migrants with complex presentation of diseases at The Migrant Health Clinic at Odense University Hospital fall into four groups (Table 15.2): (i) misinterpreted symptoms, (ii) overlooked symptoms, (iii) diagnoses that require special clinical competencies, and (iv) severe or complex compliance issues (48). A group of stigmatizing conditions of clinical importance has evolved over time: mental illness, previous child soldiers with personality disorders, women raped in hospital settings, men who have been raped or sexually tortured, patients tortured by medical doctors, urine incontinence (seen as a handicap, incontinence means you are not clean and therefore not allowed to pray), physical handicaps (shame and guilt), and sexual dysfunction (affects gender roles and hence empowerment in case of chronic illness).

Some of the tools to avoid misdiagnoses and other pitfalls are presented in Table 15.3. Medical doctors often fail to involve patients' experiences, trauma, surgical procedures, exposures, and occupational history prior to their arrival in the new country in the diagnostic and clinical decision making. Doctors should acquire basic cultural competencies and knowledge about the clinical relevance in a somatic context of how PTSD and depression affect memory and concentration and hence affects compliance in the case of chronic illness and overall care-seeking behaviour. Doctors can also improve patient compliance by trying

TABLE 15.2 Types of clinical problems encountered with examples[a]

Misinterpreted symptoms	Overlooked symptoms or health problems	Diagnoses that required specialized clinical competencies	Severe or complex compliance issues
Allergic sinusitis or tooth abscess (thought to be migraine)	PTSD (with or without secondary personality disorders)	Hemoglobinopathies Certain parasitical infections Chronic hepatitis	Refusal of MR scan because of previous incarceration or concealment in small rooms during war
Asthma (thought to be cultural symptoms without physical cause)	Schizophrenia Borderline personality disorders Adults who experienced adverse events/abuse in childhood	PTSD with somatic comorbidity (metabolic syndrome)	Refusal of colonoscopy because of exposure to similar sexual torture
PTSD (thought to be fibromyalgia or chronic fatigue syndrome) Neurogenic pain in PTSD (thought to be carpal tunnel syndrome)	Atypical anxiety disorders Sleep disorders	Tuberculosis in other organs than the lungs	Refusal of gynaecological exam because of previous rape in hospital settings
Lactose intolerance (thought to be cultural symptoms without physical cause)	Tuberculosis of the spine	Somatic illness in previous child soldiers, Khat abuse, and some personality disorders	Perceived premature ageing reduces motivation and empowerment
Tinnitus (thought to be schizophrenia) Myocardial ischaemia (interpreted as muscle ache)		Previous exposure to grenade explosions with metal splinters, brain damage, hearing loss, or substandard trauma surgery	Extensive social problems (residence, economy, children sick)
Impaired renal function (thought to be low compliance in treatment of hypertension)	Work-related conditions	Panic attacks, severe anxiety	Refusal to receive chemotherapy with severe side effects because of lacking information
Myocardial ischaemia (thought to be tiredness related to depression)	Failure to obtain clinical and exposure history during time in home country	Specific somatic consequences of certain methods in torture (such as falanga, electric torture, hanging by arms)	Refusal to receive life-saving treatment because of side effects (HIV, connective tissue disorders, cancer, surgery, diabetes)
Brain tumour or cerebral infarction (interpreted as altered personality or 'cultural inertia') Bone metastases (interpreted as 'ethnic pain')		Genetic disorders and physical handicaps (offering information misinterpreted as mutual understanding of disorder and consequences)	Chronic grieving (interpreted as temporary distress)
Connective tissue disorders (rheumatoid arthritis interpreted as 'cultural pain expression')	Connective tissue disorders	Familial Mediterranean fever (interpreted as psychosomatic pain)	Patient's/relatives' selective focus on normal blood tests or investigations in an otherwise severe condition (genetic disorder, cancer)

[a] 560 patients seen at the Migrant Health Clinic, Odense University Hospital, Denmark, 2008–2011.

TABLE 15.3 Tools to avoid or overcome difficulties in complex clinical problems with migrant patients

Misinterpreted symptoms	Think 'normal': most likely an abnormal presentation of a frequent condition.	Aim to identify diagnoses within the biomedical mindset.	'Culture', 'ethnicity', or 'strangeness' are not diagnoses or valid explanations	Develop cross-cultural communicative skills to avoid 'culturalization'	
Overlooked symptoms or health problems	Language barriers are actual barriers and need special attention	Doctors are familiar with certain expressions of symptoms but not all	Faced with a 'new' way of expressing symptoms, doctors discard them as strange or attribute them to situational/cultural factors	Think 'normal'	
Diagnoses that required specialized clinical competencies	Obtain basic knowledge of diseases that are common in the main countries of origin	Obtain knowledge about the pitfalls and sensitivities in basic genetic counselling or ask for advice with experts in the field	Understand the special circumstances surrounding physical handicaps in many cultures	Develop a set of appropriate questions to probe knowledge, attitudes, and practices regarding torture, handicaps, and genetic disorders	
Severe or complex compliance issues	Never take no for an answer – 'no' is the safe answer for an anxious, uninformed patient	What has the patient understood? What are the patient's worries? Any misconceptions?	The concept of risk is difficult for patients with low school education	The eagerness to inform patients can sometimes overload them and make them suspicious	Shame can prevent patients from revealing hidden burdens of treatment (poverty, isolation)

to understand family decision-making processes about illness perception, priorities, and medicine (Chapter 11). Having cross-cultural conversations involving medical interpreters is a challenge, but doctors should pay attention to words and concepts that are difficult to translate directly and should allow time for interpreters to explain complex concepts to patients. It is advisable to instruct the interpreter about the frame and goal of the conversation so the interpreter can, for example, help build up the plan, an explanation, or advice.

Doctors can sometimes inadvertently trivialize problems that patients see as disasters, and this discrepancy can easily be lost in bilingual communication. Likewise, doctors can communicate in a way that sounds as stigmatizing values and opinions when translated. The patient may, without the doctor knowing, feel undeserving or unworthy of the doctor's attention, or the patient may feel blamed, or that his/her symptoms are ignored. It is essential that doctors check how messages and information are received by the patient through fairly direct questions and without assumptions. The doctor has to be very clear about crucial points and conclusions as the flow of a conversation is deeply rooted in culture: some cultures are straightforward in giving difficult information, while a serious diagnosis in other cultures should be mentioned very discretely and indirectly. The meaning of pauses can also be culturally bound. The essence is to ask and listen instead of carrying on with clinical routines.

The framework the clinician sets up for the clinical encounter with migrant patients is crucial to the patient's motivation to talk about actual and difficult problems, and how detailed/sensitive information the doctor receives. If the patient has the experience that doctors are uninterested in their social or psychological challenges as a minority with language barriers, they are less communicative – even with relevant information. The communication frame is created by actively engaging the psychosocial conditions and earlier experiences of migrant patients in the clinical decision process. The patient should be invited to discuss the doctor's observations and to clarify uncertainties about unfamiliar cultural values and habits. Attempts at generalization without involving the patient should be avoided, as this creates mistrust and patient withdrawal. Respect for the individual's preconditions without cognitive bias or assumptions, clarification of ambiguities and doubt, active involvement of the life story in patient information, and a more liberal use of interpreter assistance are the pillars of a professional doctor-patient encounter with language barriers. The interpreter should be seen as the only person who has the key to a sensible cross-cultural contact that makes clinical sense and motivates the patient to disclose all relevant information, including the most private traumas and challenges. The interpreter is a cultural ambassador and mediator, not just an interpreting 'machine'. Ensuring that the patient understands given information and plans at the end of the conversation should be standard. Prejudice, convenient assumptions, and guesswork are the causes for most misunderstandings and inappropriate patient investigations. Express your doubts, create trust, obtain eye contact, be curious, and let a wider understanding of the individual patient's hidden burdens and survival strategies as a refugee or any other migrant become a clinical instrument and a health education tool.

Establishing contact, trust, and a mutual understanding of the patient's health complaints requires interpreter assistance because illness concepts, coding of values, and perceptions of bodily sensations are rooted in the maternal language. This may be even more important to remember in communication with the bilingual patient who may have a work-related second language but is often poorly equipped for complex narratives, unspecific mental health issues, or distinctions between physical and mental symptoms.

A systematic approach where the patient is given a chance to explain and unfold deeper layers of symptoms perception is necessary. This can be done through a structured life history, a full non-exclusive list of problems including health, social, economic, minority/exile issues, residence permit, identity, and network-related challenges, and finally a family and network tree. PTSD or comparable conditions such as Disorders of Extreme Stress Not Otherwise Specified (DESNOS) and personality disorders after catastrophic or traumatic events are frequent among refugees and should be ruled out early in the clinical course. PTSD affects concentration, memory, and strategic thinking while at the same time leading to pain syndromes that need to be understood in a PTSD context if present. This can be done by a series of open questions such as: 'You come from XX country and many refugees from your country have had bad or traumatic experiences. Have you ever seen or been exposed to events that you have difficulty living with, thinking about, or discussing with other people?' Follow-up questions could include: 'Do you sleep at night?' 'Do you react strongly to sudden sounds or movements?' 'Can you watch the news on TV?' or 'Do you try to avoid certain situations that make you very uncomfortable?'

SUMMARY

Migrant patients experience barriers within health care that reduce their access to and outcome of standard care, ranging from too complex written communication to use of low-quality interpreters and lack of clinical cultural competencies among health care workers. The types of barriers include professional misinterpretation of symptoms, overlooking symptoms, lack of specialized culturally competent clinical teams, and complex compliance issues. Lack of respect for language barriers, health literacy, and functional illiteracy are key drivers of inequity. Certain health conditions associated with social stigma require special hospital attention. Medical doctors and their patients would benefit from dropping anxiety about discussing or asking about sensitive issues, guessing, and engage into trustworthy conversations. If complex patients are not offered an opportunity to describe and discuss their illness and symptom perceptions, the symptoms will become ruminating and linked to high levels of anxiety provoking diffuse sensations that medical doctors fail to understand.

REFERENCES

1. Hughes CC. Culture in clinical psychiatry. In: Gaw AC, editor. *Culture, Ethnicity, and Mental Illness.* American Psychiatric Publishing; 1993. pp. 3–41.
2. Simons RC, Hughes CC. 3 Culture-Bound Syndromes. In: Gaw AC, editor. *Culture, Ethnicity, and Mental Illness.* American Psychiatric Publishing; 1993. p. 75.
3. Smith D, Mayes T, Smith R. Culture specific diagnoses. In: Sajatovic SLM, editor. *Encyclopedia of Immigrant Health.* USA: Springer Science; 2012.
4. Kressing F. Migration and health in medical education: a work in progress report from Central Europe. *J Health Cul.* 2016;1(1):38.
5. Özkan I, Belz M. Clinical diagnosis of traumatised immigrants. *Trauma and Migration.* Springer; 2015. pp. 83–93.
6. Van der Kolk B. *The Body Keeps the Score.* New York: Viking; 2014.
7. Mladovsky P. A framework for analysing migrant health policies in Europe. *Health Policy.* 2009;93(1):55–63.
8. Aragona M, Tarsitani L, Colosimo F et al. Somatization in primary care: a comparative survey of immigrants from various ethnic groups in Rome, Italy. *Int J Psychiatry Med.* 2005;35(3):241–8.
9. Kirmayer LJ, Young A. Culture and somatization: clinical, epidemiological, and ethnographic perspectives. *Psychosom Med.* 1998;60(4):420–30.

10. Fenta H, Hyman I, Rourke SB, Moon M, Noh S. Somatic symptoms in a community sample of Ethiopian immigrants in Toronto, Canada. *Int J Cult Ment Health*. 2010;3(1):1–15.
11. Haller H, Cramer H, Lauche R, Dobos G. Somatoform disorders and medically unexplained symptoms in primary care: a systematic review and meta-analysis of prevalence. *Dtsch Ärztebl Int*. 2015;112(16):279–87.
12. Harper G, Mammen O. Fulminant somatization: medical investigation in trauma survivors. *Adolesc Psychiatr*. 2014;4(3):207–11.
13. Hooper EM, Comstock LM, Goodwin JM, Goodwin JS. Patient characteristics that influence physician behavior. *Med Care*. 1982;20(6):630–8.
14. Eisenberg JM. Sociologic influences on decision-making by clinicians. *Ann Intern Med*. 1979;90(6):957–64.
15. Van Ryn M. Research on the provider contribution to race/ethnicity disparities in medical care. *Med Care*. 2002;40(1):I-140-I-51.
16. Lutfey KE, Link CL, Marceau LD et al. Diagnostic certainty as a source of medical practice variation in coronary heart disease: results from a cross-national experiment of clinical decision making. *Med Decis Making*. 2009;29(5):606–18.
17. Næss HM. Norske pasienter og innvandrerpasienter ved et legecenter. Er det virkelig forskjeller? *Tidskrift for den Norske Lægeforening*. 1992;3(112):361–4.
18. Waxman MA, Levitt MA. Are diagnostic testing and admission rates higher in non–English-speaking versus English-speaking patients in the emergency department? *Ann Emerg Med*. 2000;36(5):456–61.
19. Bäärnhielm S, Ekblad S. Turkish migrant women encountering health care in Stockholm: a qualitative study of somatization and illness meaning. *Cult Med Psychiatry*. 2000;24(4):431–52.
20. Rafnsson SB, Bhopal RS, Agyemang C et al. Sizable variations in circulatory disease mortality by region and country of birth in six European countries. *Eur J Public Health*. 2013.
21. Rhodes P, Nocon A, Wright J. Access to diabetes services: the experiences of Bangladeshi people in Bradford, UK. *Ethn Health*. 2003;8(3):171–88.
22. Webster R. The experiences and health care needs of Asian coronary patients and their partners. Methodological issues and preliminary findings. *Nurs Crit Care*. 1997;2(5):215.
23. Jolly K, Greenfield SM, Hare R. Attendance of ethnic minority patients in cardiac rehabilitation. *J Cardiopulm Rehabil Prev*. 2004;24(5):308–12.
24. Vandenheede H, Deboosere P, Stirbu I et al. Migrant mortality from diabetes mellitus across Europe: the importance of socio-economic change. *Eur J Epidemiol*. 2012;27(2):109–17.
25. Norredam M, Olsbjerg M, Petersen JH, Juel K, Krasnik A. Inequalities in mortality among refugees and immigrants compared to native Danes–a historical prospective cohort study. *BMC Public Health*. 2012;12(1):757.
26. Norredam M, Olsbjerg M, Petersen J, Bygbjerg I, Krasnik A. Mortality from infectious diseases among refugees and immigrants compared to native Danes: a historical prospective cohort study. *Trop Med Int Health*. 2012;17(2):223–30.
27. Agyemang C, Addo J, Bhopal R, de Graft Aikins A, Stronks K. Cardiovascular disease, diabetes and established risk factors among populations of sub-Saharan African descent in Europe: a literature review. *Global Health*. 2009;5(1):7.
28. Rechel B, Mladovsky P, Ingleby D, Mackenbach JP, McKee M. Migration and health in an increasingly diverse Europe. *Lancet*. 2013;381(9873):1235–45.
29. Floen SK, Elklit A. Psychiatric diagnoses, trauma, and suicidality. *Ann Gen Psychiatry*. 2007;6(1):12.
30. Momartin S, Silove D, Manicavasagar V, Steel Z. Comorbidity of PTSD and depression: associations with trauma exposure, symptom severity and functional impairment in Bosnian refugees resettled in Australia. *J Affect Disord*. 2004;80(2):231–8.
31. Mollica RF, Sarajlić N, Chernoff M, Lavelle J, Vuković IS, Massagli MP. Longitudinal study of psychiatric symptoms, disability, mortality, and emigration among Bosnian refugees. *JAMA*. 2001;286(5):546–54.
32. Mollica RF. Surviving torture. *N Engl J Med*. 2004;351(1):5–7.
33. Sareen J, Cox BJ, Stein MB, Afifi TO, Fleet C, Asmundson GJ. Physical and mental comorbidity, disability, and suicidal behavior associated with posttraumatic stress disorder in a large community sample. *Psychosom Med*. 2007;69(3):242–0.

34. Mekkodathil A, El-Menyar A, Al-Thani H. Occupational injuries in workers from different ethnicities. *Int J Crit Illn Inj Sci*. 2016;6(1):25.
35. Suurmond J, Uiters E, de Bruijne MC, Stronks K, Essink-Bot M-L. Explaining ethnic disparities in patient safety: a qualitative analysis. *Am J Public Health*. 2010;100(S1):S113–S7.
36. Crane JA. Patient comprehension of doctor-patient communication on discharge from the emergency department. *J Emerg Med*. 1997;15(1):1–7.
37. Alegría M, Nakash O, Lapatin S et al. How missing information in diagnosis can lead to disparities in the clinical encounter. *J Public Health Manag Pract*. 2008;14(Suppl):S26.
38. Sodemann MØ, AM; Kamionka S, editor. Hospital based patient coordination for ethnic minority patients–a health technology assessment. 6th European Conference on Migrant and Ethnic Minority Health; 2016; Oslo, Norway: EUPHA Migrant section.
39. Schenk L, Ellert U, Neuhauser H, editors. *Migration und gesundheitliche Ungleichheit*. Public Health Forum; 2008: Urban & Fischer.
40. Aronson J, Burgess D, Phelan SM, Juarez L. Unhealthy interactions: the role of stereotype threat in health disparities. *Am J Public Health*. 2013;103(1):50–6.
41. Van Houtven CH, Voils CI, Oddone EZ et al. Perceived discrimination and reported delay of pharmacy prescriptions and medical tests. *J Gen Intern Med*. 2005;20(7):578–83.
42. Giordano P, Plancke A, Van Meir C et al. Carrier diagnostics and prevention of hemoglobinopathies in early pregnancy in The Netherlands: a pilot study. *Prenat Diagn*. 2006;26(8):719–24.
43. Anwar WA, Khyatti M, Hemminki K. Consanguinity and genetic diseases in North Africa and immigrants to Europe. *Eur J Public Health*. 2014;24(suppl_1):57–63.
44. Roberts I, de Montalembert M. Sickle cell disease as a paradigm of immigration hematology: new challenges for hematologists in Europe. *Haematologica*. 2007;92(7):865–71.
45. Ward MM. Education level and mortality in systemic lupus erythematosus (SLE): Evidence of underascertainment of deaths due to SLE in ethnic minorities with low education levels. *Arthritis Care Res*. 2004;51(4):616–24.
46. Wekell P, Friman V, Balci-Peynircioglu B, Yilmaz E, Fasth A, Berg S. Familial Mediterranean fever — an increasingly important childhood disease in Sweden. *Acta Paediatr*. 2013;102(2):193–8.
47. Odabas AR, Cetinkaya R, Selcuk Y, Bilen H. Familial Mediterranean fever. *South Med J*. 2002;95(12):1400–4.
48. Sodemann M. Clinically important barriers to quality of hospital care for ethnic minority patients. 4th EUPHA Conference on Health of Migrants and Ethnic Minorities in Europe, Entitled 'Beyond Facts Figures Communi-Care for Migrants'. Milan, Italy. 2012.

CHAPTER 16

Cancer among migrant patients

Karolien Aelbrecht and Stéphanie De Maesschalck

LEARNING OBJECTIVES

At the end of this chapter, the reader should be able to:

- Understand barriers of cancer health care with migrant patients
- Raise awareness on the influence of language in cancer consultations
- Raise awareness of the role of emotions in cancer consultations with migrant patients
- Provide the reader with some tools to overcome barriers' for cancer care in a diversity-sensitive manner

---

INTRODUCTION

Cancer is one of the leading causes of death worldwide. In 2015, 8.8 million people died as a result of different types of cancer, representing 1 out of 6 of all deaths. Furthermore, it is estimated that these numbers will continue to increase; in 2030, more than 13 million people will die from cancer (1). Prevalence and incidence figures on cancer in migrants vary depending on the region of origin, age, migration, and personal history in addition to educational level, citizenship, socioeconomic position, and so on (2–4). The same diversity applies for risk factors, making the overall picture too complex to make general statements on the relation between migration and cancer. However, when looking at access to health care, we do see common barriers for migrants that will become even more important in an oncological setting (5). Problematic access to care for migrants is a general trend discussed in Chapter 6. When these patients suffer a life-threatening disease, such as cancer, their confusion and helplessness may grow even further. Language barriers, educational, financial, social, cultural, religious, and structural/organizational aspects may all play important roles in hampering the processes of care for migrants with cancer, resulting in a lower quality of care, a lower satisfaction with the encounter, and poorer compliance.

Findings of research on cancer screening show a clearer picture. Migrants show patterns of lower utilization of breast cancer, cervical cancer, and colorectal cancer screening tests. The same results can be found in most high-income countries, in both recently arrived newcomers and migrants who have been living in the host country for many years. A number of potential explanations for the lower screening numbers among migrants, including lower health literacy (overall and specifically about cancer [care] and cancer screening practices), low socioeconomic status, lack of health insurance, access problems such as transportation to the health care facilities, language barriers, as well as sociodemographic issues, including religion and culture, have been postulated (5).

In order to overcome these barriers, the cultural competence of health care providers and of the health care systems has been hypothesized as the necessary answer in most recent research and publications on this subject (6) (Chapter 20). However, in an increasingly super-diverse society, these cultural competences become more and more complex. Which competences do health care providers need for which patients in which situation? In the following sections, two cases are described to illustrate the complexity of care and the possible approaches to equity in oncological settings.

CLINICAL VIGNETTE 1: MR X HAS LUNG CANCER

Mr X is a 74-year-old man who migrated from Turkey in 1968 to work in the Belgian coalmines. He continued working there until the closure of the mines in 1986. After that, he worked in a car factory until the age of 65. His wife joined him in 1973. The couple has three children — two daughters and one son — and eight grandchildren. They are living in the family house in a middle-sized town close to the mines.

He has been suffering from COPD for many years. He recently received the diagnosis of lung cancer in an advanced stage. He will need radiotherapy and chemotherapy in palliative setting. He is not expected to get well; doctors have told the family that life expectancy is about 1 year.

CLINICAL VIGNETTE 2: MRS Y HAS A BRAIN TUMOUR

Mrs Y fled from Chechnya 3 years ago after having received threats from the police and local politicians, being taken into custody, and tortured because of her political oppositional activism. She came to Europe with her newborn son, leaving her other three children behind in Grozny with her husband and her mother. After having received a first negative decision in her asylum procedure, she is planning to start a new application.

Mrs Y has been suffering from severe headaches over the last year. Because of her legal status, she did not dare to see a physician as often as she would have wanted or needed to. She visited a friend's physician once under a false name; he prescribed painkillers and told her that the headaches were due to her stressful life circumstances. Last week she had an epileptic seizure after which she was admitted to emergency care, where a large brain tumour was diagnosed. After further examination it became clear that she is suffering from metastatic breast cancer. The tumour has spread to her brain and lungs.

LANGUAGE AND COMMUNICATION

In all phases of cancer care, from the initial diagnosis, to talking about end-of-life issues, communication with the patient and relatives requires special attention and a specific kind of sensitivity, even more so when the health care provider and the patient do not share the same culture and/or language (7,8). In such situations, the two most important prerequisites for achieving proper communication are (i) to become aware of the possible sensitivities and pitfalls, and (ii) to make sure there is a shared language between patient and health care provider.

Language support is not the unique solution for better communication; it is a 'condition sine qua non' for information exchange. Unfortunately, in spite of increasing numbers of physician-patient encounters with a language barrier, there is still underuse of the several sources for interpretation or language support that exist in medical settings, as explained in detail in Chapter 20. As a consequence, patients with cancer risk feeling more alienated, lonely, and ill-understood in their experience when language support is not offered, and thus the communication about diagnosis and treatment is suboptimal (7,9,10).

Nowadays, in most medical settings in high-income countries, several language support systems are offered to providers and patients. Ideally, a professional interpreter is used: either in person or by using video or audio systems (11). However, the barrier for emotional communication can also arise in the presence of an interpreter. Providers should be aware of the importance of a shared language in talking about emotional issues. And, since communication about cancer issues is often emotionally charged, interpretation by an in-person interpreter or by using video interpreting is preferred over telephone interpreting services (12).

Many providers still use informal interpreters, such as family members, acquaintances, neighbours, staff, and so on. Although in some cases they are the only available practical option, critical awareness of the risks in using informal interpreters is crucial, especially in cancer care. The lack of a guaranteed confidentiality is the first major issue. Since cancer diagnosis can be a taboo subject in some cultures, confidentiality in the patient-caregiver-interpreter triad is crucial in such encounters. When using informal interpreters, however, confidentiality cannot be completely guaranteed, resulting in a higher risk that patients will not share what really matters to them or what they actually worry about (13,14).

The second issue is that family members who are used as interpreters are confronted with a double role (Chapter 20), which might be especially burdensome when the patient has cancer. The third issue is that there is no quality guarantee on what is being translated and how, in both directions. This implicates that both provider and patient can never be certain of having a full and correct understanding of each other's message. In cancer cases, both explaining the diagnosis and discussing treatment options are often complex and demand a full and accurate translation. Finally, there are differences in role interpretation and expectations of informal interpreters by all people involved, for example patients or providers expecting their interpreters to also complete medical documents, which are often needed in oncologic settings, or interpreters using their own perspectives on cancer care in the translation of the information that is given by the doctor. These different interpretations and expectations create a high risk of frustration and misunderstandings. Tables 16.1 and 16.2 propose some tips for professional and informal language support in cancer care.

TABLE 16.1 Tips for *professional language support* in cancer care

- *Prepare* the consultation: What do you want/need to ask? What do you want/need to explain?
- *Involve the patient:* What are patient preferences on language support?
- *Structure*: These consultations need a more structured, patient-centred communication and shared decision making: What does the patients want (to know)? How much does the patient want to be involved?
- Provide a calm environment where you're not interrupted. *Privacy and confidentiality* are very important during these consultations
- Provide sufficient *time* for these consultations

TABLE 16.2 Tips for *informal language support* in cancer care

- See the bullet points in Table 16.1
- Try to understand the relationship between the interpreter and the patient, and check the patients' agreement and preferences on this type of language support
- Evaluate accurately the language proficiency of the interpreter in the lingua franca
- Evaluate your own language proficiency in the lingua franca
- Decide which language will be used
- Acknowledge the interpreter in his/her role as interpreter
- Explain your expectations to the interpreter:
  - Everything should be translated accurately
  - Privacy and confidentiality are most important
  - You will try not to give too much information at once, and/or ask too many questions at once
  - In case of a lack of clarity, the interpreter and the patient are invited to ask for more clarification
- Express your gratitude to the interpreter
- Pay extra attention to nonverbal signals, such as facial expressions, emotions, hand gestures, etc., of the patient as well as the interpreter

Mr X is not completely fluent in the language of his host country. He has been working all of his life with no time for studying, and when he arrived in the country, language courses did not exist. In his country of birth, he went to school until the age of 10. At this stage in life, Mr X is always accompanied by either his daughter or his son when consulting a physician. He is not a very active patient. The physician has limited time per consultation and is confident that the son will translate the important messages to his father. Often the son comes or calls to talk about blood results without Mr X being present. During the most recent visit, Mr X tried to ask the physician about what would happen to him. The physician couldn't really understand, and the son said he would explain everything later, at home. Mr X seemed distressed.

Mrs Y has never had anyone translating in a proper way for her. Each of the few consultations she has had was, without exception, short, and filled with anxiety because of her legal status and worry about the financial impact of possible disease. No physician ever organized a professional interpreter in any way to talk to her. Only now, she has received a telephone call from the hospital's cultural mediator saying that she will attend the next consultation with the oncologist together with the patient.

DELIVERING BAD NEWS

In European medical schools, delivering bad news to patients is being taught in a specific way. Medical students learn to deliver the diagnosis in an open and direct way, in clear and understandable language (without jargon), also leaving room for emotions. Western providers are taught to be 'honest' with their patients, not hiding any information regarding the diagnosis. Western providers use the words 'cancer', 'tumour', and so on, in a sensitive, but nevertheless direct way. While this way of communicating is believed to be the norm in the Western world, the increase of other cultures in our European societies makes it less self-evident.

In a super-diverse society, providers should reflect on whether and how patients with a different cultural background would prefer to receive bad news, and how much information they would prefer to receive (15). These preferences can be as diverse as the patients' backgrounds, depending on one's cultural, social, educational background, as well as their personal preferences and the level of acculturation in the new country. In order to know this, providers simply need to ask. Questions about the patient's background and perceptions and health beliefs on cancer, preferences on receiving health information, and so on, can be easily implemented in every bad news model. One example of a model is the SPIKES model, which is a patient-centred six-step protocol for delivering bad news in a diversity-sensitive way (16). The acronym stands for the following:

- *Setting* is the context in which the conversation will take place
- *Perception* is about getting to know the patients' and relatives' perspectives and knowledge of the medical issues at stake
- *Invitation/information* is exploring patients' and relatives' preferences on being informed
- *Knowledge* is about how to actually break the bad news in a sensitive manner
- *Empathy* is about how to deal with the emotions that are inherent to a bad news conversation
- *Summarizing* is what has been said and what the next steps in the process will be

---

In the story of Mrs Y, the social service has organized for a GP to visit her and to arrange organization of her home care. When the GP talks to Mrs Y she doesn't seem to realize the seriousness of her diagnosis. She is crying a lot. The neighbour, a man of Russian origin, is translating for the GP, and tells the GP that he suspects Mrs Y does not know she has cancer, or at least does not talk about it. The GP has no idea if the neighbour is translating accurately the words 'cancer' and 'prognosis'. The GP calls the hospital cultural mediator and they arrange a video conversation with patient, GP, and mediator. In that conversation, the GP manages to explore knowledge and expectations, worries and ideas with the patient. Mrs Y says she wants her other children to come to Belgium, or that she will return home if this is not possible. She says that she wants to do everything possible to get well again, and that this is not possible within the Chechnyan health care. She is therefore in existential doubt about what to do next.

EMOTIONAL COMMUNICATION

Health care providers are trained to deal with patients' emotions. However, in end-of-life situations such as cancer, emotions can take the lead and make both health care provider and patient feel uncomfortable. Moreover, in encounters with patients who have a different cultural background, emotional communication is often a challenge for health care providers (17,18). Compared to encounters where health care provider and patient share the same culture, in encounters with migrant patients both health care provider and patient might behave differently towards each other. In the latter, there is less affective behaviour, such as less social talk and empathy, and they are less emotionally engaged with each other. In addition,

TABLE 16.3   Tips regarding emotional communication

- Be aware of this issue
- Know that a language barrier often overshadows emotional communication; pay extra attention to nonverbal signals
- Ask the patient how he/she feels; a patient does not always know it is OK to talk about emotions during a medical encounter

both patient and health care provider communicate differently about unpleasant emotions. While migrant patients reveal fewer emotional cues, health care providers show less positive affect and a lower degree of patient-centred response with migrant patients (19). Nevertheless, migrant patients find a health care provider's display of concern, courtesy, and respect very important (20). This affectively imbalanced relationship between health care providers and migrant patients not only hinders further contact between both, but also decreases the chance of reaching a mutual understanding of the patient's health complaints and delivering an adequate treatment plan based on a shared decision. Table 16.3 gives some tips regarding emotional communication for patients with language barriers.

HEALTH LITERACY

Health literacy (Chapter 20) is discussed as an increasingly critical factor affecting communication across the continuum of cancer care. At least one-third of patients have inadequate health literacy and struggle with everyday health and health care tasks. Low health literacy is associated with diminished screening, advanced stage at diagnosis, decreased acceptance of and compliance with treatment, and decreased participation in clinical trials. Moreover, migrant cancer patients often fill in the lack of knowledge by using different, sometimes questionable strategies. Some participants use the nonverbal behaviour of the health care provider to literally fill in the missed words; other participants revert to the knowledge (e.g. on the use of certain herbs) and myths (e.g. the influence of a certain God on the disease) that exist in their country of origin, and others use Dr Google to learn more about their disease. The literature confirms the use of these strategies, which might lead to communicative misunderstandings, incomplete understanding of the disease and therapy, and even ignoring the hard truth about their health status. As a health care provider, it can be helpful to double-check or use the teach-back method, by asking the patient to repeat the messages in their own words, to make sure the patient has understood all the information that was given.

COMPLIANCE AND MOTIVATION

Migrant patients may not comply due to a lack of efficient and clear communication or due to different knowledge or cultural habits, and thus not follow the therapeutic instructions as advised (21,22). This can be problematic in cases of chronic illness or a life-threatening disease such as cancer.

As a health care provider, it is essential to:

- Explore patients' existing knowledge and information preferences.
- Give an unambiguous explanation, indicating precisely the expected behaviour; this means that it is important to leave out any medical jargon or the use of general, abstract sayings, for example 'three times a day'.

- Check for understanding regularly.
- Ask the patient and/or his carer to repeat the prescribed procedures step by step.
- Ask the patient how he/she understands the importance of the treatment, and the consequences of not following a treatment or instruction, for example oral care and chemotherapy.

In cases of noncompliance, it is crucial, as a physician, to take a step back. Patients who do not comply with the prescribed procedure give an important signal. They either did not understand what was said or why it was said. Exploring the reason(s) why the patient did not comply will give the physician an insight in their underlying thoughts and motivation. Understanding the patients' perspective allows providers to adapt their communication with the patient.

To motivate patients is also to activate them as a participant in their treatment. However, research confirms that migrant patients are often less participative in medical consultations compared to majority patients. It is thus a challenge to find effective strategies to enhance migrant patients' participation and improve health outcomes.

RELIGION AND HOPE

Previous literature suggests that religion and spirituality play a central role in the way patients cope with cancer (23,24). Providing comfort, hope, and meaning, religiosity is reported to aid patients in their struggle to cope with cancer. However, religious and spiritual beliefs may also alter patients' perceptions of their illness and symptoms and thereby influence treatment decisions. Studies also suggest that religious individuals more frequently request life-prolonging therapies. Patients with cancer who use spiritual coping to a greater extent are more likely to desire life-sustaining treatments.

As a health care provider, it is important to be aware of the role religion does or does not play in patients' lives. Physicians can explore the importance of religion (and by extension, cultural issues in dealing with cancer and end-of-life issues) by asking about it in a respectful manner. For example, 'For some patients, religion or spirituality play an important role in their lives, especially when becoming ill. I would like to learn more about your point of view on these matters. Can I ask you some questions about it? Could you tell me if and how religion plays a role in your life?' 'In your religion, what do people usually expect in this situation? What is important to you? Do you know or consult a religious counsellor? If not, would you like to ask for some religious advice?'

END OF LIFE, DEATH, AND DYING

Besides differences in communication preferences between groups of patients and health care providers who do not share the same cultural background, cultural ways of looking at and dealing with end-of-life issues may differ considerably between cultures. The difficulty, however, is that we never know in advance what the perceptions, ideas, expectations, fears, and so on, of the patient and his/her caregivers are towards the end of life. Learning about patients' and caregivers' religiosity and religious prescriptions and preferences helps physicians to provide culturally sensitive care to cancer patients. Some patients, even though religious, still feel doubts about what to do when faced with life-threatening situations. It might be a relief, and deepen the relationship between patients, family, and physician, if the latter takes the initiative to show interest and to ask how he can be of help, including helping to find religious support.

CONCLUSION: TEN TIPS FOR DEALING WITH CANCER CARE

1. *Take time, prepare yourself.*
2. *Work in a culturally sensitive way*: As explained in depth in Chapter 5, this means that we should be aware of the existence of stereotypical ideas and prejudices and try to avoid them. Culturally sensitive communication, as opposed to culturally specific communication, implicates a reflective attitude of the health care provider: when seeing a patient who might have different cultural and/or religious ideas, health care providers should be willing to explore these ideas, preferences, habits, etc., as well as being sensitive to all language issues. In addition to exploring the patient's side of the story, health care providers should also be aware of their own cultural biases.

    Reflexivity is thus the keyword here. Sometimes providers find themselves in a situation that they would deal with from a European point of view in a shared-decision, patient-centred way, but a different approach may be called for in a culturally diverse situation. Reflexivity in this context means realizing what the provider's personal cultural viewpoint on the situation is (e.g. a patient has to decide on their own health; too much family interference should be limited or avoided), exploring in depth and in an empathic way what the patient's cultural viewpoint is as well as that of the caregivers, and trying to come to a shared, and thus well informed (on both sides) decision on treatment.

3. *Use an intersectional approach* to explore the individual preferences of the patient and their family. Be aware that patients with another cultural background often have experienced different levels of problems (language, education, health literacy, gender, etc.) and discrimination. Intersectionality, a concept stemming from the black feminism movement in the 1960s in the United States, explains how different social identities, belonging to social groups that are being discriminated in the society where one lives, can pose double jeopardy to the individual belonging to these social groups (Chapter 2). For example, a patient with a migrant background, a language barrier (low language proficiency, no or little shared language with the provider), low educational level, low health literacy, and a woman, will have to deal with the risk of discrimination on different levels in life, and will develop different preferences, ideas, fears, etc., than a patient with a migrant background who has recently arrived, who is highly educated, and who came from an upper class background in the home country. We need to distance ourselves from any stereotypical ideas and prejudices that inevitably come up when meeting migrant patients for the first time, or even when we have known those patients for a while.

4. *Deal with language barriers*: See previous discussion and Chapter 20 for some tips on detecting and overcoming language barriers. Avoid using ad hoc interpreters in cases where emotions and difficult issues will be discussed. Make sure to be trained in using language support. Be aware of possibilities in language support in your local context. Provide information to patients on their rights to ask for language support.

5. *Explore patient's preferences on end-of-life issues*: How does the patient perceive the importance of autonomy? What are their ideas on life-prolonging or life-shortening interventions? What are their spiritual needs? What are their emotional needs? Who are the meaningful persons in the patient's context that

need to be around when the end is near? Are there any gender issues that need attention? Does the patient need support by a spiritual caregiver? Are there any cultural customs that come with death and dying: where does the patient prefer to die, who should be present, who should wash the patient, where does the patient want to be buried?

These issues should be discussed as soon as possible in the process. Timely discussion of possibly sensitive issues is crucial: it leaves room for building trust and exploring difficult matters without rushing or forcing things. The sooner provider, patients, and caregivers start discussing concerns broader than the pure medical issues, the better. Do not overestimate the influence of culture, but do not underestimate the influence of culture.

6. *Always first ask, then tell.*
7. *Use preventive communication*: Explore patients' ideas and preferences on communicating bad news and treatment information. Explain what you want to do, which information you need, and why you ask the questions that you do.
8. *Stress confidentiality.*
9. *Get the patient's permission* to talk about these issues with the immediate caregivers. Examples of questions to ask are:
   - Would you consider yourself religious? Do you need moral support by a religious counsellor? If so, which one; will you contact this person, or do you need support in doing so?
   - Do you have specific wishes on what we can or cannot do in the last stage of your life?
   - When you have died, what is, according to you and your family, the appropriate way of dealing with your body?
   - What will happen after you die? Are you afraid? Are there things you worry about? What are these?
   - Is there anything I can do for you?
10. *Pay attention to the caregivers*: In many cultures, taking care of ill family members is essential and cannot be denied. However, this may put a lot of stress on the often female caregivers who have, besides the caregiving role for their family member, also a family of their own, a career, etc. In addition, since caregivers in some cultures play a crucial role in the process, it is of utmost importance that health care providers learn to communicate not only with the patient but also with their relatives. Explore the patient's context and who plays which role in the (extended) family.

REFERENCES

1. WHO. Cancer. Key Facts. 2015. Available from: http://www.who. int/news-room/fact-sheets/detail/cancer
2. Arnold M, Razum O, Coebergh JW. Cancer risk diversity in non-western migrants to Europe: an overview of the literature. *Eur J Cancer*. 2010;46(14):2647–59.
3. Kristiansen M, Razum O, Tezcan-Guntekin H, Krasnik A. Aging and health among migrants in a European perspective. *Public Health Rev*. 2016;37:20.
4. Rechel B, Mladovsky P, Ingleby D, Mackenbach JP, McKee M. Migration and health in an increasingly diverse Europe. *Lancet*. 2013;381(9873):1235–45.
5. Norredam M, Nielsen SS, Krasnik A. Migrants' utilization of somatic healthcare services in Europe-a systematic review. *Eur J Public Health*. 2010;20(5):555–63.

6. Horvat L, Horey D, Romios P, Kis-Rigo J. Cultural competence education for health professionals. *Cochrane Database Syst Rev.* 2014;(5):CD009405.

7. Butow PN, Sze M, Dugal-Beri P et al. From inside the bubble: migrants' perceptions of communication with the cancer team. *Support Care Cancer.* 2011;19(2):281–90.

8. Aelbrecht K, Pype P, Vos J, Deveugele M. Having cancer in a foreign country. *Patient Educ Couns.* 2016;99(10):1708–16.

9. Zendedel R, Schouten BC, van Weert JC, van den Putte B. Informal interpreting in general practice: comparing the perspectives of general practitioners, migrant patients and family interpreters. *Patient Educ Couns.* 2016;99(6):981–7.

10. Zendedel R, Schouten BC, van Weert JCM, van den Putte B. Informal interpreting in general practice: the migrant patient's voice. *Ethn Health.* 2018;23(2):158–73.

11. Karliner LS, Jacobs EA, Chen AH, Mutha S. Do professional interpreters improve clinical care for patients with limited English proficiency? A systematic review of the literature. *Health Serv Res.* 2007;42(2):727–54.

12. Brisset C, Leanza Y, Laforest K. Working with interpreters in health care: a systematic review and meta-ethnography of qualitative studies. *Patient Educ Couns.* 2013;91(2):131–40.

13. Meeuwesen L, Twilt S, ten Thije JD, Harmsen H. "Ne diyor?" (What does she say?): Informal interpreting in general practice. *Patient Educ Couns.* 2010;81(2):198–203.

14. Silva MD, Genoff M, Zaballa A et al. Interpreting at the end of life: a systematic review of the impact of interpreters on the delivery of palliative care services to cancer patients with limited English proficiency. *J Pain Symptom Manage.* 2016;51(3):569–80.

15. Mitchison D, Butow P, Sze M et al. Prognostic communication preferences of migrant patients and their relatives. *Psychooncology.* 2012;21(5):496–504.

16. Kaplan M. SPIKES: A framework for breaking bad news to patients with cancer. *Clin J Oncol Nurs.* 2010;14(4):514–6.

17. Schouten BC, Schinkel S. Emotions in primary care: are there cultural differences in the expression of cues and concerns? *Patient Educ Couns.* 2015;98(11):1346–51.

18. Willems S, De Maesschalck S, Deveugele M, Derese A, De Maeseneer J. Socio-economic status of the patient and doctor-patient communication: does it make a difference? *Patient Educ Couns.* 2005;56(2):139–46.

19. Aelbrecht K, De Maesschalck S, Willems S, Deveugele M, Pype P. How family physicians respond to unpleasant emotions of ethnic minority patients. *Patient Educ Couns.* 2017;100(10):1867–73.

20. Koppenol M, Francke AL, Vlems F, Nijhuis A. Allochtonen en kanker. enkele onderzoeksbevindingen rond betekenisverlening, communicatie en zorg [Immigrants and cancer. Some research findings on giving meaning, communication and care]. *Cultuur Migratie Gezondheid.* 2006;3:212–22.

21. Hyatt A, Lipson-Smith R, Schofield P et al. Communication challenges experienced by migrants with cancer: a comparison of migrant and English-speaking Australian-born cancer patients. *Health Expect.* 2017;20(5):886–95.

22. Schinkel S, Schouten BC, van Weert JC. Are GP patients' needs being met? Unfulfilled information needs among native-Dutch and Turkish-Dutch patients. *Patient Educ Couns.* 2013;90(2):261–7.

23. de Graaff FM, Francke AL, van den Muijsenbergh ME, van der Geest S. 'Palliative care': a contradiction in terms? A qualitative study of cancer patients with a Turkish or Moroccan background, their relatives and care providers. *BMC Palliat Care.* 2010;9:19.

24. de Graaff FM, Mistiaen P, Deville WL, Francke AL. Perspectives on care and communication involving incurably ill Turkish and Moroccan patients, relatives and professionals: a systematic literature review. *BMC Palliat Care.* 2012;11:17.

CHAPTER 17

Migration and mental health

Rebecca Farrington

LEARNING OBJECTIVES

This chapter focusses primarily on new migrants in the host country, those at greatest need and posing the greatest challenge. This chapter will help the reader to:

- Conduct mental health assessments using a cultural sensibility approach
- Understand the universal psychological consequences of trauma and how to approach them
- Acquire special skills, considerations, and treatment options for migrants with mental health disorders

---

CLINICAL VIGNETTE 1

Fifty-six-year-old Divine is from Africa. She was referred for counselling by her GP for low mood. On being questioned by a mental health practitioner about her daily activities, she says 'I don't go out because they might be watching me. They will get my son'. The counsellor decides she is paranoid and discharges her, recommending a Community Mental Health Team (CMHT) referral. The GP goes with this diagnostic momentum and codes 'Paranoia' in her notes. Divine told her GP she could 'smell blood all the time' and he referred her to psychiatry with psychotic symptoms without exploring her migration or trauma history.

Divine worked for a national newspaper in Africa. She was threatened repeatedly following her articles on women's rights. For many years she was followed, intimidated, and beaten for her activism. She was raped, and escaped the country after a period in hiding. Divine left her son behind. He is studying law and has since received threats. He is afraid to leave their house. She feels guilty about leaving him in danger.

She has just received leave-to-remain and lives in a noisy homeless hostel. Divine finds it hard to trust anyone and has not revealed her refugee status. She manages about 4 hours of sleep, broken by nightmares. She has a strong belief that her movements in the UK are being monitored and refuses to mix with her countrymen. When she has attended voluntary groups in the past, Divine has found it hard to deal with people speaking her dialect, as it triggers flashbacks. She doesn't attend language class, as she can't concentrate.

INTRODUCTION

In addressing the mental health of migrants, it must be acknowledged they are a heterogeneous group with variable migration histories and experiences in their home and host countries. These multifactorial influences on mental health include motivation for migration, long-term access to care, different clinical presentations, and confidence in services. There are clear ethnic variations with non-Western migrants overrepresented in psychiatric emergency care (1). Ethnicity is often recorded in medical notes or research, rather than country of birth and socioeconomic circumstances, which may have more effect on culture, stigma, and variable use of alcohol and stimulant drugs (2).

Pre-existing mental illness may have been neglected or poorly assessed since arrival. Most migrants will be healthy, but some face challenges relating to migration that have a negative impact. There are significant stressors. They are usually fit on arrival, showing the well-described 'healthy migrant effect' (3); however, adversity and post-migration resettlement experiences, especially economic instability, can influence long-term health (4,5) (Chapter 2). A Swedish study found social adversity contributes to a higher risk of psychosis (6), and studies of the Afro-Caribbean community in London show lower rates of schizophrenia in countries of origin, concluding 'more attention needs to be focussed on socioenvironmental variables'.

While this chapter concentrates on the most vulnerable migrants, asylum seekers, and new refugees, it is worth mentioning that the skills in caring for them are transferable to others who face challenges with language and acculturation, are displaced from familiar settings and health systems, and suffer disparities in access to health care. Regardless of motivation to leave their country, many experience a migratory grieving process (7), and depression and anxiety are common. The concept of 'family' may have wider connotations than those to which we are accustomed (Chapter 11). Usual support systems may be distant or destroyed. Separation can provoke feelings of guilt. Shame and loyalty play bigger roles for those from collectivistic cultures.

Post-traumatic stress disorder (PSTD) is important to explain in more detail, although depression and anxiety are more prevalent. The psychological consequences of trauma are universal. 'PTSD is prevalent cross-nationally, with half of all global cases being persistent' (8). Many forced migrants will not fully develop this condition but may experience similar symptoms intermittently. They require psychological support and attention to the wider determinants of health until symptoms remit. This can include connections with multicultural support organizations and people from their original culture. Promoting a welcome from the wider host community is an essential advocacy aim. Understanding how to sensitively establish a dialogue about common mental illnesses such as depression and anxiety is useful when the presentation seems atypical for cultural reasons or a person seems reluctant to engage.

Forced migration

'Traumatic events destroy the fundamental assumptions about the safety of the world' (9). The removal of autonomy, power, and purposefulness from asylum seekers underwrites feelings of futility and illness. Contact with conflict, violence, persecution, torture, rape, and loss of governmental protection are commonly encountered before arrival. Journeys are hazardous. Losses can be numerous and include loved ones, employment, status, language, culture, and dignity (10) (Chapter 1).

Stressors revolve around detention, future insecurity, and hostile legal proceedings with life-altering verdicts. Denied permission to work, asylum seekers might de-skill, and lose self-confidence and social capital. People can experience extreme poverty. Employment and economic stability, important protective factors for migrant mental health (4), are often removed in the asylum system, which has been described in the UK as 'retraumatising and dehumanising' (11).

Distress

Distress is a normal reaction to highly abnormal circumstances: we must be mindful of 'disguising disadvantage as disease' (12). Many migrants will only require Psychological First Aid, described by WHO (13), comprising unintrusive, calm, active listening in a respectful manner. The emphasis is on acknowledging losses and strengths, providing protection without false reassurances, and maintaining dignity. Formal debriefing is not recommended as a first aid measure (14). Basic social support needs identification and action, such as keeping families together and combatting isolation and loneliness. The practitioner must be aware of vulnerabilities and discrimination on age, gender, disability, or minority group membership.

Normal reaction versus mental illness

Medicalizing experiences related to migration can be problematic, distracting from the social context and placing the focus on the individual; however, pragmatically, when symptoms are severe or persist, it is worth considering PTSD, comorbid depression, and anxiety disorders. Diagnostic labels might be seen as a limiting response but, as Boyles stresses, there are advantages for torture survivors: 'Naming the injury acknowledges that a crime has been committed' (11).

It is difficult to quantify how many migrants with traumatic experiences will suffer PTSD; risks are multifactorial and estimates from the literature cover a wide range. Kirmayer quotes 10 times the rate of the general population (4), with the biggest factor being exposure to torture. Where trauma has been intentionally inflicted, the emergence of symptoms may take longer (15). Protective factors include positive experiences of dealing with previous stressors, personality, and available support. People prepared to face traumatic consequences for their actions, such as political activists, may be less affected (16); however, as seen with Divine, the protagonist in the clinical vignette, prolonged trauma can be detrimental despite pre-existing resilience or expectation of challenge.

Many have experienced betrayal and sometimes mistrust or fear their caregivers, but at other times feel utterly dependent on them (17). In a culture of disbelief, people seeking asylum may be faced with practitioners who accuse them of deception or exaggeration for benefit in their asylum claim (10).

Practically, diagnoses can lead the way to alleviation of suffering through accessing care pathways and documenting medical evidence; however, their stigmatizing effect in mental health should not be underestimated. In Europe, we are still struggling with parity of esteem for mental illness. In some countries further afield, a label of 'crazy' has far-reaching consequences for individuals and their families. People with mental illness can be incarcerated and even chained. Families may be shunned for generations. If the presentation is related to modifiable factors, such as social isolation, the period of assessment should be prolonged if possible to rectify these before formalizing a diagnosis.

UNDERTAKING AN ASSESSMENT

Communication

GPs already possess skills to assess distressed or traumatized people, for example in domestic violence. Providing the opportunity for independent, appropriate language interpretation is essential. Be mindful of avoiding an interrogatory style and explain confidentiality explicitly. People may not understand why you are asking personal questions and what you might do with their information. Some find open questions difficult (18) and others feel talking to a stranger, or elder, about private experiences culturally uncomfortable.

Communication between doctor and patient requires self-awareness on the practitioner's part. Many factors, including privilege, education, and socioeconomic status, affect how we all perceive life. The patient's opinions may be strikingly different from your own. People may struggle, having lost faith in previously strong views. Some seemingly inexplicable or unsophisticated lay beliefs are tightly held. Explicitly showing a non-judgmental willingness to work across cultures is important. You have power as a role model for your team and local community.

Helplessness can be contagious. Beware of transference and countertransference, where the negative emotions expressed are taken on by the practitioner and reflected back to the patient. 'Chronically traumatized patients have an exquisite attunement to unconscious and nonverbal communication' (17). Awareness of body language is therefore crucial. Techniques such as mirroring are worth exploration, but require attentiveness to cultural considerations around eye contact, gestures, and touch. A good interpreter can help differentiate meanings.

Cultural sensibility

The wider cultural and sociopolitical contexts are interesting; however, assessing the individual requires consideration of their own interpretation of these, rather than making assumptions driven by knowledge-based cultural 'competency' models (Chapter 5). Divine is a well-educated, independent woman whose resources may be different from her countrywomen who are not literate and may have different gender role expectations. Background socio-geographic context can help us understand the patient's situation, and is accessible online from international human rights organizations; however, current information about your own country's asylum processes and resources in your local community to support migrants are more important than detailed knowledge of a specific country or society.

CLINICAL VIGNETTE 2

Ana and Nico migrated for work. Nico found a job in technology, but Ana, whose language skills are poor, remained unemployed. She didn't know about free contraception and became pregnant a few months after arrival. Their son, Andrei, was born prematurely. Ana blamed herself for cutting her hair before the birth. They spent a month in hospital. Ana found it hard to breastfeed but was ashamed to ask for help because she felt she ought to be able to do this.

Her mother and sister have been unable to get a visa to visit, and Ana cannot afford to go home. She calls them on the internet, especially when Nico travels with his job. They tell her Andrei looks thin and she should take him to the doctor. The midwife said she should go to the community clinic regularly for weighing and to meet other mums. Ana is not sure which bus to catch and feels her heart beating very fast when she has to go somewhere new. Anyway, Nico prefers her to stay at home and look after the house.

Ana is lonely and often tearful. She is exhausted because Andrei sleeps poorly. Ana sometimes wakes up while he is still sleeping. She is worried if she tells the doctor they will take Andrei away from her. The last time she attended, the interpreter told her that social services remove babies from families if they look neglected.

Ana bought diazepam from the internet because she thought it would help her to relax, but she just feels low. Sometimes she thinks it might be better if she was dead. She nearly told the nice new GP, but she seemed so young and Ana thought Dr Grace might be upset if she told her what she was really thinking.

A cultural sensibility (19) approach to communication respects an individual's circumstances over generalizations. It encourages 'respectful curiosity' and moves away from the 'all-knowing' clinician to a patient-centred focus. This would allow Ana, from the clinical vignette, to voice her fears that she is to blame for Andrei's prematurity. Acculturation, cultural bereavement (20), and intergenerational conflict (4) are well documented and need space to be explored (Chapter 11). Ana's family feels strongly that Andrei's care should be doctor-led, when in fact a Health Visitor is more appropriate in her new setting.

Intersectionality

The concept of an individual identifying with more than one oppressed social group is described as intersectionality (21). Gender, poverty, and migration inequalities, for example, magnify their effects when they are present for the same person. Multiple experiences of discrimination and power imbalances become intertwined. Consider a more nuanced examination of personal cultural identities including their balance between individualism and collectivism (11) with such diverse groups. Divine may feel she is missing out on care she would normally expect from her son as she becomes elderly, or feel she is neglecting her matriarchal role. Without exploration of your assumptions you could inadvertently misunderstand the patient's perception of her problems and be perceived as disrespectful.

PRESENTING COMPLAINTS

Common symptoms

The initial history is often dominated by physical symptoms. This may be the only language patients have to articulate their distress to a doctor, even when they are aware that stress or depression are contributing factors. The physical consequences of psychological trauma are evident with higher rates of chronic disease (22) including dementia (23), necessitating exclusion of physical causes despite psychosomatic symptoms being prevalent (Chapters 15 and 23).

Sleep disturbance, pain syndromes, and headache are common, alongside symptoms of anxiety: sweating, shaking, and palpitations, such as those experienced by Ana. The over-activation of the sympathetic system brings a loss of the baseline level of calm. Chest pain and a feeling of blockage in the throat occur. Gastrointestinal issues including acid reflux and diarrhoea accompany heightened anxiety.

Poor memory and concentration affect learning capacity, especially retention of information, causing frustration, especially for those like Divine who are used to previous academic achievement. Cognitive impairment affects daily function and confidence. They lack trust in their previous coping strategies. People feel overwhelmed by multiple symptoms and disorganized in their ability to articulate and control them. Some, like Ana, have concerns about causing the practitioner distress (11) or the consequences for their family.

Psychological symptoms can be transient and isolated with relapse and remission to varying degrees. An in-depth assessment over time will help to discern those who need a formal diagnosis and referral for specialist support. Continuity of care and recognizing and reacting to stressors related to the wider determinants of health are keys to success.

Post-traumatic stress disorder

WHO uses ICD-10 classification for PTSD (24). In the United States, the DSM-V is used. The differences have implications for research and insurance; however, a pragmatic approach can be taken for clinical purposes. Be aware that 'comorbidity in PTSD is the rule rather than the exception' (25) (Chapter 15).

PTSD is an anxiety disorder typified by a clinical magnification of the normal responses to danger in those who have experienced frightening events. Herman describes symptoms as Hyperarousal, Intrusion, and Constriction (17).

Hyperarousal includes hypervigilance, irritability, and agitation. Concentration is difficult and a 'flight, fright, or freeze' response is active. People fear sleep. They have low thresholds for anxiety, even with minimal provocation. They are unable to tune out repetitive stimuli and find self-soothing difficult.

Intrusion encompasses re-experiencing: flashbacks, nightmares, and unwanted thoughts. The triggers are often seemingly insignificant stimuli. Memories of trauma do not form a coherent narrative. They are vivid and fragmentary sensations and images. Van der Kolk describes their non-verbal nature as 'speechless horror' and quotes research using functional MRI showing speech areas of the brain inactive during flashbacks (26). People feel terror and rage as though the trauma is happening again.

Constriction describes shrinking of psychological range: a form of surrender with emotional numbing, detached calm, dissociation, and a sense of a foreshortened future. This restriction happens in the quest for safety. Sufferers will avoid cues: people, situations, objects, or sounds that trigger recollections. Sometimes mislabelled as 'learned helplessness', people have a 'paralysis of initiative' where they fear taking any action (17).

Psychosis can feature in PTSD and depression presentations, but real events may be misinterpreted and mislabelled — for example, paranoia, as in the case featuring Divine. Her fear triggered learned survival behaviour preventing her from leaving the house.

Sometimes flashbacks are misdiagnosed as hallucinations, as was the case in her experience of smelling blood.

Herman describes recovery from PTSD akin to 'running a marathon' needing training, endurance, and coaching (17). There may be resistance in accepting the need for treatment where the patient perceives this as a victory for a perpetrator. Reframing this as an act of courage to overcome the perpetrator's aims can be useful. Overcoming the barriers takes time and courage on the part of patient and practitioner. It is tempting just to see the disengagement rather than explore the underlying reasons. Advocacy can be a slow process. Maintaining trust involves doing what you say you will do and updating progress even when it is slow.

WHO surveys show half of PTSD cases recovered within 24 months and 77% within 10 years (27), leaving some with long-term symptoms. Stressful events trigger relapses and symptoms can recur after many years. Helping people recognize the turbulent nature of their illnesses can reassure them, for as much as symptoms return, they also remit. Reinforcing coping strategies and supporting relapses with longitudinal care is important in mental health, regardless of diagnosis.

Complex PTSD

Herman advocates the diagnosis 'complex PTSD', considering the effects of enduring prolonged exploitation: domestic violence, child abuse, prisoners of war, political prisoners, or hostages (28). While it does not feature in DSM-V, many people working in the field find it a useful distinction from trauma arising from single events such as natural disasters.

Often survivors describe not recognizing the person they have become. This dissonance is distressing. There can be a preoccupation with suicide with the absence of protective factors such as close confiding relationships, family support, homes, and jobs. Some are young men who have been exposed to violence. They ruminate, hopeless about a future they find difficult to imagine; consequently, their suicide risk is high. Many engage in inappropriate risk-taking behaviour, deliberately putting themselves in harm's way.

Barriers to meaningful care

Shared decision making and confidentiality may be alien to people from paternalistic societies. There are clear benefits to restoring control, but autonomy may require additional explanation. Patients may not understand the need to attend follow-up without you making this obvious. People have disorganized lives or give precedence to other appointments, for example with legal representatives. Sometimes another calendar is used, such as Ethiopian. The lack of work routine makes days very similar, and time is distorted or passes without note.

People worry about being charged for care when they are unable to pay. This acts as a deterrent to help-seeking behaviour even when they are entitled to free treatment. Failure to attend hospital or therapy appointments usually leads to discharge. Telephone consulting is challenging. Prolonged time on hold or language difficulties deter people from rearranging appointments.

Child and adolescent mental health

WHO uses the term 'unaccompanied and separated child', moving away from associations with the negative connotations of migration pathways (Chapters 8 and 9). These children may have had to take responsibility for themselves in adult settings for long periods. They report multiple and extreme traumatic events. Sixty-seven percent of the unaccompanied girls and 14% of boys attending a Dutch clinic had experienced sexual abuse (29). They are known to experience more PTSD symptoms than accompanied migrant children, particularly females (30), and these symptoms are persistent (31).

Children exposed to trauma can present with behavioural problems, bed-wetting, withdrawal, clinginess, acting out, violence in play, poor sleep, and nightmares. In a study of Syrian refugee caregivers, more than a third of children had clinical levels of behavioural problems on both the Paediatric Emotional Distress Scale and the Strengths and Difficulties Questionnaire (32). The term 'developmental trauma disorder' (33) takes into consideration the long-term impact of psychological trauma on children, who often end up with multiple diagnoses in adulthood with difficulty in responding to usual treatments.

The ability to play may have been lost by those who have undertaken journeys in survival mode for long intervals. Play is essential to children's normal development. Early re-engagement in normal childhood activities, especially education, is vital. A GP or community paediatrician has an advocacy role in facilitating this.

Some families are separated for years. Achieving reunion is often complicated, prolonged, and costly. Children have grown and may feel abandoned by the absent parent. Expectations of the reunion are high and sometimes unrealistic. Preparation and support for the highs and lows of the process is useful, and organizations such as The Red Cross are experts.

Children may be asked at age 18 years of age to make an asylum claim independent of their family. This can mean separation from their family to another city at a time they are trying to assimilate into a new culture. It can mean curtailment of their education. In some families, older teenagers are married young, and soon after arrival, try to secure their future.

MANAGEMENT AND TOOLS

The experience of migration is not homogenous. Many do not need counselling or high-level psychological therapies but an opportunity to rebuild their lives and reunite with family. Restoring hope, dignity, and control is key. Combatting isolation and loneliness, engaging with the host community, work, or a purposeful activity is essential for mental well-being.

Screening

Presentations of distress are not usually accompanied by frank disclosure of trauma details. This often requires prior establishment of a trusting relationship. People do, however, appreciate being asked if they have been ill-treated at some point, even if they cannot yet reveal the particulars. Genuine interest in Divine's circumstances and sensitive enquiry as to her reasons for being displaced might have opened a useful dialogue for the GP. Phrases giving invitation to disclose can be utilized, such as 'are you able to tell me something of what happened?'

The use of questionnaires is not always culturally acceptable or valid. They contribute to 'therapy bureaucracy' (11), but for example questions to start a dialogue, we recommend the Primary Care PTSD Screen (34).

In your life, have you ever had any experience that was so frightening, horrible, or upsetting that, in the past month, you:

1. Have had nightmares about it or thought about it when you did not want to?
2. Tried hard not to think about it or went out of your way to avoid situations that reminded you of it?

3. Were constantly on guard, watchful, or easily startled?
4. Felt numb or detached from others, activities, or your surroundings?

PTSD is as a diagnosis worthy of further investigation if a patient answers 'yes' to three items. They will also need a suicide risk assessment.

The person's distress can be upsetting and may deter you from enquiring. Good preparation for this work includes awareness of your current state of resilience and a clear idea of where to seek help. Psychological supervision, formal or informal, is invaluable, and limiting your exposure to detailed information is useful.

CLINICAL VIGNETTE 2: FOLLOW-UP

Grace is a newly qualified GP. Ana is coming to see her with an interpreter. She always finds this challenging. Ana is quiet and Grace suspects there is another problem, maybe even domestic violence. Grace knows Ana has no relatives in this country. She sees that her baby, Andrei, is behind with his immunization schedule.

Grace notices Ana seems flat in her affect and asks if she has any worries about her own health. The interpreter talks for longer than she expected. Ana seems to become upset, but the interpreter tells Grace that Ana is fine. Grace moves quickly to discuss the vaccinations before their appointment time is finished, as Ana must leave to catch her bus.

Over coffee Grace tells her colleague she feels uneasy about Ana but didn't know how to challenge the interpreter. She is especially worried because there is a baby at home. Grace also wasn't sure what services might be available to people who don't have good language skills.

Her colleague suggests a joint home visit with the Health Visitor. They take a new interpreter who she knows is also a good cultural broker. Ana discloses her loneliness, low mood, and anxiety and Grace negotiates a treatment plan with her. Grace is reassured Ana and Andrei are safe at home. The Health Visitor sensitively normalized the domestic violence screening questions by explaining the screening is routine in this country for all women who have recently been pregnant.

Social rehabilitation

Normalizing 'ordinary human suffering' and emphasizing the resilience people have already demonstrated can be powerful. Papadopoulos presents the concept of Adversity-Activated Development (35) — surviving adversity and becoming more resourceful. Outreach activities can link these resilient role models to their communities, sharing resources and hope. GPs are good at coordinating this kind of care and empowering self-management. It is important we recognize the effort required to assimilate and explicitly acknowledge the patients' successes.

Meeting others from their home country can be positive and supportive, but for some causes stress. Reminders of home, language, and culture could be a trigger for increased symptoms as it was for Divine in the clinical vignette. Figuring out whom to trust, and potentially meeting people who bear bad news or who have certain expectations, can be challenging.

Encouraging people to engage socially is beneficial, but be cognizant of the pitfalls. Consider companionship: being around people doing similar activities is less threatening initially than trying to 'make friends'. The International Organization for Migration advocates improving the capacity of local communities to foster integration and manage mental illness within the community rather than hiding it away; however, many patients worry about the perception of others and are conscious of stigma. The GP advocate has a role in bridging this gap.

People seeking asylum can be in situations of continuing threat. Ongoing stress about lack of a secure future can mean they are not yet stable enough for some formal talking treatment models if there is little flexibility in their delivery. The GP's role in maintaining a therapeutic connection and frequent reassessment, including suicide risk, is vital in this situation. Liaison with NGOs, highly experienced in care at this stage, can be beneficial. Merely signposting a person in the direction of help is often ineffective, as mistrust is rife. Joint consultations work better as an initial means of contact.

Practical help and advocacy, for example, to improve housing or access food parcels, is a great start to developing a therapeutic relationship. This action 'inside and outside the therapy room' (11) shows commitment and genuine care.

Grounding techniques

Involuntary intrusive thoughts provoke extreme fear. You may see people upset and unable to concentrate on the consultation. Simple techniques (36), used by psychologists and in Psychological First Aid (13) to help control re-experiencing symptoms, can be used in GP surgeries with anyone distressed, anxious, or dissociative. Grounding helps re-focus and dispel anxiety. Ask what has helped previously and pick one or two from the list to try.

- Remind people that they are in a safe place; reiterate where they are, who is with them, and that these are just memories. They are unpleasant but not injurious.
- Stimulate the senses: Use a distracting noise — for example, music; ask them to push their feet hard into the floor, touch something cold, or describe the colours of things around them.
- Count backwards, recite an alphabet, or list facts.
- Breathing exercises: Breathe in for a count of 4, pause for 1, then slowly release for 6, and repeat.

Talking treatments

For uncomplicated depression and anxiety, usual therapy is a good start: behavioural activation, cognitive behavioural therapy, and social re-engagement.

Some cultures do not share our models of psychological illness. Ideas exist of evil spirits, responsible for altered thoughts or behaviour. The expectation may not be of medical treatment to alleviate symptoms. Nor can we assume prior knowledge of what therapy entails (11). Psychoeducation before a referral is important to contextualize it. In some areas, transcultural psychiatry is being developed.

The relationship between practitioner and patient, regardless of professional training, has a therapeutic effect. Listening, bearing witness, believing, and providing explanations or normalizing symptoms are potent tools. In PTSD, no single model of therapy has been shown to be optimal (11). Traumatized people usually respond best to longer-term relationships.

The difficulty in disclosing trauma for brief interventions can mean people do not identify modifiable goals quickly and struggle to make progress. The 'paralysis of initiative' (17) can make 'homework' tasks seem impossible. The political context in the host country may be an additional barrier to overcome with risk of hate crime and discrimination, including institutional racism in health services. Sometimes people are discharged early and labelled as lacking engagement. There are also issues with insufficient time to develop trust and work effectively with interpreters. Therapists and interpreters can feel overwhelmed by the magnitude of some people's circumstances and become vicariously traumatized.

An effective therapist helps navigate a way for traumatic memories to be narrated and integrated into memory in a manageable context. They can support mourning of losses. Their aim is to recover autonomy and worth, reconnect to others, and recover aspirations and ambitions (17).

Establishing a sense of safety and strategies to self-soothe are crucial before exploring traumatic memories. These techniques may need to be frequently revisited. Mindfulness-based treatments can achieve calm states for therapy (37). Yoga is beneficial in PTSD (38).

Rehabilitation includes exercise, limiting exposure to triggers — for example, 24-hour news — and practicing prepared responses for when people ask their history. Initially encouraging and facilitating participation at the periphery of social events or in creative activities that don't require deep conversation — for example, sports, music, and art — is helpful.

Group work needs careful preparation, especially with multiple languages. It can be overwhelming and expose people to triggers and power dynamics, but if carefully facilitated can allow the chance to care for each other, exchange information, and share strategies.

Eye movement desensitization and reprocessing (EMDR) (39) is a practice that helps some people process intrusive sensory memories into their narrative memory, with consequent decreases in anxiety. Its mechanism of action is poorly understood, but it is becoming a more widely available helpful technique.

Medication management

Where depression or anxiety is uncomplicated, we advise following local prescribing guidelines, taking into consideration severity and duration of symptoms, risk factors, comorbidities, and tolerability of treatment.

Pharmacological symptom control is frequently required before people with PTSD are able to engage in talking treatments, or alongside therapy to help manage the strong emotions provoked. It is not a panacea but rather a tool. Careful explanation is needed for correct adherence and management of expectations. Weekly dosing boxes can be helpful where lives are chaotic and memory unreliable. It is worth checking that people are not also taking medication they perceive as more popular or familiar, sent from relatives in their home country, from their housemates, or from the internet.

The onset of mood stabilization takes longer in PTSD than in uncomplicated depression. Useful medications include sedating antidepressants such as mirtazapine, taken at night to aid sleep, or trazodone with some additional anxiolytic activity. SSRIs are helpful if sedation is intolerable. Discussing 'unwanted effects' is more useful than the term 'side effects', which provokes anxiety. Toxicity in overdose must be high priority when selecting antidepressants with this group, and we rarely recommend tricyclics.

For anxious patients without contraindications, beta-blockers — for example, propranolol — are recommended. This can also help as migraine prophylaxis for the ubiquitous headache. Antipsychotic medications — for example, risperidone or olanzapine — can help re-experiencing symptoms, but may need to be initiated by a specialist and require monitoring of physical health, especially cardiovascular risks. Hypnotic medicines are not useful except as very short-term interventions; however, they may be obtained from non-medical sources, such as Ana buying diazepam from the internet, unbeknownst to the practitioner.

Drugs and alcohol

Illegal drugs, smoking, and alcohol are sometimes used as self-medication for psychological and physical pain, eating into limited financial resources. Many people remain unaware of the health risks, including psychosis and lung cancer from smoking cannabis and the depressant effect of alcohol. Information about nicotine replacement and navigation of self-referral pathways to drug and alcohol services are helpful (10).

Integrated treatment is needed for mental illness, substance misuse, and physical symptoms. PTSD increases the risk of developing opioid overuse disorder (40), which should influence your analgesia-prescribing strategy. Treatment of chronic pain involves paced activity, physiotherapy, massage, psychological support, and medication. There is growing evidence that long-term opioid analgesia adds no advantage and may be harmful (41). Other drugs used for chronic pain include antidepressant and anticonvulsant medications. This complex polypharmacy requires regular review. Chaotic taking of medication can lead to discontinuation symptoms and loss of faith in their effectiveness. Suicide risk assessment needs to be frequently revisited (42).

CONCLUSION

Caring for migrants can be challenging. Their loss of agency and deprivation of the wider determinants of health can make recovery harder to reach and maintain. Integrated health and social care, including the voluntary sector, is needed alongside longitudinal relationship building and cultural sensibility. As GPs, although mindful of the risk of vicarious traumatization, standing alongside someone in their journey to adapt and be healthy in their adopted country is imperative. I feel the role of the GP is crucial in a humanitarian response that seeks societal change, and this advocacy role brings additional meaning to our work.

REFERENCES

1. Mulder CL, Koopmans GT, Selten JP. Emergency psychiatry, compulsory admissions and clinical presentation among immigrants to the Netherlands. *Br J Psychiatry*. 2006;188:386–91.
2. Report by the South East Migrant Health Study Group on behalf of the Department of Health A. Understanding the health needs of migrants in the South East region [Internet]. [cited 2018 April 12]. Available from: http://webarchive.nationalarchives.gov.uk/20140714113244/http://www.hpa.org.uk/webc/HPAwebFile/HPAweb_C/1284475770868
3. Newbold KB. Self-rated health within the Canadian immigrant population: risk and the healthy immigrant effect. *Soc Sci Med* [Internet]. 2005 March 1 [cited 2017 November 12];60(6):1359–70. Available from: http://www.sciencedirect.com/science/article/pii/S027795360400334X?via%3Dihub
4. Kirmayer LJ, Narasiah L, Munoz M et al. Common mental health problems in immigrants and refugees: general approach in primary care. *CMAJ* [Internet]. 2011 [cited 2017 Nov 12];183(12):959–67. Available from: https://www.ncbi.nlm.nih.gov/pmc/articles/PMC3168672/pdf/183e959.pdf
5. Mallett R, Leff J, Bhugra D, Pang D, Zhao JH. Social environment, ethnicity and schizophrenia. A case-control study. *Soc Psychiatry Psychiatr Epidemiol*. 2002;37(7):329–35.
6. Hjern A, Wicks S, Dalman C. Social adversity contributes to high morbidity in psychoses in immigrants–A national cohort study in two generations of Swedish residents. *Psychol Med*. 2004;34(6):1025–33.

7. Casado BL, Hong M, Harrington D. Measuring migratory grief and loss associated with the experience of immigration. [cited 2018 April 15]. Available from: http://journals.sagepub.com/doi/pdf/10.1177/1049731509360840

8. Koenen K, Ratanatharathorn A, Ng L et al. Posttraumatic stress disorder in the World Mental Health Surveys. *Psychol Med.* 2017;47(13):2260–74.

9. Janoff-Bulman R. The aftermath of victimization: rebuilding shattered assumptions. In: Figley CR, editor. *Trauma and its Wake. Vol I. The Study and Treatment of Post-Traumatic Stress Disorder.* New York: Brunner Mazel; 1985: p. 15–35.

10. Farrington R. UK refugee and asylum seeker health. In: Wroe L, Larkin R, editors. *Social Work with Asylum Seekers, Refugees and Undocumented People: Going the Extra Mile.* 1st ed. Jessica Kingsley, UK; 2019.

11. Boyles J, editor. *Psychological Therapies for Survivors of Torture.* 1st ed. Monmouth: PCCS Books; 2017.

12. Littlewood R, Lipsedge M. *Aliens and Alienists: Ethnic Minorities and Psychiatry.* 3rd ed. Penguin Books; 1982.

13. World Health Organization WLC-PD. Psychological first aid: guide for field workers [Internet]. 2011 [cited 2017 November 12]. Available from: http://apps.who.int/iris/bitstream/10665/44615/1/9789241548205_eng.pdf

14. Rose SC, Bisson J, Churchill R, Wessely S. Psychological debriefing for preventing post traumatic stress disorder (PTSD). In: Rose SC, editor. *Cochrane Database of Systematic Reviews* [Internet]. Chichester, UK: John Wiley & Sons; 2002 [cited 2017 December 30]: CD000560. Available from: http://www.ncbi.nlm.nih.gov/pubmed/12076399

15. Santiago PN, Ursano RJ, Gray CL et al. A systematic review of PTSD prevalence and trajectories in DSM-5 defined trauma exposed populations: intentional and non-intentional traumatic events. *PLOS ONE.* 2013;8(4):1–3.

16. Başoğlu M, Mineka S, Paker M, Aker T, Livanou M, Gök Ş. Psychological preparedness for trauma as a protective factor in survivors of torture. *Psychol Med.* 1997;27(6):1421–33.

17. Herman JL. *Trauma and Recovery* [Internet]. Vol. 1992, *(1992) Trauma and Recovery xi.* New York, NY, US: Basic Books; 1992: 276 pp. Available from: http://ovidsp.ovid.com/ovidweb.cgi?T=JS&CSC=Y&NEWS=N&PAGE=fulltext&D=psyc3&AN=1992-97643-000%5Cnhttp://openurl.bibsys.no/openurl?url_ver=Z39.88-2004&rft_val_fmt=info:ofi/fmt:kev:mtx:journal&rfr_id=info:sid/Ovid:psyc3&rft.genre=article&rft_id=info:doi/&rft

18. Van der Veer G, Waning A. Creating a safe therapeutic sanctuary. In: Wilson J, Drozoek B (editors). *Broken Spirits: The Treatment of Traumatised Asylum Seekers, Refugees, War and Torture Victims.* 1st ed. Hove: Brunner Routledge; 2004: 187–219.

19. Betancourt J. Cross-cultural medical education: conceptual approaches and frameworks for evaluation. *Acad Med.* 2003;78(6):560–9.

20. Eisenbruch M. From post-traumatic stress disorder to cultural bereavement: diagnosis of Southeast Asian refugees. *Soc Sci Med.* 1991;33(6):673–80.

21. Crenshaw K. Demarginalizing the intersection of race and sex: a black feminist critique of antidiscrimination doctrine, feminist theory and antiracist politics. Univ Chic Leg Forum [Internet]. 1989 [cited 2017 October 1];1989. Available from: http://heinonline.org/HOL/Page?handle=hein.journals/uchclf1989&id=143&div=10&collection=journals

22. Andersen J, Wade M, Possemato K, Ouimette P. Association between posttraumatic stress disorder and primary care provider-diagnosed disease among Iraq and Afghanistan veterans. *Psychosom Med* [Internet]. 2010 June [cited 2017 September 24];72(5):498–504. Available from: http://content.wkhealth.com/linkback/openurl?sid=WKPTLP:landingpage&an=00006842-201006000-00009

23. Yaffe K, Vittinghoff E, Lindquist K et al. Posttraumatic stress disorder and risk of dementia among US veterans. *Arch Gen Psychiatry* [Internet]. 2010 June 1 [cited 2017 Sep 24];67(6):608–9. Available from: http://archpsyc.jamanetwork.com/article.aspx?doi=10.1001/archgenpsychiatry.2010.61

24. WHO. *The ICD-10 Classification of Mental and Behavioural Disorders: Clinical Descriptions and Diagnostic Guidelines.* World Health Organization [Internet]. 1992: 1–267. Available from: http://apps.who.int/iris/handle/10665/37950%5Cnhttp://scholar.google.com/scholar?hl=en&btnG=Search&q=intitle:The+ICD-10+Classification+of+Mental+and+Behavioural+Disorders#1

25. Brady KT, Killeen TK, Brewerton T, Lucerini S. Comorbidity of psychiatric disorders and posttraumatic stress disorder. *J Clin Psychiatry*. 2000;61(Suppl 7):22–32.
26. Van der Kolk B. The body keeps score: memory and the evolving psychobiology of posttraumatic stress. *Harv Rev Psychiatry*. 1994;1(5):253–65.
27. Rosellini A, Stein M, Benedek D, Bliese P, Chiu W, Hwang I, Kessler R. Using self-report surveys at the beginning of service to develop multi-outcome risk models for new soldiers in the U.S. *Army Psychol Med*. 2017;1(13).
28. Herman JL. Complex PTSD: a syndrome in survivors of prolonged and repeated trauma. *J Trauma Stress*. 1992;5(3):377–91.
29. Batista E, Wiese P, Burhorst I. The mental health of asylum-seeking and refugee children and adolescents attending a clinic in the Netherlands. [cited 2018 April 15]; Available from: http://journals.sagepub.com/doi/pdf/10.1177/1363461507083900
30. Hodes M, Jagdev D, Chandra N, Cunniff A. Risk and resilience for psychological distress amongst unaccompanied asylum seeking adolescents. *J Child Psychol Psychiatry* [Internet]. 2008 July [cited 2018 April 15];49(7):723–32. Available from: http://www.ncbi.nlm.nih.gov/pubmed/18492037
31. Bean TM, Eurelings-Bontekoe E, Spinhoven P. Course and predictors of mental health of unaccompanied refugee minors in the Netherlands: one year follow-up. *Soc Sci Med* [Internet]. 2007 March 1 [cited 2018 Apr 15];64(6):1204–15. Available from: https://www.sciencedirect.com/science/article/pii/S0277953606005910?via%3Dihub
32. Cartwright K, El-Khani A, Subryan A, Calam R. Establishing the feasibility of assessing the mental health of children displaced by the Syrian conflict. *Glob Ment Health (Camb)* [Internet]. 2015 June 19 [cited 2015 October 17];2:e8. Available from: http://journals.cambridge.org/abstract_S2054425115000035
33. D'Andrea W, Ford J, Stolbach B, Spinazzola J, Van der Kolk BA. Understanding interpersonal trauma in children: why we need a developmentally appropriate trauma diagnosis. *Am J Orthopsychiatry*. 2012;82(2):187–200.
34. National Center for PTSD. PTSD screening instruments [Internet]. [cited 2017 September 24]. Available from: https://www.ptsd.va.gov/professional/assessment/screens/index.asp
35. Papadopoulos RK. Refugees, trauma and adversity-activated development. *Eur J Psychother Couns* [Internet]. 2007 September [cited 2017 October 1];9(3):301–12. Available from: http://www.tandfonline.com/doi/abs/10.1080/13642530701496930
36. Najavits L. *Seeking Safety: A Treatment Manual for PTSD and Substance Abuse*. Guilford Press; 2002.
37. Hopwood TL, Schutte NS. A meta-analytic investigation of the impact of mindfulness-based interventions on post traumatic stress. *Clin Psychol Rev* [Internet]. 2017 November [cited 2017 August 16];57:12–20. Available from: http://linkinghub.elsevier.com/retrieve/pii/S0272735817301551
38. Canadian Agency for Drugs and Technologies in Health. *Yoga for the treatment of post-traumatic stress disorder, generalized anxiety disorder, depression, and substance abuse: a review of the clinical effectiveness and guidelines* [Internet]. Ottawa; Available from: https://www.ncbi.nlm.nih.gov/books/NBK304564/
39. Shapiro F. Eye movement desensitization and reprocessing: basic principles, protocols, and procedures [Internet]. 2001. 472-xxiv, 472 p. Available from: http://proxy.library.nd.edu/login?url=http://search.proquest.com/docview/619595584?accountid=12874 LA-English
40. Hassan AN, Le Foll B, Imtiaz S, Rehm J. The effect of post-traumatic stress disorder on the risk of developing prescription opioid use disorder: results from the National Epidemiologic Survey on Alcohol and Related Conditions III. *Drug Alcohol Depend* [Internet]. 2017 [cited 2017 August 24]; Available from: http://dx.doi.org/doi:10.1016/j.drugalcdep.2017.07.012
41. Elsesser K, Cegla T. Long-term treatment in chronic noncancer pain: results of an observational study comparing opioid and nonopioid therapy. *Scand J Pain* [Internet]. 2017;17(October):87–98. Available from: https://doi.org/10.1016/j.sjpain.2017.07.005
42. Sareen J, Cox BJ, Stein MB, Afifi TO, Fleet C, Asmundson GJG. Physical and mental comorbidity, disability, and suicidal behavior associated with posttraumatic stress disorder in a large community sample. *Psychosom Med* [Internet]. 2007 April [cited 2017 October 21];69(3):242–8. Available from: http://content.wkhealth.com/linkback/openurl?sid=WKPTLP:landingpage&an=00006842-200704000-00004

CHAPTER 18

Multimorbidity: The complexity

Amaia Calderón-Larrañaga and Luis Andrés Gimeno-Feliu

LEARNING OBJECTIVES

After reading this chapter, the reader will be able to:

- Have a better understanding of the implications and epidemiology of multimorbidity, as well as its social and psychosocial determinants
- Gain further insight into the intersection between migration and multimorbidity and the relevance of area of origin, length of stay in the host country, and reason for migration as key modulators
- Identify key recommendations to handle migrant patients with multimorbidity in primary care and community settings, based on up-to-date evidence

---

CLINICAL VIGNETTE 1: THE CASE OF RACHID

Rachid is a Moroccan man who arrived in Spain 23 years ago, at the age of 30 years. Upon arrival, he was diagnosed with hypertension. Over the years, he has developed obesity, type 2 diabetes, dyslipidaemia, gonarthrosis, ischaemic heart disease (angina pectoris), chronic kidney disease (stage G3b), and insomnia. He is taking acetylsalicylic acid, ramipril, bisoprolol, isosorbide dinitrate, simvastatin, metformin, sitagliptin, paracetamol, naproxen for severe pain, omeprazole, and occasional lormetazepam. At his last visit to the cardiologist, it was recommended he initiate insulin therapy due to an HbA1c value of 7.6%. He was also encouraged to take high-fibre, low-glycaemic index sources of carbohydrates in his diet, to control the intake of foods containing saturated and trans fatty acids, and to walk a minimum of 150 minutes per week.

CLINICAL VIGNETTE 2: THE CASE OF AZRA

Azra is a 58-year-old Bosnian woman who arrived in Norway 15 years ago as a political refugee. She lives alone and works as an intern looking after an old woman. She spends most of her free time reading at home. She already suffered from type 2 diabetes and hypertension when she arrived in Norway. Over the years, she has developed COPD (she is a hard smoker), osteoporosis, depression, psoriasis, rheumatoid arthritis, and obesity. She has recently changed neighbourhoods and has chosen a new GP. She is currently taking thiopropion, salbutamol, salmeterol, inhaled beclomethasone, metformin, NPH insulin, gliclazide, ramipril, amlodipine, alendronate, calcium, vitamin D, paroxetine, calcipotriol, methotrexate, paracetamol, and naproxen. In the last year, she visited the endocrinologist, rheumatologist, psychiatrist, and dermatologist several times.

CLINICAL VIGNETTE 3: THE CASE OF YING

Ying is a 64-year-old Chinese woman who arrived in Italy 10 years ago and has since worked in retail trade. She suffers from knee osteoarthritis and dyslipidaemia, and was recently diagnosed with breast cancer by her private gynaecologist. She occasionally takes acetaminophen for pain. In her last visit to the private clinic, the endocrinologist prescribed rosuvastatin, given her high cholesterol levels (292 mg/dL).

MULTIMORBIDITY: AN EPIDEMIC CHALLENGING CURRENT HEALTH SYSTEMS

Chronic conditions are one of the main current and future challenges to health systems worldwide. This chronic disease epidemic has enforced a paradigm shift in health care systems. Having more than one chronic disease concurrently, known as multimorbidity, adds still another layer of complexity to the management of patients with chronic diseases, especially at the primary care level, where this type of patient is more the rule than the exception (1).

Faced with patients with multimorbidity, general practitioners (GPs) need to adapt medical decision schemes to consider antagonisms or therapeutic synergies among all interacting health problems (2). Decision making in these patients is further hampered by the fact that clinical evidence is generated for individual diseases, given that most randomized trials exclude multimorbid and older people. Consequently, clinical guidelines rarely provide clinicians with tools to prioritize recommendations for the different conditions co-occurring in this type of patient (Chapter 21). Patients with multimorbidity are thus prescribed several drugs, each of which is recommended by a disease-specific guideline, leading to high levels of treatment burden that are often difficult for them to manage and potentially harmful (3). Hence, the care of patients with multimorbidity is characterized by uncertainty and enforced trade-offs, which often challenge the daily practice of primary care physicians.

People with multimorbidity are moreover at special risk for care fragmentation and medical error given the single disease-based approach of specialist care. On the one hand, this further increases the treatment burden of these patients, as they are likely to undergo more visits to health caregivers, complementary examinations, and lifestyle change efforts, all of which lead to an unrealistic workload for patients and their carers. On the other hand, working in the context of multiple care providers requires that any possible reassessment by the GP is shared and taken over by the rest of the specialist physicians, since patients will often continue to visit them on a regular basis.

EPIDEMIOLOGY AND DETERMINANTS OF MULTIMORBIDITY

Multimorbidity is very frequent in ageing people, with a prevalence spanning from 55% to 98% (4), although it is even more common in absolute terms and increasing at a higher speed among younger people (5). Such rise in numbers goes in parallel with the boost of individual chronic diseases and the ageing of the population, but could also be related to the increasing exposure to environmental, social, and personal risk factors that enhance people's vulnerability to a variety of illnesses.

The most common way to measure multimorbidity is to count whether a person has two or more of a predefined list of chronic conditions. Three patterns of multimorbidity have been consistently suggested to be prevalent in the elderly, involving (i) *cardio-metabolic diseases*, (ii) *psychogeriatric problems*, and (iii) *mechanical and somatoform disorders* (6).

In the same way the degree of susceptibility to chronic conditions is determined by people's social context, multimorbidity is also conditioned by social factors. Poor income and/or wealth, low education, manual occupation, and lack of social assistance have all been linked to higher prevalence of multimorbidity (4). Moreover, low socioeconomic position is associated with earlier onset of multimorbidity. In a study from Scotland, it was found that populations from deprived areas present with multimorbidity 10–15 years earlier than those from the most affluent areas (1). Lower socioeconomic status was also a major risk factor for a faster accumulation of chronic diseases among middle-aged Australian women (7). The mechanisms through which socioeconomic factors impact the likelihood of multimorbidity include increased exposure to lifestyle risk factors, hindered access to health care services, and suboptimal care provision (8). An allostatic overload, whereby the organism's adaptive and restorative capacity is overtaxed by the cumulative impact of lifelong strain, could also play a role (9).

Other factors beyond a person's material circumstances have also been found to increase the risk of multimorbidity, namely, self-esteem, control over one's environment, and social network (10). Yet to what extent these psychosocial determinants act independently or are mediated by other sociodemographic factors remains uncertain.

MIGRATION AND MULTIMORBIDITY: TWO COEXISTING VULNERABILITY FACTORS

Being a migrant, which is both socially determined and a social determinant of health per se, has been increasingly studied in relation to multimorbidity. Migration and multimorbidity are both considered health care-related vulnerability factors, i.e. factors entailing higher care needs and lower health care accessibility and/or quality (11). Thus, the simultaneous study of these two phenomena is crucial if we want to move towards health services that meet the needs of the most vulnerable patients.

MULTIMORBIDITY IN MIGRANT VERSUS NATIVE POPULATIONS

Only recently has research on migration and multimorbidity been undertaken. Despite the methodological differences, most studies find a lower prevalence of multimorbidity among migrants, which increases with longer stays in the host country at an even faster speed compared to non-migrants (Table 18.1).

In a study of Canadian adults, a 70% and 30% lower risk of suffering from three or more chronic diseases was found among migrants living in the country less than and above 5 years, respectively, after taking sex and age into account (12). Similar results were found in a Swiss population-based study that reported an up to 40% excess risk of multimorbidity among those with Swiss citizenship compared to migrants, after adjusting by age, sex, and lifestyle factors (13). A nationwide register-based study of people 15 years old or older in Norway also confirmed higher rates of multimorbidity among Norwegians compared to most migrants, even after adjusting for age, sex, income level, and number of visits to primary care (14). Along the same lines, another administrative data-based study carried out in a Northern Italian region found a significantly lower age- and sex-standardized prevalence of multimorbidity among migrants compared to Italian citizens (15). More recently, a study from a North eastern Spanish region using diagnostic data from primary care electronic health records also found a lower age- and sex-adjusted prevalence of multimorbidity among migrants compared to natives, regardless of the area of origin (16). The risk of multimorbidity was double in migrants residing in the region for 5 years or longer than that of those residing for less than 5 years.

Several hypotheses have been put forward to explain why the burden of morbidity is consistently lower in migrants, and especially among those with a short length of residence in the host country. One possible explanation is the lower use of the health care services by migrants due to access problems, which would decrease the likelihood of detecting diseases. Some authors have also brought up the issue of the 'salmon bias' or 'unhealthy remigration effect', according to which severely ill migrants tend to re-migrate to their country of origin in order to be cared for by their families. Consequently, multimorbidity rates among migrants could be underestimated. Still, recently published literature seems to discard this hypothesis as the main explanation for the better health outcomes of migrants as compared to native populations (17). What is most likely is that migrants, particularly those leaving for economic reasons, are generally healthier and have better health behaviours compared not only to the native-born but also to the population from their country of origin. This phenomenon has been defined as the 'healthy migrant effect' (18) (Chapter 2).

Different authors have also reflected on the reasons why the risk of multimorbidity in migrants increases with longer lengths of stay in the host country. Under the understanding that migration constitutes a social determinant of health itself, longer exposures may contribute to a worsening of health and a loss of the before-mentioned health status advantage after a number of years. Chronic stress, lower socioeconomic status, low health literacy, barriers to health care service use, and discrimination are some of the factors associated with the post-migration experience with which migrant status can intersect, adversely affecting health outcomes (Chapter 2).

TABLE 18.1 Studies on migration and multimorbidity available in the literature

Author; country	Data source; age range; study year	Definition of migrant status (% of population)	Definition of multimorbidity	Prevalence of multimorbidity			OR (95% CI) Reference category: non-migrants (unless otherwise stated)	Adjustment by confounders
				General population	Migrants	Non-migrants		
Roberts et al. (12); Canada	Canadian Community Health Survey; ≥20 years; 2011–2012	Born in foreign country (24.3%)	Self-report of ≥2 chronic diseases from a list of 9	12.9%	LOS <5 years: 2.3% LOS ≥5 years: 11.6%	...	...	...
			Self-report of ≥3 chronic diseases from a list of 9	3.9%	LOS <5 years: 0.5% LOS ≥5 years: 3.4%	...	LOS <5 years: 0.3 (0.1–2.1) LOS ≥5 years: 0.7 (0.6–0.8)	Age, sex
Pache et al. (13); Switzerland	Cohorte Lausannois; 35–75 years; 2003–2006	Born in foreign country (39.6%)	Self-report of ≥2 chronic diseases from a list of 27	34.8%	31.4%	37.1%	1.27 (1.09–1.49) *Ref category: migrants*	Age, sex, education, provision of social help, smoking, BMI
			Diagnosis of ≥2 chronic diseases from a list of 27	56.3%	52.3%	58.8%	1.29 (1.11–1.49) *Ref category: migrants*	
			≥2 chronic diseases from the FCI	22.7%	19.7%	24.8%	1.41 (1.17–1.71) *Ref category: migrants*	
Diaz et al. (20); Norway	National Population Register + primary care claims; ≥15 years; 2008	Born in foreign country with both parents from abroad (10.4%)	Diagnosis of ≥2 chronic EDC from a list of 114	9.9%	Western countries[a]: 10.6% Eastern Europe: 6.3% Other non-Western countries[b]: 9.3%	10.1%	Western countries[a]: 0.81 (0.79–0.83) Eastern Europe: 0.64 (0.63–0.66) Other non-Western countries[b]: 0.68 (0.66–0.69)	Age, sex, income level, number of visits to primary care
Lenzi et al. (15); Italy	Hospital registers + community mental health services + residential facilities + outpatient pharmaceutical database; ≥18 years; 2003–2012	Non-Italian citizenship (11.2%)	Diagnosis of ≥2 chronic diseases from a list of 26 (defined based on Charlson index, Elixhauser measure, and Quan algorithm)	15.3%	9.3%	14.4%	...	Gender, age (standardization of prevalence rates)

(Continued)

TABLE 18.1 (CONTINUED) Studies on migration and multimorbidity available in the literature

Author; country	Data source; age range; study year	Definition of migrant status (% of population)	Definition of multimorbidity	Prevalence of multimorbidity			OR (95% CI) Reference category: non-migrants (unless otherwise stated)	Adjustment by confounders
				General population	Migrants	Non-migrants		
Gimeno-Feliu et al. (16); Spain	Primary care electronic health records; ≥15 years; 2011	Born in foreign country (13.2%)	Diagnosis of ≥2 chronic EDC from a list of 114	36.5%	Africa: 11.7%	39.9%	Africa, LOS <5 years: 0.29 (0.27–0.31)	Age, sex, number of visits to primary care
							Africa, LOS ≥5 years: 0.64 (0.61–0.67)	
					Asia: 10.0%		Asia, LOS <5 years: 0.17 (0.14–0.20)	
							Asia, LOS ≥5 years: 0.54 (0.48–0.60)	
					Eastern Europe: 10.4%		Eastern Europe, LOS <5 years: 0.27 (0.25–0.28)	
							Eastern Europe, LOS ≥5 years: 0.59 (0.57–0.61)	
					Latin America: 18.5%		Latin America, LOS <5 years: 0.47 (0.44–0.49)	
							Latin America, LOS ≥5 years: 0.87 (0.84–0.89)	
					Western Europe and North America: 21.2%		Western Europe and North America, LOS <5 years: 0.29 (0.26–0.33)	
							Western Europe and North America, LOS ≥5 years: 0.78 (0.74–0.82)	

[a] West Europe and North America.
[b] Asia, Africa, and Latin America.

Abbreviations: OR, odds ratio; CI, confidence interval; LOS, length of stay; BMI, body mass index; FCI, Functional Comorbidity Index; EDC, Expanded Diagnostic Clusters.

REASON FOR MIGRATION: ANOTHER KEY DETERMINANT OF MULTIMORBIDITY

The reason for migration is an essential feature to better understand and assess health disparities in migrant communities, given that it shapes the migration experience. A study among asylum seekers carried out in the emergency care setting of central Switzerland singled out refugees as an especially vulnerable group compared to other migrants (19). Nearly 40% of all adult asylum seekers admitted to that specific hospital had two or more from a list of 18 diseases. Refugees are indeed the greatest exponent of adverse pre-migration and post-migration experiences characterized by violent conflicts in the country of origin, hazardous journeys, and detention-like living conditions and fear of persecution in the country of asylum, all of which have a profound impact on health.

In a Norwegian multi-register-based study (20), the odds of multimorbidity were significantly lower for labour and education migrants and higher for refugees than for family reunification migrants, even after adjusting by age, sex, income level, and civil status. For all groups, multimorbidity doubled after a 5-year stay in Norway, although the negative effect of a longer length of stay was more important for labour migrants and less important for refugees than for other groups, confirming that the effects of pre-migration and migration on health extend throughout the remaining phases of the migratory process. A higher risk of multimorbidity was also found in refugees living in Denmark, although the risk became lower for all migrant groups compared to the Danish-born when adjusting for civil status and mean income (21).

PATTERNS OF MULTIMORBIDITY AMONG MIGRANTS

A study comparing multimorbidity patterns in migrant versus majority populations in Norway using primary care claims data (14) showed more similarities than differences between Norwegian-born people and migrants, confirming a common physiopathological basis of diseases. This was also the case in another Italian study on multimorbidity (15). In the Norwegian study, a picture consistent with previous literature emerged, including a *cardiovascular-endocrine* pattern comprising a variety of cardiometabolic conditions, sometimes split into two factors, a *mental health* pattern, and a *musculoskeletal pattern*. Three additional patterns of multimorbidity were identified, *malignant, haematological*, and *respiratory*. The main differences identified between natives and migrants are summarized as follows.

- The *mental health pattern* was more often associated to schizophrenia in migrants from other non-Western and East European countries and to dementia in older people from Norway and Western countries. This latter *mental-geriatric* pattern did not emerge for older men from other non-Western countries and was associated to a more complex psychosomatic pattern for older Eastern Europeans of both genders. These differences could reflect the lower proportion of dementia diagnoses among migrants from low-income countries, higher degrees of somatization among migrants, cultural differences, and social stigma attached to some diseases, as well as communication problems for some groups (Chapter 23).
- The *malignant pattern* appeared at older ages and included the most common cancer types. However, this pattern was more complex in East European and other non-Western countries. This could reflect the intricacy of cancer diagnoses and the higher number of consultations needed to refer migrant patients with cancer to secondary

health care, which may lead to increased detection rates of coexisting comorbidities and thus to a higher complexity of the pattern in these population groups.

- The *haematological pattern* appeared only in women from Eastern Europe and other non-Western countries. In accordance with the high prevalence of anaemia described among young migrants, its main components were iron deficiency and other haematological disorders, but the pattern became more complex with age, especially for Eastern Europeans. These complex patterns might reflect a higher vulnerability to disease, as explained by the concept of allostatic overload. Other explanations include GPs' difficulties categorizing disease for women from different cultural and linguistic backgrounds, and the different presentation of diseases among migrant women compared to Norwegian-born and Western women.

The epidemiological studies mentioned so far have tended to group morbidities and even migrant populations into broad categories for the sake of data manageability. Yet more nuanced analyses are essential in order to make the findings clinically relevant. Aspects such as the severity of health conditions (e.g. cancer vs hearing impairment), their impact on daily life (e.g. hypertension vs arthralgia), and/or their diagnostic accuracy (e.g. depression vs adjustment disorders) can all affect the management of multimorbidity and should be accounted for in future studies. Individual biographical pathways will also need to be considered, as discussed previously.

HANDLING MIGRANT PATIENTS WITH MULTIMORBIDITY IN PRIMARY CARE

Although universal access to health services is crucial for equitable health care, facilitating access alone does not necessarily lead to equitable health care outcomes. On the one hand, providing person-centred care, defined as care that is empathic, respectful of, and responsive to individual preferences, needs, and values, is essential when managing multimorbidity, given that multiple diseases and upstream risk factors are to be addressed and a range of outcomes are to be achieved. On the other hand, a biopsychosocial approach to care is required to contextualize people's health, considering the impact of biography on biology and thus developing the skills that enable cross-cultural interactions.

These two overarching features are linked in Betancourt's reflection about cultural competence (22): 'cultural competence has evolved from the making of assumptions about patients on the basis of their background to the implementation of the principles of patient-centred care, including exploration, empathy, and responsiveness to patients' needs, values, and preferences' (Chapter 20). Indeed, person-centred and biopsychosocial care are most needed among migrant populations where multimorbidity, although less common at arrival, becomes highly frequent with time. Migrants are moreover particularly vulnerable to the health-threatening impact of other interacting dimensions of social disadvantage.

Primary care has a key role in managing migrant patients with multimorbidity, as it is person-focussed rather than disease-focussed and continuous over time, leading to long-lasting doctor-patient relationships that enable GPs to dig into patients' social and cultural background (i.e. food tradition, health culture, religious beliefs, etc.) (23). GPs are qualified to identify and balance patients' preferences considering other non-health-related factors belonging to the socioeconomic, cultural, and/or behavioural dimensions, and optimize their care, minimizing unnecessary harm and treatment burden. Practitioners working in primary care may also play a major role in increasing the awareness of the complexity of multimorbidity among migrants during their clinical encounter. Last, primary care is ideally suited to orchestrate the multidisciplinary care needed by migrants with multimorbidity, given that it is embedded within local communities, where other social and public health agents coexist.

But this is not always straightforward for GPs due to a number of difficulties spanning system factors, the evidence base for chronic disease management, and their own communication skills in the context of multiple physician and patient agendas (24). Such difficulties may be accentuated when attending vulnerable migrant groups, given language problems, the lack of cultural awareness, and potential threats to care continuity such as lack of insurance, frequent mobility, or forced dispersal policy (25).

INTERVENTIONS AND NEW MODELS OF CARE IN THE PRIMARY CARE AND COMMUNITY SETTINGS

Despite the growing size of migrant populations, there is a relative paucity of intervention studies aimed at improving health outcomes among migrants (26). Moreover, existing interventions have mainly focussed on individual chronic and non-communicable conditions. Older migrants, whose numbers are expected to increase in the near future, have seldom been considered as the target population.

A recent systematic review on interventions to improve the management of multimorbidity found no more than 18 randomized trials with mixed and inconclusive results (27). Overall, organizational interventions targeted at the management of specific risk factors or focussed on areas where patients have difficulties (e.g. functional ability, management of medicines, etc.) seemed more likely to be effective. In contrast, interventions with a broader focus, such as case management or changes in delivery of care, or those not linked to specific functional difficulties, were less effective. Still, most studies ignored the impact of the social context, and none of them explored how the effect of interventions changed for different socioeconomic groups. The only intervention that has proved to be potentially effective and cost-effective to limit the decline in quality of life and well-being in multimorbidity patients in the context of deprivation consisted of system changes to allow longer consultations and relationship continuity, group-based training for practitioners, and self-management support material for patients (28).

Several tools have recently been developed to support decision making in patients with multimorbidity. Among these, the *Ariadne principles* deserve special attention, given their specific focus on patients in primary care consultations, who require a longitudinal and comprehensive approach (29). This model places the setting of realistic treatment goals at the centre of the multimorbidity consultation (Figure 18.1). Such goals result from a thorough interaction assessment of the patient's conditions, treatments, and context, the prioritization of health problems that take into account the patient's preferences, and individualized management to determine the best options of care to achieve these goals. Clinical Vignettes 1 and 2 serve as illustrative examples of the diversity and complexity of expressions of multimorbidity in the migrant population and the central role of primary care professionals in adapting the therapeutic objectives to the individuality of each patient.

As part of the interaction assessment, prioritization, and individualized management process, GPs should actively identify social circumstances affecting patients' health and care-seeking behaviours, given the potential of contextual factors to disrupt the balance between patients' internal capacity and their illness burden. Indeed, financial constraints, living conditions and social support, health literacy, functional autonomy, and coping strategies have all been found to moderate the self-reported health status and physical functioning

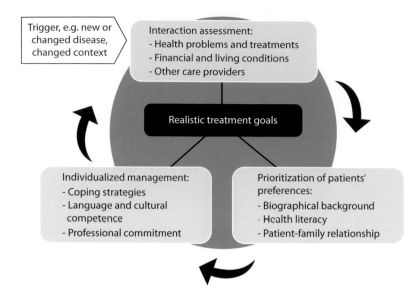

FIGURE 18.1 Ariadne principles (adapted): Core elements of an ongoing counselling process for migrant patients with multimorbidity in primary care. (Adapted from Muth C et al. *BMC Med.* 2014;12:223.)

of seniors with multimorbidity, and must accordingly be elicited and considered in clinical decision making and care planning (30). The reason for migration has been shown to intersect with many of these factors and consequently may contribute to the multilevel complexity that determines the success of any preventive and/or therapeutic intervention.

The Ariadne principles, as well as the other existing alternative consultation models, still need empirical validation, not only though pragmatic randomized controlled trials but also through qualitative and mixed methodologies, to test their applicability and effectiveness in real-world practice. On the other hand, expecting a 'one size fits all' model to support and improve the quality of care in multimorbidity is unrealistic, and even more so for migrant patients with multimorbidity, given the enormous heterogeneity behind these groups of patients. Here again, methodological pluralism and quality research are required to better identify the challenges derived from the complex care needs of these populations. In parallel, person-centred and biopsychosocial medicine, professional commitment, and patient advocacy should guide everyday primary care practice.

THE PRIMARY CARE APPROACH

THE CASE OF RACHID

Knowing about Rachid's social, biographical, and cultural background is essential to establish a consensus treatment plan. During his last consultation, which was held jointly with the GP, primary care nurse, and his wife, Rachid revealed he was working as a street vendor, that he was Muslim, and that he had recently become a legal resident, enabling him to bring his family over. Rachid manifested his reluctance to start insulin and his difficulty taking all 17 pills for which he did not know the indication. After clarifying the significance of his different diseases and treatments, his GP set realistic blood pressure and glycaemic control targets for Rachid and informed him about the convenience of avoiding the use of naproxen and benzodiazepines. It was decided to postpone insulin therapy, and to start a weight loss plan by adjusting the family's traditional diet, reducing the consumption of sweets, and adapting the physical activity recommendations to his daily schedule and his problem of gonarthrosis. He also agreed to be followed up by the nurse every 3 weeks. Rachid lost considerable weight after 3 months, which relieved his gonalgia and led to a decrease in his blood pressure and glycaemic levels, reducing his medication burden. His GP communicated these achievements to the cardiologist. The successful diagnosis and treatment of a radiologically confirmed pneumonia in his wife also contributed to improve his adherence and trust in the primary care team.

THE CASE OF AZRA

Azra is a paradigmatic case of complexity, where different health problems, care providers, and social inequality axes (i.e. political refugee, woman, precarious employment, isolation, and poverty) intersect. This scenario prompted her GP to take up a comprehensive dialogue with Azra during her first visit to the health centre. Throughout the interview, the GP realized that what interfered most with her patient's work activity was the pain and stiffness derived from her rheumatoid arthritis. Azra also stated that her depression, probably linked to her living conditions, significantly conditioned her daily life. Based on this insight, her GP established an individualized long-term care plan for Azra and stated his compromise to coordinate the work of the different specialists in order to share therapeutic goals and avoid iatrogenia. With the help of the primary care social worker, Azra was put in contact with a local reading club. The endeavour to optimize Azra's medication regime and the improvement of her depression encouraged her GP to initiate antidepressant withdrawal. The good relationship built between Azra and her GP also made it possible for the latter to start working on the cessation of Azra's smoking habits.

THE CASE OF YING

Ying rarely visits the public health service, and she is a regular user of traditional Chinese medicine. She has always followed her hometown diet and enjoys a satisfactory economic and social situation. Driven by her concern for the recent diagnosis of breast cancer, she decided to contact her primary care centre. During the consultation, her GP took advantage to explore her cardiovascular health, to discuss the risk/benefit ratio of initiating statin therapy, and to consider other non-pharmacological interventions such as increasing her daily physical activity. Regarding her breast cancer, Ying told the GP about her plans to consult with her traditional Chinese practitioner. After acknowledging her efforts to share her worries, the GP offered Ying an appointment with the oncologist, with the aim to provide her with rigorous information on the characteristics of the cancer and possible therapeutic options. The GP also encouraged her to share the oncologist's feedback with her traditional practitioner. Ying finally decided to follow the treatment proposed by the oncologist, complementing it with several Chinese herbs that were examined by the hospital's clinical pharmacology unit to avoid possible interactions. It was also decided to suspend statin therapy pending a future cardiovascular risk assessment. The GP's visit to the hospital during Ying's short stay reinforced their bond, favouring the continuity of the follow-up from primary care.

CONCLUSION

Even if multimorbidity is less prevalent among migrants at arrival, it may become highly frequent — and at an even faster speed — with time, given their greater exposure to other interacting dimensions of social disadvantage. This puts them at higher risk of increased care needs and lower health care accessibility and quality. Person-centred and biopsychosocial care, professional commitment, and patient advocacy will be crucial in order to foster primary care services that meet the needs of migrant populations with multimorbidity.

ACKNOWLEDGEMENTS

We want to thank Carlos Coscollar-Santaliestra and Carlos Calderón-Gómez for their comments and help with the chapter.

REFERENCES

1. Barnett K, Mercer SW, Norbury M, Watt G, Wyke S, Guthrie B. Epidemiology of multimorbidity and implications for health care, research, and medical education: a cross-sectional study. *Lancet.* 2012;380(9836):37–43.
2. Starfield B, Lemke KW, Bernhardt T, Foldes SS, Forrest CB, Weiner JP. Comorbidity: implications for the importance of primary care in 'case' management. *Ann Fam Med.* 2003;1(1):8–14.
3. Boyd CM, Darer J, Boult C, Fried LP, Boult L, Wu AW. Clinical practice guidelines and quality of care for older patients with multiple comorbid diseases: implications for pay for performance. *JAMA.* 2005;294(6):716–24.
4. Marengoni A, Angleman S, Melis R et al. Aging with multimorbidity: a systematic review of the literature. *Ageing Res Rev.* 2011;10(4):430–9.
5. Taylor AW, Price K, Gill TK et al. Multimorbidity — Not just an older person's issue. Results from an Australian biomedical study. *BMC Public Health.* 2010;10:718.
6. Prados-Torres A, Calderón-Larrañaga A, Hancco-Saavedra J, Poblador-Plou B, Van Den Akker M. Multimorbidity patterns: a systematic review. *J Clin Epidemiol.* 2014;67(3):254–66.
7. Jackson CA, Dobson A, Tooth L, Mishra GD. Body mass index and socioeconomic position are associated with 9-year trajectories of multimorbidity: a population-based study. *Prev Med.* 2015;81:92–8.
8. Mercer SW, Guthrie B, Furler J, Watt GCM, Hart JT. Multimorbidity and the inverse care law in primary care. *BMJ.* 2012;344:e4152.
9. Tomasdottir MO, Sigurdsson JA, Petursson H et al. Self reported childhood difficulties, adult multimorbidity and allostatic load. A cross-sectional analysis of the Norwegian HUNT study. *PLOS ONE.* 2015;10(6):e0130591.
10. van den Akker M, Buntinx F, Metsemakers JF, van der Aa M, Knottnerus JA. Psychosocial patient characteristics and GP-registered chronic morbidity: a prospective study. *J Psychosom Res.* 2001;50(2):95–102.
11. Grabovschi C, Loignon C, Fortin M. Mapping the concept of vulnerability related to health care disparities: a scoping review. *BMC Health Serv Res.* 2013;13:94.
12. Roberts KC, Rao DP, Bennett TL, Loukine L, Jayaraman GC. Prevalence and patterns of chronic disease multimorbidity and associated determinants in Canada. *Health Promot Chronic Dis Prev Can.* 2015;35(6):87–94.
13. Pache B, Vollenweider P, Waeber G, Marques-Vidal P. Prevalence of measured and reported multimorbidity in a representative sample of the Swiss population. *BMC Public Health.* 2015;15:164.
14. Diaz E, Poblador-Pou B, Gimeno-Feliu L-A, Calderón-Larrañaga A, Kumar BN, Prados-Torres A. Multimorbidity and its patterns according to immigrant origin. A nationwide register-based study in Norway. *PLOS ONE.* 2015;10(12):e0145233.

15. Lenzi J, Avaldi VM, Rucci P, Pieri G, Fantini MP. Burden of multimorbidity in relation to age, gender and immigrant status: a cross-sectional study based on administrative data. *BMJ Open*. 2016;6(12):e012812.

16. Gimeno-Feliu LA, Calderón-Larrañaga A, Díaz E et al. Multimorbidity and immigrant status: associations with area of origin and length of residence in host country. *Fam Pract*. 2017;34(6):662–6.

17. Norredam M, Hansen OH, Petersen JH et al. Remigration of migrants with severe disease: Myth or reality? – A register-based cohort study. *Eur J Public Health*. 2015;25(1):84–9.

18. Gushulak B. Healthier on arrival? Further insight into the 'healthy immigrant effect'. *CMAJ*. 2007;176(10):1439–40.

19. Pfortmueller CA, Stotz M, Lindner G, Müller T, Rodondi N, Exadaktylos AK. Multimorbidity in adult asylum seekers: a first overview. *PLOS ONE*. 2013;8(12):e82671.

20. Diaz E, Kumar BN, Gimeno-Feliu L-A, Calderón-Larrañaga A, Poblador-Pou B, Prados-Torres A. Multimorbidity among registered immigrants in Norway: the role of reason for migration and length of stay. *Trop Med Int Health*. 2015;20(12):1805–14.

21. Taleshan N, Petersen JH, Schioetz ML, Juul-Larsen HG, Norredam M. Multimorbidity and mortality thereof, among non-western refugees and family reunification immigrants in Denmark – A register based cohort study. *BMC Public Health*. 2018;18(1):844.

22. Betancourt JR. Cultural competence--marginal or mainstream movement? *N Engl J Med*. 2004;351(10):953–5.

23. Starfield B. New paradigms for quality in primary care. *Br J Gen Pract*. 2001;51(465):303–9.

24. Sinnott C, Mc HS, Browne J, Bradley C. GPs' perspectives on the management of patients with multimorbidity: systematic review and synthesis of qualitative research. *BMJ Open*. 2013;3:e003610.

25. Jensen NK, Norredam M, Priebe S, Krasnik A. How do general practitioners experience providing care to refugees with mental health problems? A qualitative study from Denmark. *BMC Fam Pract*. 2013;14:17.

26. Diaz E, Ortiz-Barreda G, Ben-Shlomo Y et al. Interventions to improve immigrant health. A scoping review. *Eur J Public Health*. 2017;27(3):433–9.

27. Smith SM, Soubhi H, Fortin M, Hudon C, O'Dowd T. Managing patients with multimorbidity: systematic review of interventions in primary care and community settings. *BMJ*. 2012;345(1):e5205.

28. Mercer SW, Fitzpatrick B, Guthrie B et al. The CARE Plus study – A whole-system intervention to improve quality of life of primary care patients with multimorbidity in areas of high socioeconomic deprivation: exploratory cluster randomised controlled trial and cost-utility analysis. *BMC Med*. 2016;14(1):88.

29. Muth C, van den Akker M, Blom JW et al. The Ariadne principles: how to handle multimorbidity in primary care consultations. *BMC Med*. 2014;12:223.

30. Bayliss EA, Bonds DE, Boyd CM et al. Understanding the context of health for persons with multiple chronic conditions: moving from what is the matter to what matters. *Ann Fam Med*. 2014;12(3):260–9.

IV

Opportunities and tools

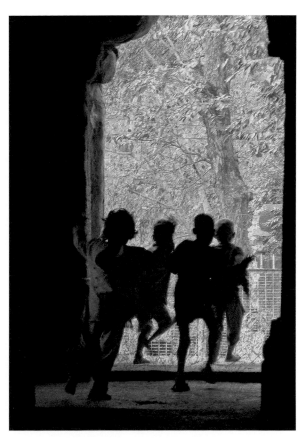

Photo credit: Sue Macartney.

Opportunities and tools when meeting migrant patients

Christine Phillips and Jill Benson

LEARNING OBJECTIVES

At the end of this chapter, the reader should be able to:

- Describe opportunities for primary health care to improve health care access and services for migrants
- Summarize skills needed by primary care practitioners who work with migrants in communication, knowledge acquisition, and cultural sensitivity
- Outline the roles of guidelines, protocols, and procedures and community engagement in delivering health care for migrants

---

CLINICAL VIGNETTE: A NEW FAMILY IN GENERAL PRACTICE

Mahmoud Hamzah is the head of a Druze Syrian family, who recently came to Australia under the humanitarian programme. He arrived with six adult family members: his daughters Rana, Mona, and Alina, his sons Faisal and Najib, and Najib's wife Luna. They lived in a camp in Turkey for the last 5 years, where they had minimal health care.

Most of the family have tertiary education and worked in professional positions in Syria before the conflict. Only Rana speaks any English. Their home had come under direct attack, and they have lost contact with the third son, Khaled, who they think has probably been killed. Mahmoud's wife had diabetes, but because of limited health care, she died soon after arrival in the camp. Mona 'disappeared' for 3 days during their escape from Syria but refuses to talk about what happened to her.

The family is taken to a mainstream general practice with experience working with refugees

BACKGROUND

It is a truism of primary health care that you don't fully understand a patient's illness until you know their history and their social world. The social world of migrants is marked by the experience of displacement and resettlement. Contained in the patient's present is always a *past* that may be historically and geographically strange to the clinician. In few other areas of primary health care must the practitioner consciously and conscientiously engage in the daily negotiation of difference.

This section addresses the organizational frameworks, skills, and collaborations to help primary care practitioners negotiate this difference. While this compendium is relevant for all patients, primary care practitioners who work with refugees and other migrants are likely to spend every consultation employing some of these. The delight of this area of practice is that practitioners become nimble at employing perspective-taking to understand different cultures, focussing on diversity as strength, using a range of assessment tools and networks, and collaborating with other practitioners.

Migrant health care is a mainstream area of primary care practice. Of Australian residents, 28.5% were born in another country (1). High rates of in-migration are found in other settler countries like Canada and New Zealand, and in the countries of the European Union.* On any day, any primary care provider is likely to treat several patients who were born outside the country. Thus, in their everyday practice clinicians need to be alert to differences in health literacy and to patterns of illness and representations of illness among migrant populations. To regard health care for migrants as a specialist area of practice is to marginalize patients in every clinician's practice.

At the same time, this area of health care does require some specialized skills. Most countries also offer specialized migrant health care services that can provide support for mainstream primary care. There are four types of specialized primary care services:

1. Services designed to respond to needs specific to some migrant populations. Examples include specialized services for women who have had female genital cutting performed when they were children (2), or for survivors of torture (3).
2. Services designed to provide on-arrival screening for newly arrived refugees and other migrants (4). These are generally short-term services that use standard screening instruments focussing on conditions of public health importance, nutrition status, and catchup immunization. Referrals may be provided for urgent surgical or psychiatric services. Sometimes these services are provided in community health services or in hospitals, and sometimes they are provided in integrated services addressing other elements of settlement, such as housing support and linking with language training.
3. Services for migrants and refugees designed to deliver comprehensive, integrated primary health care for patients with complex needs (5,6). Such services generally help patients to negotiate social services and hospitals and have connections

---

* The discussion in this section does not address the needs of temporary residents seeking cross-border health care arrangements which reflect inter-country or international legal agreements. (Wismar M, Palm W, van Ginneken E, Buse R, Ernst K, Figueras J. The Health Service Initiative: supporting the construction of a framework for cross-border care. In: Wismar M, Palm W, Figueras J, Ernst K, van Ginneken E, editors. *Cross-Border Health Care in the European Union. Mapping and Analysing Practices and Policies.* WHO, on behalf of the European Observatory on Health Systems and Policies; 2011.)

with mainstream primary health care services and integrated multidisciplinary health care. These services tend to be small and specialized, and must have clearly articulated exit policies to avoid becoming parallel primary care services.
4. Specialized health navigation. A health navigator may be a nurse or a specialized care coordinator (7,8). Their role is to personally assist the migrant to navigate the health sector in the early days of resettlement.

HEALTH CARE NEEDS FOR DIFFERENT TYPES OF MIGRANTS

Refugees and other migrants differ categorically in their mode of departure from their own country (9). Migrants choose to leave, perhaps for employment, marriage, or for family reunification. Refugees are forced to leave. This important distinction points to the nature of the past, and it likely impacts upon the present, for patients of refugee background. Increasingly, refugees' pasts include the impact of guerrilla war in civilian communities, and the sustained withholding of basic services such as education, housing, and health care from the most vulnerable, marginalized groups, or non-citizens. Most importantly, refugees are likely to have experienced firsthand significant losses within their own lives and be struggling with the burden of witness (10).

Many people — at least in Australia — argue that one of the features distinguishing refugees from other migrants is poverty. A genuine refugee, the argument runs, lives in abject poverty; those who belong to the middle class are less likely to be refugees, since they have economic resources. This confusion of cause and effect would have surprised the drafters of the 1951 Refugee Convention, which defined refugees at a time when Western Europe was facing floods of persecuted, but not necessarily impoverished, people fleeing Communist Europe (11). It is demonstrably false to assert that the middle class cannot, by reason of their class, be refugees. In fact, the middle class are often the engines of revolution, and when these revolutions fail, they can suffer disproportionately as victims of political persecution (12,13).

Other types of migrants in settlement countries, depending on their visa class, may have worse access to health care than refugees. Migrants who arrive on temporary work visas frequently struggle to access health care. In many countries with Beveridge (government managed, tax based) health financing systems, visas for newly arrived migrants who have come for specific reasons (marriage, family reunion, work) preclude or delay access to the social safety net, including health care. In countries with Bismarck (independent, insurance based) health financing systems, migrants' access to health care is determined by their ability to access health insurance, often through their employers.

While there are overlaps between the experiences of refugees and other migrants, the major practical difference relates to the need for catchup primary health care. Once protected as neutral sites, heath care services have become the targets and battle (14). The long-term impact of war in some refugee-source countries — the civil wars in Afghanistan, Sudan, and Somalia have occupied several generations — has resulted in lifetime gaps in primary health care. When the current generation of primary health practitioners began working in refugee health care, the assumption was that adult refugees had probably received their primary courses of immunizations as babies. So protracted has the humanitarian disaster been in some countries that no such assurance can now be held for many adults from refugee-source countries.

OPPORTUNITIES FOR PRIMARY HEALTH CARE

Appropriate health care for newly arrived migrants and refugees will not only improve their immediate health but is also likely to decrease the long-term health burden on the individual, their family, society, and the health system.

To be effective, health care providers for migrants need two capabilities. Firstly, they must be able to identify rapid changes in health care needs. An emerging health care issue of public health importance may not be recognized in primary care because the sample population in each clinic is too small to identify trends. Services for migrants often have to collaborate with each other to identify sentinel conditions and to pool their data (15,16).

Secondly, they must be able to meet surges in demand. Most primary care services have limited surge capacity, which they put into practice in pandemics or environmental disasters (17). Health care providers for migrants, on the other hand, must think and plan for inevitable surges in demand. When major conflicts occur, desperate people cross borders asking for protection. In 2015, 378,000 survivors of the conflict in Syria applied for asylum in countries of the European Union, a threefold increase on applicant numbers over the previous year (18). Changes in government policy towards asylum seekers or migrant workers can also result in sudden ebbs and flows of potential patient populations.

When these rapid changes in people flows occur, primary health care providers can become overwhelmed (19). With the best of intentions, they may find that their resilience to serve people in great need is exhausted. Services that do succeed in meeting surges in demand have thought ahead about what to do when a surge happens: expanding their staff, changing their model of care, using triage protocols, and systematizing their health care delivery. To be able to expand staff numbers on short notice, primary health care services need to have established relationships with other health care services and health care practitioners who would be willing to work for a short period in refugee or migrant health care. Ideally, these people would have some prior training in or exposure to migrant health care. We recommend that services which may be expected to respond to a surge in demand keep a register of clinicians who have expressed willingness to respond if required, even for short periods (Box 19.1).

Barriers to access such as finances, transport, language, adequate time to address complex issues, and the clinical skills of the health practitioners may be addressed by socially aware governments and organizations. However, more subtle problems such as lack of understanding of health procedures, protocols, or management strategies taken for granted in many Western countries require sensitive and adaptive providers and services.

Many settlement countries encourage and support some form of on-arrival assessment for refugees. In their rationale for such assessments, UNHCR states: 'as well as being a fundamental human right, optimal physical and mental health is a vital resource for integration, enhancing people's capacity to meet the inevitable challenges and stresses of the resettlement process. In contrast, poor health may act as a significant barrier to integration' (20). Although the same reasoning could be applied to all newly arrived migrants, most countries do not offer them health assessments or supported access to health care services. Asylum seekers seeking health care usually rely upon charity or volunteer-based services.

These services are usually located in the primary care sector, and clinicians who engage in this kind of work may find that at least some of their work is pro bono. Volunteer or charity-based health care has a place, particularly in an emergency, but in our view primary care practitioners should be advocating for accessible health care for all migrants. For many

BOX 19.1   RESPONDING TO SURGES IN DEMAND

One Thursday evening, Mulligan General Practice, a mid-size practice in a regional town with an existing refugee population, was told by the local authorities that 290 refugees were expected to arrive by bus over the next 3 days. They had been discharged from a remote migration detention centre and were undertaking an arduous journey across three states to arrive in the town. Accommodation had been arranged for them in the local backpacker lodge and in a convent. It was understood that they might be distressed. Many had lived for prolonged periods in the migration detention centre after arriving by boat in Australia.

All staff met on the Friday afternoon to discuss their approach. The practice principal and the administrator (who spoke the language spoken by most refugees) met the first arrivals at the backpacker lodge. Many were suffering discontinuation reactions to antidepressants that had been ceased on leaving the detention centre. Several women were heavily pregnant, and some older people with diabetes and asthma needed support and medications. Mulligan General Practice set up extra clinics for the refugees, including an outreach clinic at the backpacker lodge, inviting interested seasonal staff to increase their hours temporarily. Clinicians in other practices who had in the past expressed an interest in working with refugees were invited to contribute to the surge response. Over 3 months, the practice provided enhanced care, drawing on the capabilities of other clinicians. A collaboration of primary care and psychological services near the backpacker lodge agreed to provide health care for the refugees once their immediate health care needs were met.

The surge response did not overwhelm the day-to-day workings of the practice because leadership was delegated to another clinician in the practice, the clinical staffing was temporarily expanded using the register of clinicians who had expressed interest, the clinic established some new practice models, including nurse triage, and there were other practices to transfer them to in the long term.

migrants, accessing good health care is like leaping on stones across a treacherous stream rather than walking on a bridge. Primary health care practitioners are uniquely positioned to be able to witness, document, and speak out about the gaps between the stepping stones and the risks of not building a better bridge.

CLINICAL VIGNETTE: PRIMARY CARE FOR THE HAMZAH FAMILY

The Hamzah family are screened by a nurse in the general practice and are investigated in accordance with the Australian Refugee Health guidelines.

Luna, Najib's wife, is found to be pregnant. She has the thalassaemia trait, as does her husband. All of the women have vitamin D deficiencies with levels below 35 nmol/L, the lowest being 23 nmol/L. The two brothers and one sister have vitamin B_{12} deficiencies with vitamin B_{12} levels below 150 pmol/L and active B_{12} levels (holotranscobalamin) below 30 pmol/L. Alina, the youngest sister, has a haemoglobin level of 80 g/L with iron deficiency. She also has menorrhagia. She had a blood transfusion 3 years ago because of her anaemia and contracted chronic hepatitis B.

Mahmoud, aged 74, took medication for hypertension and hypercholesterolaemia before the conflict but has not had any medication for 5 years. His blood pressure on arrival was 180/120 and his cholesterol was 7.5 mmol/L, giving him a high absolute cardiovascular risk of >15%, using the Australian guidelines.

SKILLS

Health literacy

Primary health care systems differ between countries, far more so than hospital systems (21). In many cultures, primary health care may be reactive and be delivered through an authority figure clinician, who is a sole practitioner. The only preventive activity might be vaccination.

Migrants may find strange the concept of a primary care practitioner who cares for the whole family and offers continuity of care across the lifespan, preventive activities, follow-up, health advocacy, and liaison with other health professionals. To access the health care they need, migrants must therefore develop health system literacy — understanding the scope of primary prevention, knowing when to come to the GP rather than a hospital, using appointment systems, and understanding the concept of shared care.

Knowing the epidemiology

To address the needs of constantly changing populations of migrants, we need guidelines that can be adapted to cater to new and emerging issues (Chapter 18) (22). A great deal of attention has been devoted to diseases of public health importance and nutritional deficits in migrant health. Chronic diseases such as cardiovascular disease, diabetes, hypertension, and some cancers are increasingly frequent among newly arrived refugees and other migrant populations (23,24) (Chapter 14).

A competent primary care practitioner for migrants must have some knowledge of the prevalence and incidence of diseases in the source countries of migrant populations. This is easier said than done. Firstly, many refugee-source countries, and some migrant-source countries, have limited descriptive datasets. These are often drawn from hospital clinic cohorts, which tend to capture sicker cohorts, and specialized conditions catered to by hospital outpatient clinics. Secondly, we should be wary of assuming that rates of diseases or other conditions in migrant-source countries will be replicated in settlement countries. Using such an approach for chronic diseases would grossly underestimate the rates of diseases which tend to increase after settlement or in second generations, such as diabetes. It also leads us to overestimate rates for conditions which tend to undergo attrition after migration. For example, the rate of female genital mutilation (FGM)/cutting in developed countries is not the same as it is in developing countries. Applying rates from refugee-source countries to migrant populations can lead to significant overestimation of the 'at-risk' population.*

Using interpreters

As a matter of health equity, GPs should ensure that they use interpreters when they are needed (Chapter 20). Migrants who are new to the settlement country and who have just

---

* See for example (25), where an alarming risk of FGM is erroneously estimated for Australian refugee populations from Africa by applying rates from North Sudan to South Sudanese populations and assuming zero rates of post-migration attrition in the practice.

begun to learn its dominant language are unlikely to fully grasp what they need to know, even if they can hold a basic conversation. This is particularly important in stressful situations when patients are more likely to forget their second language. High-stakes situations where clinicians need to ensure of the quality of communication, and therefore may need an interpreter, are summarized as the 'three Cs': complexity, consent, and any uncertainty about the patient's competence to make decisions (26).

Despite the preference of many clinicians for on-site interpreters, telephone interpreters should not be regarded as the second-best option for communication. This mode of interpreter is easier to organize, it can often be arranged on the spot, and the communicative skills are easily learned by clinicians. Many refugees and migrants, particularly those in small communities, prefer to use remote interpreters whom they do not personally know (27).

Speech-to-speech machine translation, such as Google Translate, may offer effective communication support in the future — particularly with consultations that focus on information transmission such as consent — but there are currently no studies demonstrating the quality and safety of speech-to-speech translation in medical settings.

Cultural sensitivity

Even when interpreters are used, there are many health concepts that may not have a direct translation into another language. The words *depression, anxiety, resilience, dreams, hope,* or *self-worth* may have no direct translation, or only one that carries a cultural, religious, or relational connotation (28). The experience of pain is not understood and expressed in the same away across languages and cultures (29); it may be organized into syndromic expressions that often have quite specific networks of semantic meaning (30). Any detailed exploration of a patient's presentation with pain and distress, as with other presentations of illness, should include a set of questions to try to understand the patient's explanatory model, using the following eight questions, as outlined by Kleinman, Eisenberg, and Good (31).

1. What do you think has caused the problem?
2. Why do you think it started when it did?
3. What do you think the sickness does? How does it work?
4. How severe is the sickness? Will it have a long or a short course?
5. What kind of treatment do you think you should receive?
6. What are the chief problems the sickness has caused?
7. What do you fear most about the sickness?
8. What are the most important results you hope to get from treatment?

CLINICAL VIGNETTE: NAJIB'S EXPLANATORY MODEL OF PAIN

Najib presented to his GP with increasing concern about his back pain. The pain had been present for about 10 days, after lifting some heavy boxes. The pain was only present during the day and was sometimes accompanied by pain radiating down the back of one leg.

The GP assessed his explanatory model, and Najib attributed it to heavy lifting (Q1). He had had the pain previously, when he'd carried his wife from their bombed house and dug through rubble to find his mother (Q2). Najib felt that his back pain was a sign of a permanent problem with a damaged disc (Q3). The problem was very severe, as evidenced by the level of pain and its recurrence (Q4). Such a problem should be treated by an operation on the disc. He regarded advice for pain management and exercise as failing to address the central part of his problem, which was derangement of the anatomy of his spine. The fact that he was not being advised to have an operation reflected racism on the part of Australian doctors, as he believed that this would be offered to Australians (Q5). The problem in his disc would inevitably lead to problems with walking (Q6). He feared ending up in a wheelchair (Q7). He wanted to be assured of a capable future in which he would no longer have back pain (Q8).

Understanding Najib's explanatory model leads us to focus on why an approach other than surgery might help his back, and to emphasize that back pain is not necessarily a sinister sign. Being alert to cultural differences also helps us to recognize and respond to psychological behaviours and responses that do not fit the culture model of the receiving country.

CLINICAL VIGNETTE: CROSS-CULTURAL PRESENTATIONS OF GRIEF

Noting that Mahmoud Hamzah seemed less concerned and sad than this children about the loss of his wife and son, the GP sought to understand how he viewed death, and how loss might be expressed. Mahmoud said he took comfort from his belief, as a Druze, in bodily reincarnation. Mahmoud is certain that his son Khaled and his wife were living in reincarnated form in a safe country. His children do not share his devotion to religion, and they feel the loss of their family members more keenly.

Some migrants may consciously avoid the diagnosis of illnesses that have been untreatable in their country of origin. This is likely to include, but is not limited to, cancer, HIV, hepatitis B, deafness, congenital problems, and mental illness. Communicating such diagnoses must be done with the utmost sensitivity and support, as patients may be reluctant to be screened and slow to understand the implications of management.

TOOLS

GUIDELINES: THE LIVED IMPACT OF CONFLICT AND DISPLACEMENT

The Hamzah family are reluctant to have a face-to-face interpreter but agree to a confidential telephone interpreter.

Mona, the sister who 'disappeared' for a period of time, is severely depressed and anxious. She struggles to leave the house or to help with household chores. She sleeps only 4 hours a night and is constantly worried about the well-being of everyone in the family, is often irritable and angry, and cries easily. She was previously an accountant and would like to go back to this work but is struggling with learning English as she is unable to concentrate and has panic attacks in class.

Alina left behind her fiancé in the camp. He only rarely gets internet access. She has started a process of getting a visa for him but has been told it will take at least 3 years if it is successful. Like Mona, Alina also cries a great deal. She is shocked to find out she has hepatitis B. It takes many consultations with an interpreter for the GP to convince her that sexual and vertical transmission is preventable. With the help of the GP and a telephone interpreter, she tells her fiancé and he is able to ask his own questions and discuss his need for hepatitis B vaccination. She continues to have her hepatitis B monitored every 6 months. The GP vaccinates the rest of the family for hepatitis B.

Rana has found work in a restaurant. She is the only family member with work, and her English is rapidly improving. However, she is unable, because of her work hours, to provide a great deal of emotional support for her sisters.

Guidelines are compendia of evidence to help clinical decision making. Guidelines that are relevant for the mainstream population may not address the most pressing health problems for migrants. The migrant health sector, like mainstream primary care, has a dearth of guidelines for comorbid illnesses, especially for comorbid chronic illness and psychological illness.

New and emerging issues in migrant health are very difficult to research, and studies in this area tend to be underfunded (32). Migrants are a 'hidden population' in national data-sets in settlement countries as their numbers are low in population terms and are not readily distinguished or enumerated from the majority population (33). There is no international consensus on what is needed for screening, reflecting variations across populations in disease patterns. There is, however, general agreement that screening should address diseases of public health importance (e.g. tuberculosis, hepatitis B), nutritional deficiencies, infectious diseases prevalent in the country of origin, reproductive and sexual health, and chronic diseases. Guidelines for refugee health screening all broadly reflect these categories (22,34).

PROTOCOLS AND PROCEDURES

Health procedures, protocols, or management strategies taken for granted in many Western countries may be unfamiliar for those who come from developing countries or countries in chaos. For instance, antenatal care, dental care, counselling, and physiotherapy will need adequate explanation about the roles of the practitioners, their preventive nature, and the importance of patient involvement in monitoring and self-care. Some of the standard assessment tools used in clinical practice have been extensively validated across languages and cultures (35,36), but others have not (37,38).

CLINICAL VIGNETTE: LUNA AND ANTENATAL CARE

Luna does not understand the concerns of the staff at the hospital antenatal clinic that her baby may have a 'blood disease', especially as the antenatal clinic staff repeatedly forget to book her an interpreter. She is taken aback when the hospital explains the risks of chorionic villus sampling and amniocentesis as investigations for fetal thalassaemia. Luna declines both of these investigations. As the pregnancy advances and she is unable to catch public transport to the hospital by herself, she comes to the general practice instead of the hospital when her antenatal appointments are due. The GP rings the hospital for advice on these occasions and speaks to the midwife or the obstetrician. She uses a phone interpreter with her mobile phone lying in front of the desk phone so that the midwife can speak to the mother. Her son is finally born fit and healthy, carrying the thalassaemia trait.

COMMUNITIES OF IDENTITY AND PRACTICE

We conclude by focussing on the most important opportunity and resource of all: communities. Migrants move within and between multiple social networks: people who have migrated with them, people from their town or settlement, people from their country, people who share religious and cultural practices, and people who emerge in all civil societies to help resettled migrants, to name a few. All these networks create and reinforce identity (39), enabling the person who has left or been forced to leave one country to gather the resources they need to navigate strange systems and customs in the next.

For some migrants, locating oneself in a web of people from similar backgrounds helps mitigate the strangeness of the new country. Community activities — sporting groups, artistic or religious gatherings — all help to foster cohesiveness and identity formation in a new country. We should, however, be wary of ascribing a romanticized notion of 'community' to all population groups who share pasts, or countries of origin. The expectations and norms of cultural or ethnic communities may be experienced as a straitjacket by the children of migrants. Although public health research suggests that newly arrived migrants have lower rates of intimate partner violence than long-term residents (40,41), clinicians have a responsibility to ensure that victims of family violence are informed and supported. Refugees may be suspicious of people from their home country, particularly if they have experienced betrayal by friends who became enemies (42).

Nevertheless, being a member of a strong community is one of the determinants of successful resettlement (43,44). Working with a particular community in order to understand their barriers to health care is likely to be the most successful way of ensuring that migrants attain health equity.

Innovative experience-based co-design approaches involving patients and health service staff are now well established in hospital settings (45). Smaller primary care services are well placed to develop and use rapid co-design methods with their patient communities, perhaps using oral narrative, or community storytellers. This is a potential site of growth in patient-centred service design, and for primary care for refugees and migrants.

CONCLUSION

Two years after arrival, Rana is managing a new branch of the restaurant and training to be a chef. Alina has undertaken a transitional course to go to university, where she plans to study mathematics. Mona never discloses what happened to her, but with the help of a psychologist, she learns some strategies to calm her anxiety. After Luna's baby is born, Mona enjoys helping her sister-in-law with the baby, and slowly over the next year, her anxiety settles.

Faisal had been a dentist in Syria before the crisis. He works hard at learning English at the free English classes and earns a job working part-time in a dental surgery. The dentist teaches him the technical language needed in dentistry, and after 3 years he sits the dental exams and passes. He is able to work as a dentist under supervision for another 2 years with the same dentist and then, when he is fully registered, continues in the same practice.

Najib had previously been a lawyer. He finds it difficult to find the time to work at learning English to the level needed to practice law here, and he also realizes that the law is very different in his new country. He retrains as an aged care worker, and 5 years after arrival secures a job in an aged care facility.

There is no 'typical' migrant story, but the Hamzah family share with many other newly arrived refugee families the experiences of sustained loss, and sometimes extreme violence. Their health care involved catchup health care, seeking to rectify years of stopgap or non-existent health care. Their decisions about their health care took into consideration other survival needs. In providing care, their GPs used screening protocols, navigation of health systems, and communication support. At the same time, as in the case of Mona, who never spoke about what had happened to her, there was a need to customize care around individual needs. The Hamzah family did not mix with other Syrian refugee families when they arrived; they were the only Druze family and did not feel a sense of community with others. However, they did form some strong connections with several families of migrants from Morocco, whom Rana met through her work.

Most of the Hamzah family will never return to the careers they held before they fled the country, but they diligently sought to find employment. Their GPs found themselves advocating through philanthropic organizations for them to receive support to access medications, and to receive specialized training. Although some of this seems outside the remit of the work of general practice, such work may be the most helpful and therapeutic that we can do for newly arrived migrants.

REFERENCES

1. Australian Bureau of Statistics. *Migration, Australia, 2015–2016. ABS Cat 3412, 2015–2016.* Canberra: ABS; 2017.
2. Family Planning Victoria. *Improving the Health Care of Women and Girls Affected by Female Genital Mutilation/Cutting.* Melbourne: FPV; 2014. Available at: http://www.fpv.org.au/assets/resources/FGM-ServeCoOrdinationGuideNationalWeb.pdf
3. McGorry P. Working with survivors of torture and trauma: The Victorian Foundation for Survivors of Torture in perspective. *Aust N Z J Psychiatry.* 1995;3:463–72.
4. Joshi C, Russell G, Cheng IH et al. A narrative synthesis of the impact of primary health care delivery models for refugees in resettlement countries on access, quality and coordination. *Int J Equity Health.* 2013;12:88.
5. Kay M, Jackson C, Nicolson C. Refugee health: a new model for delivering primary health care. *Aust J Prim Health.* 2010;16(1):98–103.
6. Phillips C, Hall S, Elmitt N, Bookallil M, Douglas K. People-centred integration in a refugee primary care service: a complex adaptive systems perspective. *J Integr Care.* 2017;25(1):26–38.
7. Drennan VM, Joseph J. Health visiting and refugee families: issues in professional practice. *J Adv Nurs.* 2005;49(2):155–63.
8. Riggs E, Davis E, Gibbs L, Block K, Szwarc J, Casey S, Duell-Piening P, Waters E. Accessing maternal and child health services in Melbourne, Australia: reflections from refugee families and service providers. *BMC Health Serv Res.* 2012;12:117.
9. United Nations High Commissioner for Refugees. Migrant definition. In: *UNHCR Emergency Handbook.* 4th ed. Geneva; 2015. Available from: https://emergency.unhcr.org/entry/44938/migrant-definition
10. Voogt E. S/citing the camp. In: Norris A, editor. *Politics, Metaphysics and Death: Essays of Giorgio Agamben's Homo Sacer.* Durham, NC: Duke University Press; 2005:74–106.
11. Ginsburgs S. The Soviet Union and the problem of refugees and displaced persons 1917–1956. *Am J Int Law.* 1957;51(2):325–61.
12. Harris K. The brokered exuberance of the middle class: an ethnographic analysis of Iran's 2009 Green Movement. *Mobilization.* 2012;17(4):435–55.
13. Yoruk E. The long summer of Turkey: the Gezi uprising and its historical roots. *S ATL Q Journal.* 2014;113(2):419–35.

14. International Committee of the Red Cross. *Health Care in Danger: Sixteen-Country Study.* Geneva: ICRC; 2011. Available at: https://www.icrc.org/eng/resources/documents/report/hcid-report-2011-08-10.htm

15. Phillips CB, Smith MS, Kay M, Casey S. Refugee Health Network of Australia: towards national collaboration on health care for refugees. *Med J Aust.* 2011;195(4):185–6.

16. Benson J, Phillips C, Kay M et al. Low vitamin B12 levels among newly-arrived refugees from Bhutan, Iran and Afghanistan: multicentre Australian study. *PLOS ONE.* 2013;8(2):e57998.

17. Simonsen KA, Hunskaar S, Sandvik H, Rortveit G. Capacity and adaptations of general practice during an influenza pandemic. *PLOS ONE.* 2013;8(7):e69408.

18. Pew Research Center. Number of Refugees to Europe Surges to Record 1.3 Million in 2015. August 2016.

19. Johnson DR, Ziersch AM, Burgess T. I don't think general practice should be the front line: experiences of general practitioners working with refugees in South Australia. *Aust N Z Health Policy.* 2008;5:20.

20. United Nations High Commissioner for Refugees. *Refugee Resettlement: An International Handbook to Guide Reception and Integration.* Geneva: UNHCR; 2002. Available from: http://www.unhcr.org/4a2cfe336.html (accessed July 2016).

21. Berman P. Organization of ambulatory health care services: a critical determinant of health system performance in developing countries. *Bull WHO.* 2000;78(6):791–802.

22. Chaves NJ, Paxton G, Biggs BA, Thambiran A, Smith M, Williams J, Gardiner J, Davis JS; on behalf of the Australasian Society for Infectious Diseases and Refugee Health Network of Australia Guidelines writing group. *Recommendations for Comprehensive Post-Arrival Health Screening for People from Refugee-Like Backgrounds.* 2nd ed. Melbourne: ASID; 2016.

23. Redditt VJ, Graziano D, Janakiram P, Rashid M. Health status of newly arrived refugees in Toronto, Ontario. Part 2: Chronic diseases. *Can Fam Physician.* 2015;61(7):e310–5.

24. Kunst A, Stronks K, Ayemang C. Non-communicable disease. In: Rechel B, Maldovsky P, Deville W, Rijks B, Petrova-Benedict R, McKee M, editors. *Migration and Health in the European Union.* World Health Organization 2011 on behalf of the European Observatory on Health Systems and Policies. New York: Open University Press; 2011.

25. Mathews B. Female genital mutilation: Australian law, policy and practical challenges for doctors. *Med J Aust.* 2011;194(3):139–41.

26. Phillips CB. Using interpreters: a guide for GPs. *Aust Fam Physician.* 2010;39(4):188–95.

27. Phillips C. Remote telephone interpretation in medical consultations with refugees: meta-communications about care, survival and selfhood. *J Refug Stud.* 2013;26(4):505–15.

28. Benson J, Thistlethwaite J. *Mental Health Across Cultures. A Practical Guide for Health Professionals.* Oxford: Radcliffe Publishing; 2008.

29. Goddard C, Ye Z. Exploring 'happiness' and 'pain' across languages and cultures. *Int J Lang Cult.* 2014;1(2):131–48.

30. Coker CM. 'Traveling pains': embodied metaphors of suffering among Southern Sudanese refugees in Cairo. *Cult Med Psychiatry.* 2004;28(1):15–39.

31. Kleinman A, Eisenberg L, Good B. Culture, illness, and care: clinical lessons from anthropological and cross-cultural research. *Ann Intern Med.* 1978;88:251–88.

32. Renzaho A, Polonsky M, Mellor D, Cyril S. Addressing migration-related social and health inequalities in Australia: call for research funding priorities to recognise the needs of migrant populations. *Aust Health Rev.* 2016;40(1):3–10.

33. Sulaiman-Hill CM, Thompson SC. Sampling challenges in a study examining refugee resettlement. *BMC Int Health Hum Rights.* 2011;11:2.

34. Swinkels H, Pottie K, Tugwell P, Rashid M, Narasiah L; Canadian Collaboration for Immigrant and Refugee Health (CCIRH). Development of guidelines for recently arrived immigrants and refugees to Canada: Delphi consensus on selecting preventable and treatable conditions. *CMAJ.* 2011;183(12):e928–32.

35. Zubaran C, Schumacher M, Roxo MR, Foresti K. Screening tools for postnatal depression: validity and cultural dimensions. *Afr J Psychiatr.* 2010;13(5):357–65.

36. Naqvi RM, Haider S, Tomlinson G, Alibhai S. Cognitive assessments in multicultural populations using the Rowland Universal Dementia Assessment Scale: a systematic review and meta-analysis. *CMAJ.* 2015;187(5):e169–75.

37. Mendonça B, Sargent B, Fetters L. Cross-cultural validity of standardized motor development screening and assessment tools: a systematic review. *Dev Med Child Neurol.* 2016;58(12):1213–22.

38. Chorwe-Sungani G, Chipps J. A systematic review of screening instruments for depression for use in antenatal services in low resource settings. *BMC Psychiatry.* 2017;17(1):112.

39. Akhbar S. *Immigration and Identity: Turmoil. Treatment and Transformation. Lanham*, MD: Rowman and Littlefield; 1999.

40. Hymen I, Forte T, Du Mont J, Romans S, Cohen MM. The association of length of stay in Canada and intimate partner violence among immigrant women. *Am J Public Health.* 2006;96(4):654–9.

41. Yoshihama M. Appendix B: Literature review on intimate partner violence in immigrant/refugee communities. Review and recommendations. In: Runner M, Yoshihama M, Novick S, editors. *Intimate Partner Violence in Immigrant and Refugee Communities. Challenges, Promising Practices and Recommendations.* Princeton, NJ: Robert Wood Johnson Foundation; 2009.

42. Halpern J, Weinstein HW. Rehumanizing the other: empathy and reconciliation. *Hum Rights Q.* 2004;26(3):561–83.

43. Colic-Peisker V, Tilbury F. 'Active' and 'passive' resettlement: RHE influence of host culture, support services, and refugees' own resources on the choice of resettlement style. *Int Migr.* 2003;41:61–91.

44. Colic-Peisker V. Visibility, settlement success and life satisfaction in three refugee communities. *Ethnicities.* 2009;9(2):175–99.

45. Robert G. Participatory action research: using experience-based co-design to improve the quality of healthcare services. In: Ziebland S, Coulter A, Calabrese JD, Locock L, editors. *Using and Understanding Health Experiences: Improving Patient Care.* Oxford: Oxford University Press; 2013, 138–149.

CHAPTER 20

Bridging cultural and language discordance

Esperanza Diaz and Bernadette N. Kumar

LEARNING OBJECTIVES

At the end of this chapter, the reader should be able to:

- Recognize and reflect upon the relevance that both the patient and doctor have cultural backgrounds that might be of importance in a given consultation
- Recognize and reflect upon the importance of adequately addressing language and cultural challenges and the consequences of not doing so
- Understand how to use interpreters, including:
  - Pros and cons of professional versus non-professional interpreters
  - Basic rules of using interpreters
  - Differences between interpreters and cultural brokers

Being a GP with a migrant background myself (Diaz), serving patients with migrant and non-migrant backgrounds similar to and different from myself is a unique position. It provides me with the opportunity to reflect about my own beliefs and cultural standpoint, cross-cultural communication systems, and organization of services. In fact, this was the very reason I first became interested in migration and health many years ago: why did I, a Spanish-born GP, have so many more patients than my Norwegian-born colleagues, not only from Latin America, but also from the Congo or Afghanistan in my list? It sparked my curiosity...

INTRODUCTION

The aim of most countries in Europe is to provide equitable health care services to their citizens regardless of their ethnicity, religion, country of origin, and other characteristics (1). However, a large body of literature describes the challenges in providing health care across cultures for doctors and other health care professionals (2,3). Furthermore, European health professionals are not at ease providing adequate health care in multicultural societies, and in many countries they have yet to receive systematic training to tackle this new and complex situation (4).

Linguistic and intercultural challenges are often attributed to the migrant patients alone; however, they should also be connected to the health professionals themselves. Although international recommendations to improve cross-cultural care exist (5), health professionals' performance when meeting migrant patients varies considerably regarding the diagnostic procedures that are undertaken (6,7), the number of consultations required for referral to secondary care (8,9), and the specificity of diagnoses provided or treatments given (10,11), including for children of migrants (12) compared to non-migrants. Professional interpretation services are largely underutilized (13), and health providers often feel they lack the knowledge, skills, or competence necessary to provide equitable health care to a growing number of migrant patients (14,15). Not surprisingly, migrants from low- and middle-income countries in Europe seem to be less satisfied with health care services than the majority population (16,17).

CLINICAL VIGNETTE

Marcelo is 60 years old and originally from Argentina. He is married and has no children. He lived for many years as a migrant in Spain but migrated to Norway 10 years ago after losing his job during the financial crisis. He has worked as a cook in a tapas restaurant since then. His Norwegian skills are poor, and he does not speak fluent English either.

His wife phones to the GP office to make an appointment for him very early one Monday morning. She speaks Norwegian a little better than he does and has more experience with health services in Norway, but still cannot manage a full conversation in Norwegian. According to what the secretary understands, Marcelo attended the emergency room (ER) on Saturday because of acute abdominal pain. After a relatively short consultation there, without an interpreter, he was asked to contact his Spanish-speaking GP as soon as possible because he had 'stones in his stomach'. He is anxious and will not wait for a scheduled appointment a couple of days later, despite not being in pain any longer. The secretary would not have given the last available 'acute' appointment today to a patient without acute symptoms, but she thinks it is difficult to understand the patient's wife and afraid of overseeing something important. She also knows from previous experience that patients from Latin America sometimes have problems understanding the different types of appointments in Norway when she tries to explain on the phone. She calls the patient's Spanish-speaking GP and explains the situation, and the GP agrees to give the patient the appointment today, asking the secretary to remind the patient's wife that this is a short consultation.

INTERPRETERS: THE NEED, AVAILABILITY, AND ORGANIZATION OF APPOINTMENTS

Marcelo has 12 years of school education from his country of origin; he migrated to Spain at the age of 35 years and moved to Norway when he was 50 years old. He did not need to learn a new language for the many years when he was a migrant in Spain. For Marcelo, Norwegian is not an easy language to learn; however, he is a smart guy and manages the everyday life at work well. Though his Norwegian vocabulary is adequate for a cook, it comes to a standstill when he has to express himself in Norwegian about his body or what he feels. Thus, the first obvious problem when he gets ill is his inability to express himself in Norwegian.

Unfortunately, this was not picked up at the ER, or at least not to the extent that should have triggered Marcelo's right to an interpreter. Underutilization of interpreters, as expressed in several places in this textbook, might be the greatest challenge encountered by migrant patients not fluent in the language of the host country. A GP, regardless of all other skills and qualifications, cannot be a good one when he or she and the patient do not understand each other.

The rights and entitlements to interpreters vary among countries. For countries where the services are available, the responsibility to make accessible information about professional interpreters, such as telephone numbers and instructions to make appointments, lies with the system. When several GPs work together in areas with a relatively high proportion of migrants, the administrative personnel become more experienced in the procedures for making appointments with interpreters and thus use them more often (18). As in Marcelo's case, this usually is set up before the consultation so that procedures can commence and no time is wasted after the patient arrives at the clinic. It is extremely important that the staff making the appointments is familiar with the procedure for using interpreters at that particular clinic. In addition, some general knowledge about hiring interpreters is necessary, like exact information about language, and not only country of origin, as well as allowing for longer consultations with interpreters, given the time taken for repeating everything twice. While preparing for the interpretation session, it is important to consider the following: type (trained professional interpreter, family member, or bilingual health care staff) and mode (face-to-face, telephone, or video) of interpreting. Furthermore, in some cases it might be important to consider the interpreter's ethnic origin, religious background, or gender (19).

The availability of professional interpreters also varies depending on the country, the area, and the time of the day. Professional interpreters might be available in person during the day in areas with many migrants, while interpreters through the telephone or video might be a better alternative in more remote places, or for out-of-hours appointments or less-frequently known languages. For languages with fewer speakers, like Norwegian, where almost everybody speaks English, creative solutions such as using services from English-speaking countries might be considered in special situations. This kind of information has to be known well in advance for the person making the appointments. For Marcelo, an interpreter was not needed at the clinic because his GP speaks his own language. However, the lack of understanding by the staff at the telephone at the clinic ended in the 'wrong' type of appointment, probably leading to a suboptimal use of resources, as the last 'acute' appointment for other patients was given away. In fact, although in this special situation the consultation could be managed in Spanish, possibly sparing system cost in the short run, generally speaking, multiplying the number of consultations when language is not addressed from the beginning is probably not cost-effective for the system at large and over time, and definitely not for the patient given that it increases costs for the patient in terms of transport, time, and out-of-pocket contributions. Furthermore, it is ethically questionable to accept systematic suboptimal communication based on lack of knowledge at the first point of contact or a lack of willingness to enable patient's rights within the system level.

Marcelo seems undisturbed when he arrives at the GP clinic with his wife, who also was with him at the ER. He already feels relieved the moment he enters the room by being able to express his symptoms and fears in Spanish. He expects his GP to understand him, but also to explain what happened at the ER, what is wrong with his stomach, and the results for a number of blood tests that were taken there but that he does not have any information about.

THE SPECIAL ROLE OF CULTURALLY CONCORDANT GPs

It is natural and human to feel safe amidst the same kind or type of persons as one's self. The GP-patient relationship is strengthened when patients share similar characteristics with their physicians such as gender, personal beliefs, values, and communication. Perceived similarity, primarily described through race or ethnic concordance in culturally concordant studies, is associated with higher ratings of trust, satisfaction, and intention to adhere (20). A classical study from the United States described that race-concordant visits were longer and were characterized by greater positive affect. In this 2003 study, Cooper and colleagues advocate for increasing ethnic diversity among physicians as the most direct strategy to improve health care experiences for members of ethnic minority groups (21). Although this is a sensible proposal with many advantages, it is worth pointing out that this option should concur along with the enhancement of cultural awareness and competence among *all* GPs and health professionals, and not replace it.

In countries with free selection or choice of GP, migrant patients often prefer GPs who share their language and culture (22). In fact, it is not only the common language that migrant patients appreciate, it is also the feeling of having a 'common experience in being migrants' which makes patients from one part of the world choose GPs from another part of the world even if they do not share the same original language. Migrant GPs, for this same reason, feel a special commitment towards migrant patients. However, these consultations also challenge their roles as GPs, especially when patients expect them to be doctor, interpreter, and advocate for the system all in one (23). The extra burden that GPs with migrant backgrounds carry often goes unnoticed or unacknowledged. Therefore, it is imperative that all GPs improve their knowledge, capacity, and skills to deal with intercultural consultations, without undue reliance on migrant GPs. A higher degree of cultural awareness and humility as well as an improvement of cultural competence for all GPs will be a better and more sustainable strategy than trying to recruit GPs from abroad (24).

WHAT DO PHYSICIANS DO WHEN THEY DO NOT UNDERSTAND THEIR PATIENTS?

Marcelo wanted information about the complementary tests that were taken at the ER. In fact, there are several studies showing that when communication is at stake, GPs try to make sure that they are not 'missing anything' by taking more blood tests (7). Furthermore, invasive tests with a potential of damaging patients, like lumbar puncture, have been performed more often among migrant patients presenting, for example, with headache at the ER, even with milder forms of headache, as compared to the non-migrant patients (6). This was the same strategy that the clinic staff deployed with Marcelo, giving him an acute appointment so as to not miss anything. Another GP strategy is to give extra appointments, with or without interpreters, to make sure that the patient is given additional care, especially when the perception is that communication has been compromised. This in turn is described in the literature as the migrants being 'frequent attender' patients (25), which might be perceived by stakeholders as a fault of the patient, or as if the patient was unhealthy or overusing the system rather than a shortcoming of the system. Although these strategies are well meant by caring health personnel, we should ask ourselves if they represent appropriate and relevant care for migrant patients, or if health personnel should advocate for a system that addresses language issues in a professional way from the first possible moment.

The GP explains that he does not have any information from the ER yet but invites Marcelo to tell him what happened in a chronological way: what took him to ER, what happened there, and how has he felt afterwards. The patient reports acute abdominal pain that started some hours after a family celebration including a heavy meal. The pain was too intense to go to work and he needed a sick leave since he was supposed to work during the weekend. Thus he went to the ER, quite in pain, and was given some injection that made him feel better. He states that several blood tests were taken and he was told at the ER that he had *piedras en el estómago* ('stones in his stomach') and that it was not dangerous, and he should contact his GP. The GP begins then to ask more specific questions about symptoms that could indicate kidney stones, gallbladder stones, and all the 'stones' he can think of in medicine, but he cannot make any sense of that description. Then an idea crosses the GPs mind: 'Marcelo, could the ER doctor have said that your stomach was 'hard as a stone' (*duro como una piedra*)?, which was followed by a confirmatory simultaneous response from the couple: 'Yes, that is exactly what the doctor said!'

CHALLENGING CONSTELLATIONS: PATIENTS, FAMILY MEMBERS, INTERPRETERS, AND HEALTH PROFESSIONALS

Consultations increase in complexity when other persons apart from the patient and the GP are together at the clinic. Migrants often visit the doctor with one or more family members, and an interpreter is often in the room. The possibilities for miscommunication or difficult situations that have to be tackled increase exponentially with the number of persons in the room. However, this might still be the best way to get information if the GP manages to organize the consultation in a professional manner.

Chapter 3 describes that the patient's migrant background in itself does not necessarily lead to a good or bad consultation. Several factors affect perceived similarities, including physicians' use of patient-centred communication (20). Asking patients for their stories and their perceptions about disease and recovery is as, if not more, important when we lack a common understanding. However, it is very hard to achieve if there is a language barrier. An interesting observation is that many physicians underestimate the patient's desire to use interpreters and rely on poor-quality common language communication even when interpreter services are available. Some obvious explanations attributable to this are increased workload and additional use of time (26), and the additional cost to the system of professional interpreter services (13). Other less known reasons might be as important, and these should be actively considered and further explored in our encounters with migrant patients.

Patients often come with family members or friends to help with language difficulties and because they might have a better understanding and skills to navigate the health care system, that is, better health literacy. Patients bring these informal interpreters because they might not be aware of their rights to professional interpreters or because the system does not organize the interpreters the patient is entitled to. The evidence suggests that health professionals rely far too much on patients' knowledge of their rights regarding interpreters. Fryer et al. explored the process of decision making of older people with limited English proficiency about using a professional interpreter during their health care after stroke, and reported that patients were happy without interpreters if they 'understood the major things', thereby opening the door for several misunderstandings and adverse events. The authors concluded that health professionals have 'an opportunity and a mandate to demonstrate leadership in the interpreter decision by providing knowledge, opportunity and encouragement for people with limited English proficiency, to use an interpreter to engage in, and understand their health care' (27). As explained in Chapter 8, we should also inform patients that children should not be used as interpreters, the only exception being in case of emergencies and for the shortest time possible.

In a few cases, non-professional interpreters coming along with the patient have their own agenda, and they misuse their position as interpreters to decide which information should be given or not both from the patient to the doctor and the other way around. Rarely, family members or other persons coming along as informal interpreters, typically husbands in marriages arranged before the subjects know each other, can abuse the patients after consultation as a form of payment for their help as interpreters. Furthermore, a small minority of patients bring someone along to translate who does not have the patient's best interests at heart (28). GPs should be especially aware of these situations — be careful when you suspect that the patient may be caught in human trafficking, in a forced marriage, or with females and elderly patients in vulnerable positions with little or no social network. In such cases, the use of family members or other ad hoc options should be avoided.

Most often, informal interpreters have good intentions and do help the patient and the doctor bridge the language gaps and sometimes the cultural gap. In those cases, a trio is created that makes the consultation complex, and often longer than scheduled. Good planning and logistics from the start can avoid delays in the timetable for the day. A Turkish study compared the perspectives of the informal interpreters, the patients, and the GPs, and might provide some of the reasons as to why these consultations are complex. 'In line with family interpreters' perspective, patients expected the interpreters to advocate on their behalf and felt empowered when they did so. GPs, on the contrary, felt annoyed and disempowered when the family interpreters took on the advocacy role. Family interpreters were trusted by patients for their fidelity, that is, patients assumed that family interpreters would act in their best interest. GPs, on the contrary, mistrusted family interpreters when they perceived dishonesty or a lack of competence'. The authors state, 'GPs should be educated to become aware of the difficulties of family interpreting, such as conflicting role expectations and need to be trained to be able to call on professional interpreters when needed' (29).

INFORMAL VERSUS PROFESSIONAL INTERPRETERS: TRUST, CONTROL, AND POWER

The eternal question is if an informal interpreter is good enough or even better than a professional one, and in which circumstances. Guidelines usually recommend professional interpreters as the option of choice based on evidence suggesting that untrained interpreters are more likely to make errors, violate confidentiality, and increase the risk of poor outcomes (30). On the other hand, migrants, who have more experience in using interpreters than their GPs, often prefer to have somebody of their choice with them.

As stated, patients relatively often express their preferences for informal interpreters instead for professional interpreters, mainly for fidelity reasons. Patients assume that informal interpreters act in their best interests, and feel empowered by their presence (31). On the other hand, the presence of an informal interpreter decreases the amount of patients' expression of emotional concerns and cues. Furthermore, informal interpreters might add substantial amounts of information and cues of their own, becoming active participants in triadic medical encounters, thus disturbing the consultation (32). Trust, control, and power seem to be the three key elements to an optimal consultation with an interpreter (33). These elements should be acknowledged and balanced when choosing the type of interpreter along with the patient. As responsible actors in the consultation, patients must be heard regarding their preference. In order to remedy and improve interpreter services, patients must be effective partners and can only do so when they are aware of their rights and feel that the GP office is not trying to skip their duty of organizing the interpreter services (34).

PROFESSIONAL INTERPRETERS

Interpretation as a profession varies from country to country. Although this is improving, there is a real danger that even professional interpreters lack professional competence either in terms of language skills or regarding confidentiality or other guidelines. For small communities with only one interpreter, confidentiality, trust, and professionalism are especially challenging and important. In these cases, a given interpreter knows nearly all patients from the same area, and very often accompanies them to the doctor or any other service, including police or administration. Despite his or her knowledge of the individuals, and because of his or her special position in the community, it is even more important that consultations with these interpreters begin with one short sentence reminding all the persons in the room about confidentiality. Often, the interpreter him or herself will do this, but if it is not the case, the GP should use the first 30 seconds to do so. The interpreter should refer to him or herself as 'the interpreter' and translate absolutely everything that is said in the room, strictly following the interpretation rules. In this way, the interpreter will probably be respected and trusted within the community. The Norwegian rules provided in Table 20.1 are probably similar to rules in other countries that should regularly be used by all interpreters and GPs.

TABLE 20.1 Norwegian guidelines for good interpretation

- The interpreter will interpret what is said and not omit, add, or change any of the content.
- The interpreter should be impartial in the conversation and cannot contribute his or her own opinions or advice.
- Users of the interpretation are responsible for the content and the flow of the conversation.
- Users of the interpretation should refer directly to each other and not to the interpreter. That is, do not say 'ask him if he wants …' but ask directly. 'Do you want?' and the interpreter translates in the same form.
- If the interpreter does not perceive or understand any of what you say, the interpreter will ask you to repeat or explain and then translate your explanation.
- The interpreter is subject to strict confidentiality and cannot talk to anyone about the information gained through interpretation. The conversation between you will therefore be considered confidential.
- The interpreter's notes will be shredded at the discretion of the parties.
- The interpreter refers to himself as the 'interpreter'.

An interpreter should translate everything that is said in the room. A good interpreter very often takes notes, as hardly anybody can remember more than one sentence at a time verbatim. Thus, GPs should be sceptical when interpreters come without a notebook or do not follow the guidelines in other ways. Omissions and alterations in the process of translation are unavoidable but can be minimized. Interpreter alterations are likely to occur in utterances longer than 20 words. Therefore, sentences should be as short as possible to minimize interpreter alterations. Physicians should check the patient's understanding regularly and ask interpreters to interrupt in order to facilitate accurate interpretation (35). For Marcelo, using a metaphor 'hard as a stone/stone hard' was key to a misunderstanding that could have been avoided by using plain, straightforward language. The problem and the beauty are that we need to reflect about our mother tongue to realize that we are using metaphors and difficult sentences. This is one part of the learning about ourselves in contact with migrants!

Last but not least, as with any other patient, it is important with translation to make sure that there is an agreement and mutual understanding on the way forward at the end of the consultation. This can and should also be done in consultations with interpreters, using questions that the patient does not feel as disempowering. Some examples are: 'What are you going to explain at home regarding the diagnosis/treatment we have talked about today?' or 'What is the most important for you from our conversation today?' or 'It is important that we make sure that we have understood each other; can you tell me how you are going to use the medication?' Be aware, however, that some interpreters might find these counter-check methods unusual or even feel uncomfortable using them. In such cases, it might be worthwhile to provide information (with translation) about the reasons for asking those types of questions.

NON-PROFESSIONAL INTERPRETERS

Most GPs have experienced that the presence of family members in any consultation can be a blessing or a curse. The situation might become even more challenging when a friend or family member acts as a non-professional interpreter, as commented on previously and in Chapter 11. The GPs should be aware that non-professional interpreters not only provide in general poorer quality of translation as compared to professional ones, but are confronted with a double role: being a relative, and thus being emotionally close to the patient, at the same time as being an interpreter. This double role is challenging given that it comes with the responsibility of conveying correct information between patient and provider in a neutral, non-partisan manner. This is especially important in situations that might be culturally sensitive, as the relationship between the patient and the family member might either impede proper communication or be jeopardized after sharing information that was not supposed to be known for the family member. Several situations come to mind that illustrate these challenges: A 19-year-old boy translating for his perimenopausal mother is, for example, probably problematic for both the mother and the son. What information can she disclose? If she does talk about intimate issues, how are they going to deal with that after the consultation? Be especially careful when misunderstandings can put life in danger or have severe negative consequences for the patient, as any error in translation will be a long-lasting burden for the family member in addition to being negative for the patient. On the other hand, non-equivalent interpretation is common, and not always innocuous, when a professional interpreter is used, and some studies suggest that there may remain a role for family also in the presence of professional interpreters (36).

ESPECIALLY CHALLENGING SITUATIONS WITH AND FOR THE INTERPRETER

Some situations are, by their very nature, even more challenging to deal with when there are language barriers. This should not lead to less use of interpreters, but to a deeper reflection specific to the use of interpreters. Some of these consultations have been discussed in different chapters in Sections II and III of this book. We will outline a few challenges and some tips as to how to deal with them.

Any consultation that includes physical examination of genitalia has to be dealt with special sensitivity and respect (Chapter 13). Many women, regardless of their background, prefer a female provider for such consultations. This might be even more pronounced for women depending on their religious or cultural backgrounds. In some cases, having a female provider might be the best solution, but male physicians can also deal with these consultations when the women accept their medical competence and get to trust them. However, the interpreter's gender might be of utmost importance, as that person is not perceived to have the specific medical competence needed for the situation, as opposed to the physician. Possible strategies to manage these situations might be the use of telephone interpreters, the appointment of professional female interpreters in advance, or the use of female non-professional interpreters. As stated previously, the GP should be aware of control and power mechanisms in these consultations and try to empower women in vulnerable positions.

Cancer is still taboo in many societies, as explained in Chapter 16, and a cancer diagnosis is perceived as a threat, disregarding cultural background. In the same way as clinicians, interpreters are part of societies and are not immune to the content of the consultation. In a recent study of consultations in the transition of oncology to palliative care, four key themes emerged as problematic for interpreters: the challenges of translating the meaning of 'palliative care', managing interpreting in the presence of family caregivers, communicating and expressing sensitivity while remaining professional, and interpreters' own emotional burden of difficult clinic encounters between doctor and patient negotiations (37). Reflection on the interpreters' experiences of stress, as they probably have not been trained with coping skills, should be given due consideration. A short debriefing after the consultation might be in place and does not need to take a long time. Sometimes acknowledging with a last sentence that the GP and the interpreter are 'on the same side' in this respect might suffice.

HEALTH NAVIGATORS, PEER NAVIGATORS, AND CULTURAL BROKERS

Learning a language is a complex issue and requires several steps. Language was the first obvious barrier for Marcelo, but it is not the only one. Health literacy refers to people having the appropriate skills, knowledge, understanding, and confidence to access, understand, evaluate, use, and navigate health information and services in order to take action on the factors influencing their health. This concept relates both to the characteristics and knowledge of the individual as well as those of the system. Marcelo managed to use the health care system in Spain, although it was different from the one he grew up with, because of comprehending the language, it being the same in both countries. In Norway, the system changed, with for example different types of consultations, but this time he does not understand the language either. Although Marcelo's wife does not speak the language much better than he does, she is the one who navigates the system better. Family members, especially younger members and females, usually have this role for other members in the family, also for the majority population.

One approach to overcoming health care system barriers and facilitating timely access to health care for migrants from different systems and with low competence in the majority language, is through a patient navigator. 'A patient navigator is a trained person who individually assists patients, families, and caregivers to navigate the health care system barriers efficiently and effectively at any point along the care continuum, improving patient care at all levels of an organization' (38). Patient navigators are often, but not always, peers, especially trained for one specific group. They have been used mostly in the United States and, although generally positive, the studies are few (38) or show mixed results. A study in the United States using hospital-based community health workers as patient navigators, for example, showed decreased readmission to hospitals among older patients, while increasing readmissions among younger patients (39).

In some countries the figure of a cultural broker/mediator exists as a complement or as a substitute for interpreters. These persons facilitate or mediate between persons of different cultural backgrounds to reduce conflict or promote health change.

CONCLUSION

Patients with linguistic and cultural backgrounds different to those of the health provider and the system can be an enriching opportunity to learn about people with different ways of expressing their symptoms and different expectations, but also to learn about the system in which one works, and, not the least, about oneself.

Language and cultural backgrounds have to be addressed in intercultural communication from the very first point of contact of the patient with the system. One of the keys to success in communicating with migrants who do not have a high degree of proficiency in the majority language is the use of interpreters. In this regard, several steps have to be considered and taken. First, the health care systems have to be prepared to implement the patients' rights. Second, health care professionals need to acquire the knowledge to organize appointments with interpreters and the skills to perform these consultations, with both professional and non-professional interpreters. Lastly, user involvement is important; patient preferences regarding who should be in the room must be taken into account. It is important that patients know their rights and that the system is in fact devoted to organizing the use of professional interpreters whenever necessary.

ACKNOWLEDGEMENT

Thanks to Farhat Thaj for her help in reviewing the literature used for this chapter.

REFERENCES

1. Migrant Integration Policy Index. 2015. Available from: http://www.mipex.eu/health
2. Varvin S, Aasland OG. Legers forhold til flyktningpasienten [Physicians' relation to refugees]. *Tidsskrift Norske Legeforening.* 2009;129(15):1488–90.
3. Debesay J, Harslof I, Rechel B, Vike H. Facing diversity under institutional constraints: challenging situations for community nurses when providing care to ethnic minority patients. *J Adv Nurs.* 2014;70(9):2107–16.
4. van den Muijsenbergh M, van Weel-Baumgarten E, Burns N et al. Communication in cross-cultural consultations in primary care in Europe: the case for improvement. The rationale for the RESTORE FP 7 project. *Prim Health Care Res Dev.* 2014;15(2):122–33.

5. Teunissen E, Gravenhorst K, Dowrick C et al. Implementing guidelines and training initiatives to improve cross-cultural communication in primary care consultations: a qualitative participatory European study. *Int J Equity Health.* 2017;16(1):32.
6. Royl G, Ploner CJ, Leithner C. Headache in the emergency room: the role of immigrant background on the frequency of serious causes and diagnostic procedures. *Neurol Sci.* 2012;33(4):793–9.
7. Sandvik H, Hunskaar S, Diaz E. Immigrants' use of emergency primary health care in Norway: a registry-based observational study. *BMC Health Serv Res.* 2012;12:308.
8. Lyratzopoulous G, Neal RD, Barbiere JM, Rubin GP, Abel GA. Variation in the number of general practitioner consultations before hospital referral for cancer: findings from the 2010 National Cancer Patient Experience Survey in England. *Lancet Oncol.* 2012;13(4):353–65.
9. de Bruijne MC, van Rosse F, Uiters E et al. Ethnic variations in unplanned readmissions and excess length of hospital stay: a nationwide record-linked cohort study. *Eur J Public Health.* 2013;23(6):964–71.
10. Gimeno-Feliu LA, Calderón-Larrañaga A, Prados-Torres A, Revilla-López C, Diaz E. Patterns of pharmaceutical use for immigrants to Spain and Norway: a comparative study of prescription databases in two European countries. *Int J Equity Health.* 2016;15(32).
11. Hakonsen H, Lees K, Toverud EL. Cultural barriers encountered by Norwegian community pharmacists in providing service to non-Western immigrant patients. *Int J Clin Pharm.* 2014;36(6):1144–51.
12. Jimenez N, Jackson DL, Zhou C, Ayala NC, Ebel BE. Postoperative pain management in children, parental English proficiency, and access to interpretation. *Hosp Pediatr.* 2014;4(1):23–30.
13. Ramirez D, Engel KG, Tang TS. Language interpreter utilization in the emergency department setting: a clinical review. *J Health Care Poor Underserved.* 2008;19(2):352–62.
14. Bregård IM, Hjelde KH. *Veiviser for undervisning av helsepersonell i migrasjon og helse.* Oslo, Norway: NAKMI; 2013.
15. Hjörleifsson S, Hammer E, Díaz E. General practitioners' strategies in consultations with immigrants in Norway – practice-based shared reflections among participants in focus groups. *Fam Pract.* 2017.
16. Harmsen JA, Bernsen R, Bruijnzeels M, Meeuwesen L. Patients' evaluation of quality of care in general practice: what are the cultural and linguistic barriers? *Patient Educ Couns.* 2008;72:155–62.
17. Suurmond J, Uiters E, de Bruijne MC, Stronks K, Essink-Bot M-L. Negative health care experiences of immigrant patients: a qualitative study. *BMC Health Serv Res.* 2011;11:10.
18. Kongshavn T, Aarseth S, Maartmann-Moe K. Allmennlegers bruk av tolk [GPs' use of interpreters]. *Utposten.* 2012;5:25–8.
19. Hadziabdic E, Hjelm K. Working with interpreters: practical advice for use of an interpreter in healthcare. *Int J Evid Based Healthc.* 2013;11(1):69–76.
20. Street RL, O'Malley KJ, Cooper LA, Haidet P. Understanding concordance in patient-physician relationships: personal and ethnic dimensions of shared identity. *Ann Fam Med.* 2008;6(3):198–205.
21. Cooper LA, Roter DL, Johnson RL, Ford DE, Steinwachs DM, Powe NR. Patient-centered communication, ratings of care, and concordance of patient and physician races. *Ann Intern Med.* 2003;139:907–15.
22. Diaz E, Hjørleifsson S. Immigrant general practitioners in Norway: a special resource? A qualitative study. *Scand J Public Health.* 2011;39(3):239–44.
23. Diaz E, Raza A, Hjorleifsson S, Sandvik H. Immigrant and native regular general practitioners in Norway. A comparative registry-based observational study. *Eur J Gen Pract.* 2014;20(2):93–9.
24. Diaz E, Kumar BN. Health care curricula in multicultural societies. *Int J Med Educ.* 2018;9:42–4.
25. Diaz E, Gimeno-Feliu LA, Calderón-Larrañaga A, Prados-Torres A. Frequent attenders in general practice and immigrant status in Norway: A nationwide cross-sectional study. *Scand J Prim Health Care.* 2014;32(4):232–40.
26. Flynn PM, Ridgeway JL, Wieland ML et al. Primary care utilization and mental health diagnoses among adult patients requiring interpreters: a retrospective cohort study. *J Gen Intern Med.* 2013;28(3):386–91.
27. Fryer CE, Mackintosh SF, Stanley MJ, Crichton J. 'I understand all the major things': how older people with limited English proficiency decide their need for a professional interpreter during health care after stroke. *Ethn Health.* 2013;18(6):610–25.

28. Bonvoisin T. Healthcare professionals need more training about human trafficking and the safe use of interpreters. *BMJ*. 2017;357:j2671.
29. Zendedel R, Schouten BC, van Weert JC, van den Putte B. Informal interpreting in general practice: comparing the perspectives of general practitioners, migrant patients and family interpreters. *Patient Educ Couns*. 2016;99(6):981–7.
30. Juckett G, Unger K. Appropriate use of medical interpreters. *Am Fam Physician*. 2014;90(7):476–80.
31. Zendedel R, Schouten BC, van Weert JCM, van den Putte B. Informal interpreting in general practice: the migrant patient's voice. *Ethn Health*. 2018;23(2):158–73.
32. Schouten BC, Schinkel S. Turkish migrant GP patients' expression of emotional cues and concerns in encounters with and without informal interpreters. *Patient Educ Couns*. 2014;97(1):23–9.
33. Brisset C, Leanza Y, Laforest K. Working with interpreters in health care: a systematic review and meta-ethnography of qualitative studies. *Patient Educ Couns*. 2013;91(2):131–40.
34. Lor M, Xiong P, Schwei RJ, Bowers BJ, Jacobs EA. Limited English proficient Hmong- and Spanish-speaking patients' perceptions of the quality of interpreter services. *Int J Nurs Stud*. 2016;54:75–83.
35. Sinow CS, Corso I, Lorenzo J, Lawrence KA, Magnus DC, Van Cleave AC. Alterations in Spanish language interpretation during pediatric critical care family meetings. *Crit Care Med*. 2017;45(11):1915–21.
36. Butow PN, Goldstein D, Bell ML et al. Interpretation in consultations with immigrant patients with cancer: how accurate is it? *J Clin Oncol*. 2011;29(20):2801–7.
37. Kirby E, Broom A, Good P, Bowden V, Lwin Z. Experiences of interpreters in supporting the transition from oncology to palliative care: a qualitative study. *Asia Pac J Clin Oncol*. 2017;13(5):e497–505.
38. Ranaghan C, Boyle K, Meehan M, Moustapha S, Fraser P, Concert C. Effectiveness of a patient navigator on patient satisfaction in adult patients in an ambulatory care setting: a systematic review. *JBI Database System Rev Implement Rep*. 2016;14(8):172–218.
39. Balaban RB, Galbraith AA, Burns ME, Vialle-Valentin CE, Larochelle MR, Ross-Degnan D. A patient navigator intervention to reduce hospital readmissions among high-risk safety-net patients: a randomized controlled trial. *J Gen Intern Med*. 2015;30(7):907–15.

CHAPTER 21

Evidence-based guidelines and advocacy

Kevin Pottie

LEARNING OBJECTIVES

At the end of this chapter, the reader should be able to:

- Describe examples of guidelines and programmes that address health literacy and social determinants of health for migrant populations
- Identify ways in which primary health practitioners are well situated to advocate for the right to health for migrant populations
- Discuss key elements that support the development of community-based migrant responsive health systems

---

INTRODUCTION

Many cities, communities, and primary health clinics around the world now include culturally, linguistically, and religiously diverse persons (1). Given the diversity of migrant backgrounds and the differences between health systems, it is plausible that some of these people have limited health literacy and insufficient knowledge of the workings of the local health system (2). At the same time, members of the receiving society, including practitioners, may have limited knowledge, skills, and attitudes to support the health settlement or integration of newly arriving migrant populations (3,4). This chapter discusses societal and practitioner misconceptions around migrants, evidence-based migrant health guidelines, health literacy and mental health services, and finally, health advocacy.

Migrant populations include heterogeneous groups as described in Chapter 1. Society's fear and intolerance of migrant populations may escalate into racism, negative politics, and anti-migrant actions (Chapter 5). According to *The Lancet*, deaths among migrants are the direct result of premeditated violence and structurally racist societies that 'create unsafe, isolated, and abandoned ethnic enclaves' (5). Fear and misunderstanding of migrant populations may operate at the community and political levels, including family physicians/general practitioners (GPs) and public health officials. *The Lancet* calls on leaders, scientists, and health practitioners to work with the values of 'peace, equity, solidarity, diversity, community, and social justice' (5). Some authors have written about the importance of emancipation of migrant populations in Europe (6), however, certain social constructs, such as 'structural violence', impede this health equity process. Structural violence refers to the historic deep-seated inequities that affect the lives and the health of oppressed people (7), such as many migrants. Therefore, primary care practitioners, informed on health issues regarding migration, may sometimes find themselves in an advocacy role within their profession seeking improved health care and enhanced cultural communication skills (8).

Many primary care practitioners believe that they lack the medical training necessary to care for the myriad tropical diseases that they fear accompany migrants from low- and middle-income countries (4,9). This may have been true in the past. However, we now are able to identify more precisely which migrant populations are at an elevated risk for infectious diseases, such as HIV and chronic hepatitis C, and understand that this is related to their country of origin, their social economic class, and their migration transit countries (10). Migrant infectious diseases, however, are not nearly as extensive as the tropical medicine experts once purported. Many infections may resolve themselves once a migrant has left the endemic zone. For instance, asymptomatic intestinal worms and parasites imported from tropical countries, and tropical 'red eye' which causes concern among family physicians, typically resolve and do not progress once migrants have arrived in a country where these diseases are not endemic (10). Instead, chronic diseases and mental illness may be a more pertinent concern (10).

It is important to acknowledge that migrants face different challenges, depending on their age, gender, health literacy, and the type of potential illness with which they are afflicted. Oftentimes migrants are young, travelling with children, and soon after arrival to a new country it is typical for families to continue having more children. In this context, living without health insurance and access to timely medical care is a major stressor, especially for women's health (11).

EVIDENCE-BASED MIGRANT-SPECIFIC GUIDELINES

In recent years, there has been a movement toward tailored detection and disease prevention with the use of migrant-specific evidence-based guidelines for primary care (12–14). A national consensus among primary care practitioners in Canada identified the following key supports in order to deliver quality primary care to migrants: (i) evidence-based migrant-specific guidelines, (ii) interpretation services, (iii) mental health services, and (iv) engagement with migrant communities (9). Consensus processes with practitioners in Europe also identified access to care, empowerment, culturally sensitive health services, and respect to migrants (4) as necessary components of primary care. Along with evidence-based medicine, global health competencies that include communication, advocacy, professionalism, and leadership can assist in the training of medical students and primary care practitioners (15). For example, a country-level evidence-based migrant health checklist, e-learning, and community service learning site provides excellent opportunities to share resources and innovative programmes (16).

Evidence-based guidelines can help develop networks of practitioners committed to improving the health care of migrants. Such health professional networks can enable practitioners to share evidence-based guidelines and best practices. During times of mass migration, such as with the Syrian refugees, previously established networks facilitated the dissemination of Syrian refugee guidelines (17) and helped collect reports of conditions such as the prevalence dental pathologies and birth accidents. When there are unexpected infectious diseases, the network can service as a sentinel to detect epidemics and communicate with public health officers to develop an appropriate course of action.

Evidence-based guidelines can support both public health and primary health care in the detection and care of infectious diseases, mental health conditions, and chronic diseases. Gender, age, country of origin, forced migration, and living conditions are important variables to consider when planning disease screening (14) (see Table 21.1). Cultural values and rights are also relevant to consider in the development of migrant guidelines. At the time of writing this chapter, Scientific Advice Public health guidance on screening and vaccination for infectious diseases in newly arrived migrants within the EU/EEA is forthcoming.

As expressed previously, several guidelines specific for migrants have been developed during the last years, especially regarding infectious diseases. For example, the recent ECDC public health guidance (18) suggests chest x-rays for populations coming from a tuberculosis (TB)-endemic country and consideration of Mantoux tests when latent TB is a moderate to high risk. Informed consent is strongly recommended before screening high-risk populations for HIV, either in the clinic, or in the community through the use of rapid counselling and testing. For populations at high risk of hepatitis B/C, these two tests can be done together, often with HIV testing when appropriate. In order to protect children and adolescents from hepatitis B infection, in addition to other common childhood illnesses, it is recommended that the appropriate vaccinations be administered. For common childhood illnesses, providing (re)vaccination without records is recommended rather than attempting serology. However, serology screening for parasitic infections, such as strongyloidiasis or schistosomiasis, is recommended particularly for migrant populations coming from parasite-endemic countries (13).

Migrant populations also need strong community-based support, a focus on practical needs such as acquiring and maintaining employment, language, and literacy training, as well as access to quality primary health care (19). The guidance also shows the importance of considering migrant values, which encompass health, social and economic attributes, as well the acceptability and accessibility of public health options. Factors to consider include perceived disease susceptibility, benefits of testing, and value for potential infectious disease outcomes. Public health programmes will have to adapt their communication and approaches to align with migrant populations. For example, coupling the rapid HIV testing technology with pre-test counselling can dramatically improve uptake of testing. Multiple disease test approaches are often relevant and preferred by migrants, as many migrant populations require serology tests for diseases such as hepatitis A and B, HIV, strongyloidiasis, and schistosomiasis. Serology testing for asymptomatic parasites has emerged as an effective and more acceptable approach to screen migrant populations from parasite endemic regions (18).

Refugees value strong relationships with community-based primary care practitioners and medical students (20), as most refugee care takes place in communities rather than hospitals. Recruiting and training active community family physicians to accept refugees has been an

TABLE 21.1 Illustrative non-infectious disease recommendations for migrant populations

Condition	Recommendations	Migrant group
Contraception	Screen migrant women of reproductive age for unmet contraceptive needs soon after arrival to Canada. Provide culturally sensitive, patient-centred contraceptive counselling (giving women their method of choice, having contraception on site, and fostering a good interpersonal relationship).	Female youth and women of reproductive age
Dental disease	Screen all migrants for dental pain. Treat pain with nonsteroidal anti-inflammatory drugs and refer patient to a dentist. Screen all migrant children and adults for obvious dental caries and oral disease and refer to a dentist or oral health specialist if necessary.	Children and adults
Diabetes	Screen migrants and refugees >35 years of age from ethnic groups at high risk for type 2 diabetes (those from South Asia, Latin America, and Africa) with fasting blood glucose.	High-risk ethnic groups
Depression	If an integrated treatment programme is available, screen adults for depression using a systematic clinical inquiry or validated patient health questionnaire (PHQ-9 or equivalent). Individuals with major depression may present with somatic symptoms (pain, fatigue, or other nonspecific symptoms). Link suspected cases of depression with an integrated treatment programme and case management or mental health care.	Adults
PTSD	Do not conduct routine screening for exposure to traumatic events, because pushing for disclosure of traumatic events in well-functioning individuals may result in more harm than good. Be alert for signs and symptoms of PTSD (unexplained somatic symptoms, sleep disorders, or mental health disorders such as depression or panic disorder).	Adults
Vision	Perform age-appropriate screening for visual impairment. If presenting vision <6/12 (with habitual correction in place), refer patient to an optometrist or ophthalmologist for comprehensive ophthalmic evaluation.	Adults

Source: Pottie K et al. *CMAJ [Internet].* 2011 Sep 6 [cited 2018 Jul 4];183(12):E824–925, http://www.cmaj.ca/content/183/12/E824.

ongoing challenge (3). This has been documented in systematic reviews in Australia (21). Primary care practitioners report that they worry about loss of income, fear of tropical diseases, and communication challenges. However, practitioners who do work with refugees report feelings of satisfaction in contributing to the well-being of refugee patients, and enjoy the challenge of treating patients from around the world (3).

MENTAL HEALTH GUIDELINES AND SERVICES
Regarding mental health, a national migrant health guideline Delphi consensus with primary care practitioners ranked PTSD, depression, and anxiety disorders within the top five

conditions in need of evidence-based guidelines (22). Models of collaborative care between primary and specialist health professionals as well as trained community health practitioners can enhance the delivery of care (23). Evidence-based migrant guidelines may increase the skills and comfort of primary health practitioners in identifying and managing mental health problems. In many cases, routine screening for PTSD is not standard practice, but practitioners should watch for distressing symptoms and disability (14).

Peer support workers provide emotional and social support to migrants, who share a common experience (9). Peer support is intended to complement traditional clinical care, and vice-versa. Such outreach services involve meeting clients in their own environments. Indeed, mental health assessments are beginning to take place in migrant homes or newcomer shelters, and public health practitioners are using rapid HIV tests to reach marginalized migrant communities living with HIV-related stigma. Notwithstanding some regional variance, most migrants seek health care in primary health centres. However, migrants often prefer care for mental illness in community-based settings (22,23). The utilization of this community-level engagement allows clinics to offer programmes in homes, workplaces, schools, or other settings, thus improving accessibility (23). More specifically, community health workers assist in increasing the capacity of mental health services available to patients in participating clinics. Drop-in programmes, mobile treatment services, and street contacts can also increase access to services by providing flexible hours of care in accessible locations. To improve access to existing health care resources, it is important to consider supports for transportation, interpreters, and cultural brokers.

HEALTH LITERACY AND PATIENT PREFERENCES

Large national cohort studies in Canada and Australia have shown that refugees, visible minorities, and those with low official language proficiency face a rapid decline in health status compared to other migrants (2). Health literacy may be defined as the degree to which individuals have the capacity to obtain, process, and understand basic health information and services needed to make appropriate health decisions (https://health.gov/communication/literacy/quickguide/factsbasic.htm). Migrants with limited health literacy and language barriers initially seek care from community members or retired physicians who share the same culture and language. But as health literacy increases and barriers to access fall away, migrants prefer qualified health professionals with established links to the health system (24). In this context, interpreters may play a supportive role in the delivery of care, for example to provide care to Arabic-speaking Syrian refugees (17). Evidence-based guidelines, training programmes, and networks can support the scaling up of such services to improve care for migrant populations (12).

Migrant preferences will vary due to cultural and traditional medical beliefs and past experiences with health care systems (25). For example, migrant populations coming from TB-endemic countries may have less concern over a latent TB diagnoses than a person from a non-endemic TB zone (26), thus posing a challenge in disease detection. In 2016, a discrete choice experiment looked at refugees from 11 developing countries within 3 months of arrival and found that face-to-face encounters were preferred when language was a barrier, but accepted telephone support services when these provided language interpreters. Wait times for an appointment and out-of-pocket expenses are also important factors for migrants seeking primary care. As with anybody else, the likelihood that migrants will seek care is dependent on factors such as migrants' perceived susceptibility to illness, severity of disease, and perceived benefits of intervention (11), all of which can differ from the majority population. Acceptability of seeking and accepting treatment depends on migrants' relationships with health care practitioners as well as their knowledge of the disease and the potential for disease-related stigma (26).

The acceptability of infectious disease interventions influences the readiness of migrants and clinicians to incorporate recommendations into practice, as seen in the case of HIV testing (27). Insufficient knowledge about the acceptability of interventions may also inhibit practitioners from offering screening to migrants (26). How patients value the disease-related outcomes of interventions (e.g. perception of risk of disease, diagnoses, symptoms, or disease resolution), or other outcomes (e.g. time away from work, stigma, side effects, or adverse events) can create barriers to the uptake of guideline recommendations. For example, one qualitative study on developing decision aids for HIV testing for newly arrived sub-Saharan African women to Canada demonstrated how the provision of accurate HIV information can reduce stress (28).

Disenfranchised migrants, who may be victims of structural racism, often face a range of stigma related to mental health conditions. As a result, they tend to prefer home-based care or community-based care, which may lead to shared care models where specialists work in a primary care context (11). Awareness of the range of preferences relevant for migrant populations may improve access to and implementation of care. Trust, cultural sensitivity, and taking the time to engage with the individual can improve interactions with migrant patients. Despite certain perceptions that migrants do not heed the advice of practitioners, evidence shows that recommendations from practitioners play a significant role in the acceptance of both infectious disease and chronic disease interventions (24,26).

HEALTH ADVOCACY

Despite well-intentioned government policy, a universal health system does not always ensure access and quality of care for migrants (29). Migrant health often falls outside of the health system, and service fees and medication barriers limit access to care for this vulnerable population.

Advocacy is fundamental in the interplay between policy, research, and evidence-based practices (12). When a system faces stresses, anti-migrant policies may place migrant populations and migrant-serving practitioners at a significant disadvantage. During these times, advocacy remains a unique and essential strength for primary care practitioners who may be needed. For example, in 2012, the Canadian Doctors for Refugee Care emerged as a national advocacy group to fight government cuts to health care for asylum seekers and refugees. This 'white-coat' advocacy group confronted government officials, held national rallies, and charged the government for unlawful cuts to refugee programmes on route to reversing cuts (30). Even when the health system is working well and is supported by positive policy, migrant services remain as fragile as the population they serve, and constant monitoring is needed to maintain the quality of health services and ensure health equity (31).

Evidence-based guidelines, practitioner networks, and service learning are valuable tools to improve the health of migrants. International social accountability programmes now exist in many medical schools worldwide (32). One successful programme has emerged from the Canadian Collaboration for Migrant and Refugee Health. Beginning at the University of Ottawa, this refugee health community service learning opportunity has introduced nearly

2000 medical students across Canada to refugees in shelters, apartments, and homes. The students learn cross-cultural communication and interpreter skills as they assess medication needs, help set up internet services, and share meals with their assigned refugee families.

Responsive primary health care systems and services must be at once comprehensive and nimble. Policy makers may wish to believe existing health systems effectively care for all populations equally, including refugees (31). However, we know that migrants may require a health equity approach, one in which all levels of government, all types of health practitioners, and even the public sector participate to ensure access to effective primary health care.

Public health is another valuable component of a responsive health system. Public health supports universal vaccinations, collaborates with primary care for TB and HIV programmes, and may initiate chronic disease prevention and management programmes, for example culturally appropriate diabetes screening and education. Primary care and public health have an important immediate role to play in improving the health and social determinants of health for newly arrived migrant populations. Developing prevalence-targeted, culturally sensitive community outreach programmes provides important health system leadership for both specialists and primary health care providers.

Primary health care is the front line for most health systems. A responsive health care system needs primary health care and health advocacy to remain comprehensive and sustainable (31).

Responsive primary health care systems should include interpreter services, evidence-based guidelines, specialist physicians, cultural and political profiles, and interdisciplinary collaboration. Furthermore, ensuring all migrants receive a health card soon after arrival, which allows for utilization of health care, is at the forefront of access to health services.

We also know that newly arriving refugees and other migrants may require an enhanced health equity approach — an approach where all levels of government, all types of health practitioners, and even the public sector participate to ensure access to evidence-based primary health care (31).

CONCLUSIONS

Primary health care, together with public health and other specialties, can help provide a clinically effective and supportive (medical) home for newly arriving migrants. Equipped with cultural communication skills, evidence-based prevention and disease guidelines, and equity and social justice values, primary care practitioners can play an active role against racism and inequities. Trust and cultural sensitivity, especially in the context of low health literacy, have implications for public health interventions and practitioner education. Recommendations from health care providers play an important role in the acceptance of infectious disease and chronic disease interventions. A community-based approach following evidence-based guidelines and using programmes to address social determinants of health are necessary to improve access to and ensure quality of care for refugees and other migrants. Evidence-based guidelines and solidarity and can lead to the development of primary care migrant networks, provide a foundation for advocacy, and identify areas in need of further research.

In particular, more global research is needed to continue to document the burden of diseases such as PTSD and mental illness, chronic diseases such as dental disease and diabetes, intestinal parasites, HIV, hepatitis, and xenophobia in migrant populations. This will provide further evidence for developing more migrant-specific guidelines. In addition, there is an ongoing need to improve acceptability of primary health services. For example, combining priority tests such as anemia, diabetes mellitus, HIV, and hepatitis B/C, and improve linkage to care. Finally, countries must consider research and innovations in community-based care and migration programmes to empower migrants, as well as technologies to support communication.

ACKNOWLEDGEMENT

I would like to acknowledge the expert editing and technical support of Nicole Pinto.

REFERENCES

1. International Organization for Migration (IOM). 2015. *World Migration Report. Migrants and Cities: New Partnerships to Manage Mobility.* [cited 2018 Jul 4]; Available from: www.iom.int

2. Ng E, Pottie K, Spitzer D. Official language proficiency and self-reported health among immigrants to Canada. *Health Rep [Internet].* 2011 Dec [cited 2018 Jul 4];22(4):15–23. Available from: http://www.ncbi.nlm.nih.gov/pubmed/22352148

3. Mota L, Mayhew M, Grant KJ, Batista R, Pottie K. Rejecting and accepting international migrant patients into primary care practices: a mixed method study. *Int J Migr Health Soc Care [Internet].* 2015 Jun 15 [cited 2018 Jul 4];11(2):108–29. Available from: http://www.emeraldinsight.com/doi/10.1108/IJMHSC-04-2014-0013

4. EUGATE. European best practices in access, quality and appropriateness of health services for immigrants in Europe. Project report on Delphi process on best practice of health care for immigrants. Utrecht; 2011.

5. Horton R. Offline: Racism – The pathology we choose to ignore. *Lancet [Internet].* 2017 Jul 1 [cited 2018 Jul 4];390(10089):14. Available from: https://www.sciencedirect.com/science/article/pii/S0140673617317464?via%3Dihub

6. Laurence J. In: Eichelman DF, Norton AR, editors. *The Emancipation of Europe's Muslims: The State's Role in Minority Integration.* Princeton, New Jersey: Princeton University Press; 2012.

7. Farmer P. On suffering and structural violence social and economic rights in the Global Era. In: *Pathologies of Power: Health, Human Rights, and the New War on the Poor.* 4th ed. Los Angeles: University of California Press; 2003: 1–14.

8. Gruner D. AGM 2014: The state of refugee health: a prognosis for public justice in Canada. In: *CPJ's 2014 Annual General Meeting.* 2014.

9. Pottie K, Batista R, Mayhew M, Mota L, Grant K. Improving delivery of primary care for vulnerable migrants: Delphi consensus to prioritize innovative practice strategies. *Can Fam Physician [Internet].* 2014 Jan [cited 2018 Jul 4];60(1):e32–40. Available from: http://www.ncbi.nlm.nih.gov/pubmed/24452576

10. Gushulak BD, Pottie K, Hatcher Roberts J, Torres S, DesMeules M, Canadian Collaboration for Immigrant and Refugee Health. Migration and health in Canada: health in the global village. *CMAJ [Internet].* 2011 Sep 6 [cited 2018 Jul 4];183(12):E952–8. Available from: http://www.ncbi.nlm.nih.gov/pubmed/20584934

11. Seedat F, Hargreaves S, Friedland JS. Engaging new migrants in infectious disease screening: a qualitative semi-structured interview study of UK migrant community health-care leads. Marsh V, editor. *PLOS ONE [Internet].* 2014 Oct 15 [cited 2018 Jul 4];9(10):e108261. Available from: http://www.ncbi.nlm.nih.gov/pubmed/25330079

12. Pottie K, Gruner D, Magwood O. Canada's response to refugees at the primary health care level. *Public Health Res Pract [Internet].* 2018 [cited 2018 Jul 5];28(1). Available from: http://www.phrp.com.au/?p=37322

13. Buonfrate D, Gobbi F, Marchese V et al. Extended screening for infectious diseases among newly-arrived asylum seekers from Africa and Asia, Verona province, Italy, April 2014 to June 2015. *Eurosurveillance [Internet].* 2018 Apr 19 [cited 2018 Jul 6];23(16):17–00527. Available from: https://www.eurosurveillance.org/content/10.2807/1560-7917.ES.2018.23.16.17-00527

14. Pottie K, Greenaway C, Feightner J et al. Evidence-based clinical guidelines for immigrants and refugees. *CMAJ [Internet]*. 2011 Sep 6 [cited 2018 Jul 4];183(12):E824–925. Available from: http://www.ncbi.nlm.nih.gov/pubmed/20530168

15. Redwood-Campbell L, Pakes B, Rouleau K et al. Developing a curriculum framework for global health in family medicine: emerging principles, competencies, and educational approaches. *BMC Med Educ [Internet]*. 2011 Dec 22 [cited 2018 Jul 4];11(1):46. Available from: http://bmcmededuc.biomedcentral.com/articles/10.1186/1472-6920-11-46

16. CCIRH – CCIRH Main website [Internet]. [cited 2018 Jul 4]. Available from: http://www.ccirhken.ca/

17. Pottie K, Greenaway C, Hassan G, Hui C, Kirmayer LJ. Caring for a newly arrived Syrian refugee family. *CMAJ [Internet]*. 2016 Feb 16 [cited 2018 Jul 11];188(3):207–11. Available from: http://www.ncbi.nlm.nih.gov/pubmed/26755669

18. European Centre for Disease Prevention and Control. Public health guidance on screening and vaccination for infectious diseases in newly-arrived migrants within the EU/EEA. Stockholm: ECDC; 2018.

19. Beach MC, Price EG, Gary TL et al. Cultural competence: a systematic review of health care provider educational interventions. *Med Care [Internet]*. 2005 Apr [cited 2018 Jul 4];43(4):356–73. Available from: http://www.ncbi.nlm.nih.gov/pubmed/15778639

20. Pottie K, Hostland S. Health advocacy for refugees. *Can Fam Physician*. 2007;53(11).

21. Joshi C, Russell G, Cheng I-H et al. A narrative synthesis of the impact of primary health care delivery models for refugees in resettlement countries on access, quality and coordination. *Int J Equity Health [Internet]*. 2013 Nov 7 [cited 2018 Jul 5];12(1):88. Available from: http://www.ncbi.nlm.nih.gov/pubmed/24199588

22. Swinkels H, Pottie K, Tugwell P, Rashid M, Narasiah L; Canadian Collaboration for Immigrant and Refugee Health (CCIRH). Development of guidelines for recently arrived immigrants and refugees to Canada: Delphi consensus on selecting preventable and treatable conditions. *CMAJ [Internet]*. 2011 Sep 6 [cited 2018 Jul 4];183(12):E928–32. Available from: http://www.ncbi.nlm.nih.gov/pubmed/20547714

23. Becker AE, Kleinman A. Mental health and the global agenda. *N Engl J Med [Internet]*. 2013 Jul 4 [cited 2018 Jul 4];369(1):66–73. Available from: http://www.nejm.org/doi/10.1056/NEJMra1110827

24. Dahal G, Qayyum A, Ferreyra M, Kassim H, Pottie K. Immigrant community leaders identify four dimensions of trust for culturally appropriate diabetes education and care. *J Immigr Minor Health [Internet]*. 2014 Oct 8 [cited 2018 Jul 4];16(5):978–84. Available from: http://www.ncbi.nlm.nih.gov/pubmed/23471673

25. Helman C. *Culture, Health, and Illness*. Hodder Arnold; 2007: 501 p.

26. Driedger M, Mayhew A, Welch V et al. Accessibility and acceptability of infectious disease interventions among migrants in the EU/EEA: A CERQual systematic review. *Int J Environ Res Public Health*. 2018 Oct 23;15(11):pii: E2329. doi: 10.3390/ijerph15112329

27. Pottie K, Lotfi T, Kilzar L et al. The effectiveness and cost-effectiveness of screening for HIV inmigrants in the EU/EEA: A systematic review. *Int J Environ Res Public Health*. 2018; 15(8,1700):1–23. doi: https://doi.org/10.3390/ijerph15081700

28. Mitra D, Jacobsen MJ, O'Connor A, Pottie K, Tugwell P. Assessment of the decision support needs of women from HIV endemic countries regarding voluntary HIV testing in Canada. *Patient Educ Couns [Internet]*. 2006 Nov 1 [cited 2018 Jul 13];63(3):292–300. Available from: https://www.sciencedirect.com/science/article/pii/S0738399106001248?via%3Dihub

29. Pottie K, Gruner D, Magwood O. Canada's Response to Refugees at the Primary Health Care Level. *Public Health Research and Practice*, 2018;28(1):1–4. doi: https://doi.org/10.17061/phrp2811803

30. Gruner D, Cleveland J, Demirdache L, Pottie KC. Community resilience and activism addressing needs of refugees in sites of arrival. In: Pashang S, Gruner S, editors. *Displacement, Migration and Trauma*. Rock Mill Press; 2015.

31. Pottie K, Hui C, Rahman P et al. Building responsive health systems to help communities affected by migration: an international Delphi consensus. *Int J Environ Res Public Health [Internet]*. 2017 Feb 3 [cited 2018 Jul 4];14(2):144. Available from: http://www.ncbi.nlm.nih.gov/pubmed/28165380

32. Frenk J, Chen L, Bhutta ZA et al. Health professionals for a new century: transforming education to strengthen health systems in an interdependent world. *Lancet [Internet]*. 2010 Dec 4 [cited 2018 Jul 4];376(9756):1923–58. Available from: http://www.ncbi.nlm.nih.gov/pubmed/21112623

Diversity-sensitive versus adapted services for migrants: The example of dementia care in Germany

Oliver Razum and Hürrem Tezcan-Güntekin

LEARNING OBJECTIVES

At the end of this chapter, the reader should be able to:

- Learn how diversity-sensitive care is characterized, using the example of dementia care for migrants
- Understand what implications dementia can have for migrants and their relatives
- Help health professionals understand the situation of migrants with dementia and their family caregivers
- Provide practical tools that can be used in primary health and nursing care by professionals to implement diversity-sensitive care

---

CLINICAL VIGNETTE

In the early 1960s, Mr O migrated from Turkey to Germany. He has a son and two daughters. At the age of 72 years he started forgetting things. He became more and more aggressive when he couldn't find things at places where he thinks he has put them. His son — a social worker — is now about 60 years old and recognizes that something 'is wrong' with his father. He brings him to the family doctor who has known him for decades. The family doctor tells father and son that the father has developed dementia. With this diagnosis (which the doctor arrived at without the help of standard diagnostic instruments because of the father's low reading skills) the life of the son and the daughter-in-law changes. Due to the increasing aggressiveness of the father, the sons' wife decides to leave the son. The symptoms of dementia increase, and the father can no longer live in his flat alone anymore. The son decides to take him to his own flat. The reason for this decision is that the son thinks his father needs help. As he is the oldest child, he feels responsible for his father's well-being. They live together for about 1 year, but the symptoms of the disease become worse. The situation starts to affect the relationship of the son and his wife. They finally decide that the care situation has to be changed.

The son searches for a nursing home but cannot find one which meets his expectations. He wants his father to live in a place where he can go out and enjoy nature; a place where he does not feel like being in a 'factory' and which is near to the place he lived before. He tries to visit a few nursing homes with his father, but the father refuses even to leave the car. The son starts to look for alternative living forms for people with dementia and finds a professionally supervised living group for people suffering from dementia. The living group was recently established, and they are among the first clients. Thus it is possible to choose the room the father should get. The father accepts this place and the professionals allow the son to stay with his father for the first week and help him to get used to his new home. The son and his wife are very happy about this solution.

Turkish friends and neighbours, however, deplore the son's decision to 'give his father away' to an institution for nursing care. The son invites them to visit the father in the living group to see that it is not like a 'care factory' but more like a real home. But only few come to visit the father in his new home. Most continue to dismiss the son's decision. These reactions are very burdensome for the son.

MIGRANTS IN NEED OF CARE

People migrate to other countries for very different reasons; for example, to seek work, to re-unite with their family, or as refugees. The number of older migrants in northern and Western European countries is rising, and this development will continue in the next years (1,2). Large numbers of people migrated from southern Europe and North Africa to north-Western European countries as part of the labour recruitment in the 1960s and 1970s. Only an unexpectedly small proportion returned to their countries of origin, while many stayed in the countries they migrated to even after retirement. For example, in Germany in 2014, 3% of all migrants 65 years and older returned to their country of origin (3).

Ageing migrants bring along new challenges (see Chapter 10). Many older migrants are not familiar with the medical and nursing care system of the receiving countries, especially when they have not been in need of care before. Most of the migrants have not seen the day-to-day consequences of their own parents getting old because of the geographical distance to the countries of origin. As a result, they often lack concepts of getting old or being in need of care. Neither the migrants in need of care nor the medical/nursing care systems of the receiving countries are adequately prepared for this challenge that comes along with an ageing migrant population.

Three observations from Germany, also relevant for other countries, show that there is an urgent need to take action:

1. Migrants are in need of nursing care earlier compared to the host population (4). This difference is only partly explained by the younger age structure of the migrant population; the fact that many migrants worked under difficult conditions contributes.

2. The intensity of care needed by migrants is often higher than the level required by members of the native population (5).

3. Migrants in need of care are more often cared for at home than native Germans, and more often receive care through family caregivers (6). In many migrant communities, taking care of a family member is understood as a family matter, and as a duty. Fewer migrants in need of care and their family caregivers accept care help by professionals, compared to native Germans.

DEMENTIA AND MIGRATION: LOSS AND FOREIGNNESS

Dementia is a common reason for being in need of nursing care — both for migrants and non-migrants. About 47 million people were living with dementia globally in 2015 and it is to be expected that the number will triple by 2050 (7). The prevalence of dementia in migrant populations in European countries is not yet well documented. One reason for that is the high number of people with dementia without a diagnosis (1), especially among migrants (8). Dementia in migrants may differ from dementia in the majority population not only in quantitative terms, but also qualitatively (refer to Chapter 9). Persons suffering from dementia are confronted with different types of foreignness: the foreignness of getting older and the foreignness of the disease dementia applies to both migrants and non-migrants with dementia. But the foreignness of the migration and the foreignness resulting from losing the language of the country of residence — mostly acquired as a second language later in life — creates an additional burden specific to migrants. As a consequence, migrants are at multiple risk of social exclusion. In addition, in countries such as Turkey, dementia is often not understood as a disease but as a punishment by God, with a tabooing of the symptoms and isolation of the family caring for a member with dementia.

Caring for a person with dementia is a challenge for any family. However, there are specific problems experienced by migrant families faced with this challenge. Caregivers tend to accept little help from formal providers of health and nursing care. Reasons are cultural adaptation and communication problems due to low language fluency in the majority language, shame, and fear of negative consequences (including the misconceived worry that the family member in need of care might be removed from the family and taken to a nursing home). When families with migration background are sceptical towards majority care institutions, the person suffering from dementia may not receive professional medical or nursing care in time and the families caring for their relatives single-handedly will often be overburdened. Studies have shown that the care of a family member with dementia can frequently cause psychological problems and even mental diseases like depression among the family caregivers (9). If these family caregivers do not seek and accept help, the risk of mental illness is high. In addition, the psychological burden for migrants of both first and second generation when facing the cultural discordance between the two countries regarding the care of the elderly is probably even higher than for the majority populations.

Family caregivers also experience feelings of loss and foreignness, that of living with a once close person with dementia who might no longer respond to them or even recognize them (10). Moreover, they have to combine their roles as wife/husband or child of the person with dementia with the new role as a family caregiver. Being in need of care goes along with loss of autonomy and almost inevitably with changes of long-established hierarchic structures in relationships — for example, in the case of family caregivers as surrogate decision makers (11). Relationships have to be reflected and defined anew. This necessitates the competence to reflect on one's own situation, which not all caregiving relatives are capable of, or willing to do. But the definition of the new role is one of the key preconditions for creating strong self-management competencies. Other important elements contributing towards a constructive way of living with a person with dementia are to accept the incurability of the disease and to communicate about it openly with relatives, friends, and neighbours, thereby reducing isolation. Through these strategies, self-management competencies can be created and strengthened. They also help to increase acceptance of the use of nursing care services or of accommodating relatives in supervised living groups. How each of these challenges is perceived and coped with varies depending on many individual and social factors, including cultural and religious, which might or might not be different for some migrant families.

THE NEED FOR DIVERSITY-SENSITIVE NURSING CARE SERVICES

One reason to choose a certain nursing care service over another is the degree of its need orientation. But what does 'need orientation' mean in the context of care for migrants? To define 'need orientation' in terms of concrete measures is difficult because the needs of people requiring care (with and without migration background) and of their relatives are heterogeneous. It is still subject to debate whether services should respond to assumed 'culture-specific' needs or if they should be rather 'culturally sensitive' in order to reach patients with different cultural backgrounds.

Considering the heterogeneity of the European population as well as that of the migrant population residing in Europe, the second option seems to be more appropriate. Existing medical and nursing care structures (for example outpatient nursing care services, inpatient care services) should be modified so they respond to different needs of the people requiring care and of their relatives. In the course of such 'intercultural opening' of nursing care structures, several steps are necessary: firstly, the population's heterogeneity should not be reduced to cultural background. The primary reason for differences in health and in access to health care are socioeconomic: people with higher income and better education have better health and better access to health care, irrespective of their culture and migration background. But 'culture' should not be overemphasized in other respects as well. Importantly, other diversity characteristics besides 'culture' should be kept in mind while thinking about answering different needs of a diverse community. Examples are language spoken and religion, which influence the needs of people. Equally relevant for the nursing care setting are traumatic experiences, sexual identity, sexual orientation, special features of family culture, or intergenerational relationships. Diversity-sensitive care should be sufficiently competent to take several different diversity characteristics into account and not only focus on migration background. This is presumably the best way to satisfy heterogeneous needs in the context of nursing care. Moreover, such services would cater equally well for *all* members of a population, not only for specific subgroups.

When setting up diversity-sensitive nursing care services, the following levels have to be addressed:

- On a *political level*, decisions have to be made to enable the professional nursing care staff to invest more time for a diversity-sensitive and individual care.
- At the *management level*, it is important that the management of a nursing care service strives to provide a service appropriate for a heterogeneous community.
  - This should start with the personnel policy: staff should be representative of different diversity characteristics. Especially in the case of dementia and the loss of the acquired second language, native-speaking staff or nursing care staff who speak at

least a few sentences in the native language of the person with dementia is essential. Nursing care services should try to recruit staff with different language skills.

- Diversity-sensitive training for staff already working in the institution is indispensable and should be offered also to professionals with a migration background, because they are not inherently familiar with diversity-sensitive care. Sensitivity towards diversity cannot be learned only in theory lessons but has to be implemented into the attitude of the person through lifelong learning. Thus diversity (re-)training should be offered periodically.

- At the *service provision level*, the most important aspects of diversity-sensitive nursing care are:

  - Being open-minded towards, and interested in, people with different diversity characteristics.
  - Readiness to be attentive of different needs, even if this is a time-consuming process.
  - Constructive approach towards one's own fears and prejudices — one should not ignore them but work with them. This means, for example, to consult other people in situations of uncertainty to find out how to deal with the needs and reflect about possibilities to fulfil them.
  - Reflection of one's own culture and attitude towards other cultures or characteristics as a lifelong process.
  - Reflection of experiences and feelings in context with diversity and/or nursing care in the nursing care team. Through constructive discussions a diversity-sensitive attitude can be developed and internalized, so that it can subsequently be remembered even under time pressure when providing care.
  - The willingness to learn a few sentences in different languages, especially when caring for people with dementia. In addition, nonverbal communication is important to calm, and interact with, patients independent of their language competencies.

WHAT THIS MEANS IN PRACTICE

The vignette of Mr O shows that family caregivers of migrants with dementia often perceive feelings of foreignness — for different reasons, for example because of shame about the disease or feelings of isolation. They react differently to this feeling. Some caregivers increase the isolation from society; others are able to cope with the diagnosis and with the new situation, as the son of Mr O did. Being able to advance from a feeling of powerlessness to an attitude of activity — despite the new situation — is decisive. This paradigm shift can be supported by a user-oriented and in-depth information about the disease by the physician and the acceptance of the disease by family caregivers. It enables the family caregivers to accept the new role and remain active in society. But the case of Mr O also shows that it does not suffice for the individual caregivers to change their attitudes. There is also a need for the migrant community to change: they need to accept dementia as a disease, rather than a punishment. And they need to accept that there are several differing but acceptable models of organizing care for a relative with dementia.

If family caregivers and patients feel respected and taken seriously by professional care providers — as was the case in the vignette of Mr O — they will be more willing to accept help from professional care services. It is helpful if professional care providers understand the process of migration and the emotions migrants experience before, during, and after the migration act.

Even though many family caregivers in migrant communities prefer to care for their relative with dementia themselves, they are increasingly willing to accept supportive professional care structures when the disease progresses. Later, they usually feel that it was a good decision to accept professional help. It is important to support families in this decision-making process by helping them to find solutions that fit into their lifeworlds and individual family cultures. The family culture – and often the need to manage the nursing care in the family – and the indispensable care work the relatives are providing should be recognized and appreciated by the care professional (refer to Chapter 11). Nevertheless, helping structures should be offered repeatedly, because the challenges of the nursing care for family caregivers change permanently – mainly due to the changing nature of the dementia disease. The example of the vignette shows that the inclusion of the family caregiver in choosing a room for the father and the possibility to stay with the father for a week until he got used to the new setting answered the needs of both the family caregiver and the father in an appropriate way.

SUMMARY: PRACTICAL TOOLS/RECOMMENDATIONS FOR DIVERSITY-SENSITIVE SERVICES

From the perspective of the general practitioners, the psychiatrists, and the neurologists

For diagnostic purposes, culture- and/or language-sensitive or -neutral instruments should be used to ensure a correct diagnosis (refer to Chapter 23) (12). Primary care practitioners should be aware of their role as gatekeeper to nursing care services and other specialist services. Often they are the first and most important person who can explain to the families what dementia and other diseases that might be differently interpreted imply not only for the patient, but also for the family, and also how the family caregiver can get help in the health care and nursing care systems.

From the perspective of professional nursing care persons

Professional nursing care staff, irrespective of whether they are working in hospitals, in inpatient nursing care services, or ambulatory care, should be aware that the relatives of the patient may perceive dementia disease or other serious conditions as threatening and shameful. Dementia, the case that we have studied as an example, is often not understood as a medical condition and symptoms may be (mis-)interpreted as usual characteristics of getting older. If the person with dementia is then admitted to a hospital or nursing care institution and brought to a ward for people with psychiatric diseases, the families are often shocked and shamed. Understanding the situation of the family caregivers and sensitive handling of the situation can help to start a communication process with the family about the nature of the disease, and to find ways to organize the nursing care setting (at home or in an institution) suitable to the needs of the patient and his/her family members. In an understanding atmosphere, compromises can be found, even if not all needs of the family may ultimately be fulfilled.

Professional nursing care persons working in outpatient nursing care services should be aware that not all families understand nursing care as a professional activity – especially the basic nursing (e.g. washing the body of a person) in contrast to technical nursing (e.g. injection or wound treatment). If professional nursing care persons know about the different ideas of what nursing is about, they can openly talk with the family members about the possibilities and limits of nursing care. An open dialogue about closeness and distance between staff and family members will help to find an appropriate and acceptable way to collaborate.

Professional nursing care persons should reflect their own adherence to culture(s) to work with a diversity-sensitive and open-minded attitude — whether they personally have a migration background or not.

From the educational and institutional perspective

At the institutional level, diversity-sensitive care should be implemented into the curricula of health care training and further education. Health care policies should allow creation of conditions that make it possible to implement diversity-sensitive health care — which implicates for example a reduction of time pressure in nursing care systems. Diversity-sensitive care needs time — time to perceive and understand individual needs and lifeworlds so to get the chance to fulfil the patient's and the caregivers' wishes and expectations.

REFERENCES

1. Alzheimer Europe. *Dementia in Europe–Yearbook*. 2013. Available from: http://www.alzheimer-europe.org/Publications/Dementia-in-Europe-Yearbooks (accessed 12 September 2017).
2. Friedrich-Ebert-Foundation (FES). Auswirkungen des demografischen Wandels im Einwanderungsland Deutschland. [Effects of the demographic changes in the immigration country Germany]. 2015. Available from: http://library.fes.de/pdf-files/wiso/11612.pdf
3. Federal Statistical Office in Germany. Population and Employment. Series 1 Volume 2.2. Wiesbaden. 2015.
4. Federal Ministry of Health in Germany (Bundesministerium für Gesundheit). Daten aus der Studie zum Pflege-Weiterentwicklungsgesetz. TNS Infratest Spezialforschung. 2011. Available from: https://www.bundesgesundheitsministerium.de/fileadmin/dateien/Publikationen/Pflege/Berichte/Abschlussbericht_zur_Studie_Wirkungen_des_Pflege-Weiterentwicklungsgesetzes.pdf (accessed 26 June 2017).
5. Kohls M. Pflegebedürftigkeit und Nachfrage nach Pflegeleistungen von Migrantinnen und Migranten im demographischen Wandel. [Demographic changes, need of care and demand for nursing care benefits by immigrants]. Forschungsbericht Nr. 12, Bundesamt für Migration und Flüchtlinge (Hrsg.) Nürnberg. 2012. Available from: http://www.bamf.de/SharedDocs/Meldungen/DE/2012/20120302-forschungsbericht12.html
6. Okken PK, Spallek J, Razum O. Pflege türkischer Migranten. [Nursing care of Turkish immigrants]. In: Bauer U, Büscher A. (Hrsg.) *Soziale Ungleichheit und Pflege. Beiträge sozialwissenschaftlich orientierter Pflegeforschung*. Wiesbaden: VS Verlag für Sozialwissenschaften; 2008: 369–422.
7. Livingston G, Sommerlad A, Orgeta V et al. Dementia prevention, intervention, and care. *Lancet*. 2017;390(10113):2673–734.
8. Diaz E, BN Kumar, K Engedal. Immigrant patients with dementia and memory Impairment in primary health care in Norway: A National Registry study. *Dement Geriatr Cogn Disord*. 2015.
9. Garcia-Alberca JM, Cruz B, Lara JP, Garrido V, Lara A, Gris E, Gonzalez-Herero V. The experience of caregiving: the influence of coping strategies on behavioral and psychological symptoms in patients with Alzheimer's disease. *Aging Ment Health*. 2013 Feb 22.
10. Moyle W, Edwards H, Clinton M. Living with loss: dementia and the family caregiver. *Aust J Adv Nurs*. 2002;19(3):25–31.
11. Berry B, Apesoa-Varano EC, Gomez Y. How family members manage risk around functional decline: the autonomy management process in households facing dementia. *Soc Sci Med*. 2015;130:107–14.
12. Nielssen TR, Vogel A, Phung TK, Gade A, Waldemar G. Over- and under-diagnosis of dementia in ethnic minorities: a nationwide register-based study. *Int J Gertatr Psychiatry*. 2011;26(11):1128–35.

BIBLIOGRAPHY

Covinsky KE, Newcomer R, Fox P, Wood J, Sands L, Dane K, Yaffe K. Patient and caregiver characteristics associated with depression in caregivers of patients with dementia. *J Gen Int Med*. 2003;18(12):1006–14.

Fetherstonhaugh D, McAuliffe L, Bauer M, Shanley C. Decision-making on behalf of people living with dementia: how do surrogate decision-makers decide? *J Med Ethics.* 2017;43(1):35–40.

Jox RJ, Denke E, Hamann J, Mendel R, Förstl H, Borasio GD. Surrogate decision making for patients with end-stage dementia. *Int J Getriatr Psychiatry.* 2012;27(10):1045–52.

Papastavrou E, Kalokerinou A, Papacostas S, Tsangari H. Caring for a relative with dementia: family caregiver burden. *J Adv Nurs.* 2007;58(5):446–57.

Richardson T, Lee S, Berg-Weger M, Grossberg G. Caregiver health: health of caregivers of Alzheimer's and other dementia patients. *Curr Psychiatry Rep.* 2013;15:367.

CHAPTER 23

Assessment tools for dementia and depression in older migrants

T. Rune Nielsen and Marie Nørredam

LEARNING OBJECTIVES

At the end of this chapter, the reader should be able to:

- Understand the challenges associated with cross-cultural assessment of dementia and depression
- Learn about the implications of language, culture, and educational bias on commonly used dementia and depression screening tools
- Provide examples of cross-culturally validated screening tools for dementia and depression that can be used in primary care

---

CLINICAL VIGNETTE

Ms A is a 67-year-old woman of Turkish origin who came to Denmark as a 'guest worker' in the 1970s. She has 2 years of schooling from a rural school in Turkey but in practice she is illiterate. In Denmark she has had different unskilled jobs until her retirement.

Ms A meets at GP consultation with her adult son. She only speaks and understands a little Danish and the clinical information is largely obtained from her son. He explains that his mother has had progressive memory problems for some years and that she is 'losing her Danish'. Her husband died 4–5 years ago, after which she has been very sad and periodically in antidepressive treatment. She has increasingly been supported and cared for by the children and daughter-in-law, and also been living with relatives in Turkey some months every year.

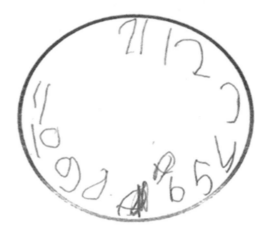

FIGURE 23.1   Clock Drawing Test performance. The patient was requested to insert the numbers in a pre-drawn circle and make the clock indicate the time 11:10.

With help from her son, Ms A explains that she forgets many things and has trouble finding her way around. Consequently, she never leaves the home on her own. Also, she has diabetes and hypertension, and complains about chronic back pain and muscle fatigue. She feels very ill and dependent on help from the family.

Based on the clinical presentation, the GP suspects dementia but also considers the possibility of depression and decides to administer the Mini-Mental State Examination (MMSE), the Clock Drawing Test (CDT), and the Geriatric Depression Scale (GDS). Ms A obtains an abnormal score of 20/30 points on the MMSE and has an abnormal CDT indicative of cognitive impairment (see Figure 23.1). Also, she scores 16/30 points on the GDS indicative of depression.

Clinicians suspecting dementia or depression in patients with migrant backgrounds may encounter challenges in communicating about this with the patients and may experience that the available screening tools are inappropriate for assessment of cognitive functioning and depressive mood, as most available screening tools do not validly portray true cognitive or emotional status when used across cultures and languages. Making efforts to bypass language barriers and using cross-culturally validated screening tools is often necessary for valid assessment of dementia and depression in patients with migrant backgrounds.

DEMENTIA AND DEPRESSION IN MIGRANT POPULATIONS IN WESTERN EUROPE

As in other European countries, in Denmark dementia is estimated to affect 7% of people older than 60 years (1), while 12% are estimated to suffer from depression (2). However, the prevalence of both dementia and depression has been found to be higher in migrant populations (3,4). Due to demographic ageing, dementia prevalence in Europe will increase significantly over the coming decades (1). This trend is even more dramatic among ethnic minority populations, where up to a sevenfold increase in dementia prevalence is expected by 2050 (www.alzheimers.org.uk). This is a significantly bigger leap than the twofold increase expected in the general population, and is related to the fact that people who migrated between the 1950s and 1970s are reaching an age where dementia is becoming a issue. Despite this, older people with migrant backgrounds remain underrepresented in dementia care in terms of diagnosis, treatment, and use of social services (5).

A number of factors may explain the underrepresentation of migrants in dementia care. In many European countries, a sizeable part of the older migrant population originates from non-European countries. As mentioned in Chapters 3 and 20, culture plays a significant role in shaping individuals' health perceptions, including how members of a given culture conceptualize a disease, recognize its symptoms, and determine help-seeking behaviour (6). Cultural understanding and stigma relating to dementia may be major reasons for the delay in diagnosis and treatment typically seen among ethnic minority groups (7,8). It is important to note, however, that in addition to knowledge and perception of dementia, numerous linguistic, economic, and other cultural factors may also hamper access to services among migrants (6). Not least, language problems may represent complex barriers for conducting clinical assessments even among migrants who have lived in the receiving country for decades (5).

Although several biomarkers for Alzheimer disease and other dementias have been developed, at the present time the use of biomarkers in the diagnostic evaluation is secondary to the clinical evaluation of cognitive impairment and loss of function. Psychiatric disorders are common differential diagnoses to dementia. Therefore, in the clinical evaluation of dementia it is important to rule out that change in cognition, mood, and behaviour are not better explained by psychiatric disorders. Depression may present with different clinical features in patients with migrant backgrounds (9), which may make it even more difficult to differentiate between psychiatric disorders and dementia. Also, somatic disorders may represent differential diagnoses, including high blood sugars due to diabetes, metabolic diseases, and drug side effects.

LANGUAGE BARRIERS TO DIAGNOSING AND TREATING DEMENTIA AND DEPRESSION

Barriers to communication between clinicians, patients, and caregivers with migrant backgrounds may lead to poor expression and recognition of symptoms of dementia and depression (10). A significant part of older non-European migrants in European countries have little or no fluency in the language of the host country (11). Although many older migrants have mastered the language of the host country earlier in life, many revert to their mother tongue as they grow older and no longer need to speak the language of the host country at work (10). Also, bilinguals with progressive dementia tend to have asymmetrical language impairment with preferential deterioration of the last acquired language (12). Therefore, ensuring efficient communication between clinicians, patients, and caregivers with migrant backgrounds is vital for the outcome of the clinical interview, and it may also have consequences for the communication of information about available treatment and services (9,10).

Improvements in communicating with older patients can be achieved through different methods. Ideally, the clinician assessing the patient has the same cultural background as the patient. This allows for ascertainment of symptoms of dementia and depression by a clinician with direct knowledge of the patient's culture (10). However, in clinical practice this is rarely possible (Chapter 20). Thus it will often be necessary to use an interpreter. The general inherent difficulties and limitations in using interpreters have been well described. There may be difficulties in eliciting the appropriate anamnesis of dementia and depression when using non-professional interpreters and professional interpreters who lack formal training. This may lead to inaccurate interpretation of the content of questions and answers. Some non-formal interpreters, especially relatives and friends of the patient, may convey their own opinions rather than facts, and they may be emotionally biased. Moreover, patients may be cautious in revealing signs and symptoms of dementia and depression because they may not feel reassured about confidentiality. Although similar difficulties can occur with professional interpreters, they are generally less common (10).

CHALLENGES IN CROSS-CULTURAL ASSESSMENT OF COGNITIVE DYSFUNCTION

Performance on cognitive tools is one of the most important pieces of data considered in the clinical evaluation of dementia. However, the vast majority of cognitive tools have not been properly validated for use with migrant populations (10), and cognitive testing of older patients with migrant backgrounds may be challenging, as cognitive tests designed for dementia standardized in one cultural group may not be appropriate for use in another. For instance, an older migrant woman from a rural area in Turkey may excel at cooking, sewing, growing vegetables, tending farm animals, caring for children, and getting along with members of her extended family. All of these reflect good cognitive abilities, yet she is likely to score in the 'impaired range' on commonly used cognitive screening instruments for dementia, such as the Mini-Mental State Examination (MMSE) and the Clock Drawing Test (CDT). The factors responsible for differences in performance between and within cultural groups on the MMSE, CDT, and other commonly used cognitive tests have repeatedly been demonstrated to be related to cultural, linguistic, and educational differences.

Impact of culture

The basic cognitive processes are universal, including the foundations for forming memories, problem solving, developing language skills, and navigating your surroundings. However, cultural differences exist in the situations to which cognitive processes are applied. Culture prescribes what should be learned, and at what age, and by which gender. Consequently, different cultural environments lead to the development of different patterns of abilities. Cognitive abilities usually measured in cognitive tests represent, at least in their content, learned abilities the scores of which correlate with the subjects' learning opportunities and contextual experiences throughout a life course. Cultural influences have been described on a variety of cognitive abilities, including perceptual abilities, spatial abilities, memory, language, abstraction, and attention (13).

The specific content and stimuli used in cognitive tests also may disadvantage older migrants. Culture-dependent elements are evident in many commonly used cognitive tests. For example, the Boston Naming Test includes naming a line drawing of a beaver, an acorn, and a pretzel. These items are familiar to most Europeans and North Americans. However, they may be unfamiliar or virtually unknown to people from different geographical areas.

Culture-specific questions about national royalty or political leaders may also disadvantage certain migrant groups (14), and differing concepts of orientation in time and place in different cultures and preferential use of the Western or traditional calendar may also influence performance on cognitive tests (13).

However, although older non-Western migrants grew up in another country, they have typically lived in the host country for a large part of their lives. Therefore, they will to various degrees have acquired knowledge of the host culture and adopted some of the knowledge, values, beliefs, and practices of this culture. *Acculturation* has proven to be a significant correlate of performance on a wide range of cognitive tests (15). Acculturation here refers to the dynamic and multidimensional process whereby the attitudes and behaviours of a person from one culture are modified as a result of contact with a different culture (16) (Chapters 3, 20).

Impact of Language

As previously described, efficient communication between clinicians and patients with migrant backgrounds is vital for the process of clinical evaluation of dementia and depression. This may be even more crucial when performing cognitive testing. However, it is not uncommon that cognitive testing of patients with migrant backgrounds takes place in the second, or even third, language, which may affect test performance (17), and test instructions are often given in a formal language, which may be very difficult to understand for patients with limited educational experience (13).

Interpreters may be used during cognitive testing. In these circumstances, problems appear when the interpreter does not accurately and completely convey statements made by the clinician and the patient. The interpreter may feel the need to assist the patient in making a response. When this happens, the true response of the patient remains unknown and the test is invalid. Likewise, the interpreter may feel the need to simplify the patient's response, making an interpretation to the clinician, resulting in the elimination of critical or missed information. Even easy and accurate translation between two languages does not necessarily result in test items of comparable difficulty. For instance, reciting the months of the year backwards is a much easier task in several East Asian languages compared to Indo-European languages, because in these languages the 12 months are simply called 'month one', 'month two', 'month three', and so on (18).

In addition, languages conceptualize the world in different ways and differ in phonology, lexicon (semantic field of the words), grammar, pragmatic, and reading systems. These differences may affect cognitive test performance (13). For instance, phonological fluency tasks requiring production of words beginning with a particular letter is not possible in non-alphabetical languages (e.g. Arabic and many Asian languages) as there are no letter-equivalent linguistic units in these languages. The choice of letter may also affect the results in phonological fluency because of differences in word frequency for each letter in different languages (13).

Impact of education

Empirical findings have repeatedly shown that higher education is associated with better performance on most kinds of cognitive tests (19). Many older non-Western migrants in Europe have a lower socioeconomic status compared to the general populations, as they came to Western European countries to perform unskilled labour work and had little or no formal education. Illiteracy is frequently higher in women due to cultural attitudes found in some countries. This is more pronounced in older women, as it is generally easier and considered more important to attend school today than it was several decades ago (13). Most cognitive tests have been developed and validated in educated populations in Western countries, and knowledge of the normal range of test performance in people with very limited or no education is often unavailable. This makes it extremely challenging to interpret test results from people without formal education, as they are likely to perform like patients with brain damage on commonly used tests (19).

The effect of education on cognitive test performance is not linear but rather represents a negatively accelerated curve tending to a plateau (20). As illustrated in Figure 23.2, performances increase rapidly between the lowest education groups of 0 years to 1–5 years of education, less rapidly between the education groups 1–5 years to 6–8 years of education, and little further beyond 9 years of education. Also, the length, quality, and content of the school day and year may vary considerably from country to country and even from school to school (19). It may not be fair to compare the educational level of someone who has completed 9 years of education in a rural Koranic school in Pakistan with someone with an equivalent period of education in London or Copenhagen. Consequently, it may be hard to make assumptions about the normal or expected level of cognitive test performance in patients with less than 9 years of education in a school system that differs greatly from the Western ones.

Education not only imparts specific knowledge and skills, but also enhances information-processing proficiency and test-taking skills in general (19). Noticeably low scores on cognitive tests in uneducated patients can be due to differences in learning opportunities of those abilities tested (i.e. calculation, reading, writing), but also due to the fact that uneducated people are not *test-wise*; that is, they are not used to being tested, and may not know how to behave in a test situation (13). A striking example is copying of line drawings (e.g. copying

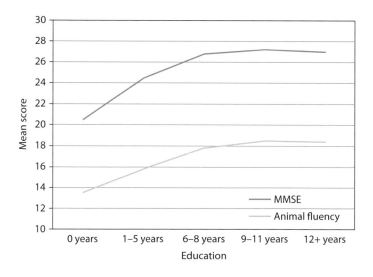

FIGURE 23.2 Mean MMSE and animal fluency scores for middle-aged and older Turkish migrants in Berlin and Copenhagen (n = 235). (Unpublished data.)

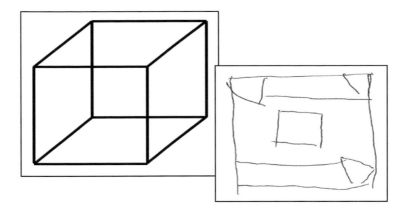

FIGURE 23.3   Example of a cognitively intact illiterate person's copy of a cube. The copy clearly illustrates that the person did not perceive the gestalt of a cube but rather a meaningless juxtaposition of two-dimensional shapes (a square, some triangles, and line segments).

a cube or overlapping pentagons) that may be extremely difficult for people without school experience. This is caused by difficulty in both manual control and in perceptual analysis (21). Individuals who are inexperienced with using a pen or pencil tend to hold the instrument in an awkward manner and have trouble drawing straight lines toward intended directions. In addition, many illiterate people are unable to interpret figures represented on a paper in three dimensions (see Figure 23.3). For individuals who have not studied geometry, these figures may appear to be a meaningless juxtaposition of line segments of two-dimensional shapes.

CHALLENGES IN CROSS-CULTURAL ASSESSMENT OF DEPRESSION

This section elaborates on depression due to it being an import differential diagnosis to dementia. Emotional expression in different cultures can be influenced by several overlapping concepts: the context of disclosure, available vocabulary and language of emotional expression, selective expressions of emotion, and definitions of self (22). For instance, the vocabulary and language required to express emotional symptoms is not equivalent and is variable between cultures (9). Also, the style of expressing existential, biological, and physical symptoms of depression varies in different cultures. People in high-income countries typically present with predominant symptoms of sadness and low mood as well as feelings of insufficiency during depression. People from low-income countries with traditional cultures are more likely to experience and express depression without the associated existential problems found in Western cultures, because the non-Western collective identity encourages the understanding and expression of depression in interpersonal or somatic domains, including symptoms of pain (Chapter 15). The result is that complaints of personal meaninglessness, worthlessness, helplessness, guilt, and suicidal thoughts are reduced or absent (9).

Because different cultures experience and express mood disorders in different ways, the diagnostic procedures designed for the general population in migration countries may not be as readily applied to patients with migrant backgrounds. Three of the most commonly used depression screening tools are the Center for Epidemiological Studies Depression Scale (CES-D), the Hamilton Depression Rating Scale (HDRS), and the Geriatric Depression Scale (GDS).

While these tools have been used as standards for depressive experience across ethnic and cultural groups, their validity remains in question. These tools are generally based on symptom criteria that are geared to patients from Western cultures. As a result, use with patients from non-Western cultures may result in faulty diagnoses because they do not sample culturally relevant symptoms and idioms of distress. Although the CES-D, HDRS, and GDS have proven to be sensitive to depression across several cultural, migrant, and patient groups, there are cultural differences in the responses to several of the questions included in the tools (23,24). For instance, patients from non-Western cultures may be less likely to have affirmative responses to questions such as 'Have you dropped many of your activities or interests', 'Do you often get bored?' or 'Do you prefer staying at home rather than going out and doing new things?' due to different cultural expectations of the activity level of older people in collectivist cultures (23). In Western individualistic cultures, successful aging is generally associated with an independent and active lifestyle, whereas aging in more collectivist cultures is generally associated with increasing family interdependence and a main aspect of life is 'staying at home'.

CHALLENGES IN CROSS-CULTURAL ASSESSMENT OF FUNCTIONAL IMPAIRMENT

Diagnostic criteria for dementia include functional impairment in social and occupational functioning, usually referred to as activities of daily living (ADL), as one of the requirements. Although people with depression may also experience challenges with handling everyday activities, this is most frequently related to changes in mood and loss of interest rather than loss of function per se.

Members of different ethnic or cultural groups may have different thresholds for cognitive impairment to impact on ADL due to different expectations of its older members (9). For example, for an older European couple who live by themselves in an urban setting, many complex skills are needed in their daily life, such as cooking, driving or using public transportation, banking, shopping, using the telephone, and operating a variety of appliances. Impairment in any of these skills may draw attention and cause concern, so they are often included in ADL assessment tools. On the other hand, for older migrants from more collectivist cultures who live with their extended family, most of the chores of managing daily life may be taken care of by the younger generations. Mild or even moderate deteriorations in cognitive abilities or social behaviour may be unnoticed (25,26) or accepted as signs of normal aging (27) and thus not be a cause of concern that is communicated at clinical consultations or properly assessed by ADL screening tools.

CROSS-CULTURALLY VALIDATED TOOLS FOR DEMENTIA AND DEPRESSION

Strategies for overcoming some of the challenges associated with conducting assessments of migrants include the use of cross-culturally validated tools. Strategies employed in the development of such tools can be broadly grouped into three general areas: (i) norm development – development of norms and cutoff values for tools in different ethnic groups, (ii) modification of existing tools – translation and adaption of existing tools for different linguistic, cultural, and educational groups, and (iii) de novo test construction – construction of new tools specifically designed for cross-cultural purposes. In the following, examples of these strategies are presented for two tools: a Turkish adaption of the GDS and the Rowland Universal Dementia Assessment Scale (RUDAS).

Rowland Universal Dementia Assessment Scale (RUDAS)	
Item	Points
Body orientation	5
Praxis (alternating hand movements)	2
Drawing (copying of a cube)	3
Judgment (in relation to crossing a busy road)	4
Memory (4-item grocery recall)	8
Language (animal fluency)	8
Total score	30

FIGURE 23.4   Items in the Rowland Universal Dementia Assessment Scale.

The original version of the GDS has been translated and adapted for several languages and cultural groups. The scale consists of 30 yes/no questions. Each question is scored as either 0 or 1 points. Generally, the cutoff used for depression is 9/10. In the Turkish adaption, two questions had to be reworded due to conceptual difficulties in the Turkish cultural context (23). Overall, the Turkish GDS has satisfactory diagnostic accuracy for depression. However, as discussed previously, several of the questions are associated with cultural bias due to collectivist aspects of Turkish culture, which probably contributes to the recommendation of a higher cutoff for depression of 13/14 in the Turkish context (28).

The RUDAS (27) was specifically designed to be a cross-cultural alternative to the MMSE for cognitive screening of multicultural populations. The RUDAS contains six items, and like the MMSE, it has 30 points and is portable and easy to administer (see Figure 23.4). Unlike the MMSE, the RUDAS does not contain any items requiring reading, writing, or calculation skills, and it is gaining credibility due to improvements in sensitivity, and decreasing susceptibility to cultural, language, and educational biases. The RUDAS has been validated in several countries, languages, and minority groups without the need to change the wording of any of the items. The most frequently cited cutoff for dementia is 22/23 (29).

WHAT THIS MEANS IN PRACTICE

Returning to the vignette of Ms A, a number of issues may have affected the outcome of the clinical consultation and the applied cognitive and depression screening tools. For instance, the son acted as an interpreter for Ms A and most information was obtained directly from him. As he is likely to explain the situation based on his own experience, knowledge, and emotions, this may have affected both how he explains his mother's situation and how he interprets during the consultation. Thus, we probably did not get access to Ms A's personal account. Also, with the son in the in the room, Ms A may have been reluctant to share personal experiences or thoughts relevant to the clinical anamnesis if she believed these would upset the son or burden the family. Finally, during assessments with screening tools we do not know whether Ms A's answers are interpreted accurately and completely by the son. Thus, there is a great risk that important information has been lost.

Several of Ms A's cognitive, emotional, somatic, and functional complaints could very well be related to a progressive dementia disorder, depression, or a somatic condition such as unregulated diabetes, metabolic disease, or drug side effects. There is also the likely possibility that two or more of these conditions are present at the same time. Thus, the results from screening tools may provide important cues to understanding the symptoms and for making the correct diagnosis. However, as discussed throughout the chapter, the results from the applied cognitive and depression screening tools are very likely to be biased by cultural, language, and educational factors. As Ms A has just 2 years of schooling and Danish versions of the MMSE and GDS were applied using the son as interpreter, it is hard to know whether the scores are valid indications of cognitive impairment and depression.

As illustrated in Figure 23.2, the mean MMSE score of someone with 1–5 years of education is approximately 24 points, and of someone without any education is just 21 points. So, even without counting the language bias it is questionable whether Ms A's score of 20 points is abnormal due to her limited schooling and illiteracy. Although applying the nonverbal CDT may remove some of the language and cultural bias, this does not eliminate the bias from Ms A's limited schooling. As discussed, drawing has proven to be a highly school-dependent skill. Many of the same biases apply to the results from the GDS. Several of the

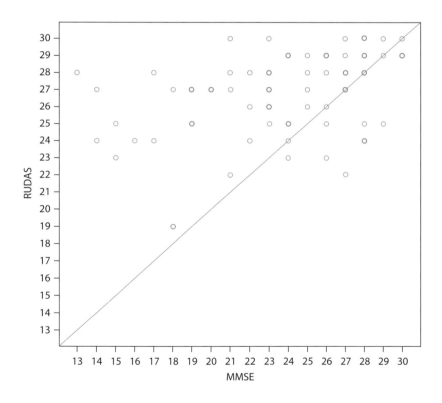

FIGURE 23.5 Scatterplot diagram of RUDAS and MMSE scores in elderly Turkish migrants. Dots above the oblique line indicate higher scores on the RUDAS compared to the MMSE, whereas dots below the oblique line indicate higher scores on the MMSE. (Reproduced from Storey JE et al. *Int Psychogeriatr* 2004 March;16(1):13–31 (30).)

more emotional terms and nuances may be hard to translate into other languages, especially when administered using a non-professional interpreter, and she may be reluctant to disclose depressive symptoms with her son in the room. Also, several of the questions are associated with cultural bias, which may require that a different cutoff for depression is used.

Applying the RUDAS and the Turkish adaption of the GDS using a professional interpreter may have given more certainty about the validity of the results. As illustrated in Figure 23.5, low-educated cognitively intact people generally obtain much higher RUDAS compared to MMSE scores. Actually, it is not uncommon that someone with a MMSE score of 20 would have a corresponding RUDAS score of 27 — a score well within the normal range. With the GDS, applying the Turkish adaption may certainly have secured a more precise and culturally relevant wording of the questions. This may have changed Ms A's score a few points in either direction, but as her original score was 16 points this would still be indicative for depression, even if using the alternative cutoff of 13/14. So, in summary, unless results from blood tests or other assessments indicate otherwise, the results from culturally validated screening tools indicate that Ms A most likely suffers from depression. Consequently, relevant treatment and monitoring of this should be initiated before considering any further dementia assessment.

SUMMARY – PRACTICAL TOOLS/RECOMMENDATIONS FOR ASSESSMENT OF DEMENTIA AND DEPRESSION IN MIGRANT PATIENTS

Conduct assessments using professional interpreters

In spite of the known limitations of working with interpreters, including the varied quality of professional interpreters' services and the fear patients and relatives often express about confidentiality not being respected, relatives without professional training in interpretation should never be the preferred method used for interpretation. Not only is there a risk of poor communication due to inaccurate interpretation of content of questions and answers, but relatives may also be emotionally biased and interpret their opinions rather than facts. Thus, when the clinician and patient do not speak the same language, assessments of dementia and depression using screening tools should be conducted with the help of professional interpreters.

Conduct assessments with validated tools

When suspecting dementia or depression, clinicians should always consider whether the adopted cognitive or depression screening tests are appropriate for assessment of patients with diverse cultural and linguistic backgrounds, particularly in the case cognitive screening of patients with limited education. If assessments are conducted with tools that have not been validated in the relevant migrant populations, clinicians need to be careful in their interpretation of the results.

Most commonly used cognitive screening tools suffer from cultural, language, and educational test bias. However, the RUDAS is proposed as a cross-culturally validated alternative to tools such as the MMSE, as the RUDAS has proven to be relatively unaffected by cultural, language, and educational test bias across several cultural and migrant groups.

Many depression screening tools also suffer from cultural and language bias as expression of emotions, and the vocabulary for emotional states differ across cultures. Further, in the case of older migrants, differences in cultural expectations of the activity level of older people may also affect responses on some of the questions typically included in the tools. Depression screening tools such as the commonly used GDS seem to validly assess depression in several cultures and migrant groups, but it may be necessary to use translated and adapted versions and apply alternative cutoffs.

REFERENCES

1. Prince M, Bryce R, Albanese E, Wimo A, Ribeiro W, Ferri CP. The global prevalence of dementia: a systematic review and metaanalysis. *Alzheimers Dement.* 2013;9(1):63–75.
2. Copeland JR, Beekman AT, Braam AW et al. Depression among older people in Europe: the EURODEP studies. *World Psychiatry.* 2004;3(1):45–9.
3. Parlevliet JL, Uysal-Bozkir O, Goudsmit M et al. Prevalence of mild cognitive impairment and dementia in older non-western immigrants in the Netherlands: a cross-sectional study. *Int J Geriatr Psychiatry.* 2016;31(9):1040–9.
4. van der Wurff FB, Beekman AT, Dijkshoorn H et al. Prevalence and risk-factors for depression in elderly Turkish and Moroccan migrants in the Netherlands. *J Affect Disord.* 2004;83(1):33–41.
5. Nielsen TR, Vogel A, Riepe MW et al. Assessment of dementia in ethnic minority patients in Europe: a European Alzheimer's Disease Consortium survey. *Int Psychogeriatr.* 2011;23(1):86–95.
6. Iworth-Anderson P, Gibson BE. The cultural influence of values, norms, meanings, and perceptions in understanding dementia in ethnic minorities. *Alzheimer Dis Assoc Disord.* 2002;16(Suppl 2):S56–S63.
7. Nielsen TR, Vogel A, Phung TK, Gade A, Waldemar G. Over- and under-diagnosis of dementia in ethnic minorities: a nationwide register-based study. *Int J Geriatr Psychiatry.* 2011;26(11):1128–35.
8. Diaz E, Kumar BN, Engedal K. Immigrant patients with dementia and memory impairment in primary health care in Norway: a national registry study. *Dement Geriatr Cogn Disord.* 2015;39(5–6):321–31.
9. Lindesay J. Diagnosis of mental illness in elderly people from ethnic minorities. *Adv Psychiatr Treat.* 1998;4(4):219–29.
10. Shah A. Can the recognition of clinical features of mental illness at clinical presentation in ethnic elders be improved? *Int J Geriatr Psychiatry.* 2007;22(4):277–82.
11. Lindesay J, Jagger C, Hibbett MJ, Peet SM, Moledina F. Knowledge, uptake and availability of health and social services among Asian Gujarati and white elderly persons. *Ethn Health.* 1997;2(1–2):59–69.
12. Mendez MF, Perryman KM, Ponton MO, Cummings JL. Bilingualism and dementia. *J Neuropsychiatr Clin Neurosci.* 1999;11(3):411–2.
13. Ardila A. Cultural values underlying psychometric cognitive testing. *Neuropsychol Rev.* 2005;15(4):185–95.
14. Bhatnagar K, Frank J. Psychiatric disorders in elderly from the Indian sub-continent living in Bradford. *Int J Geriatr Psychiatry.* 1997;12(9):907–12.
15. Baird AD, Ford M, Podell K. Ethnic differences in functional and neuropsychological test performance in older adults. *Arch Clin Neuropsychol.* 2007;22(3):309–18.
16. Berry JW. Psychology of acculturation. In: Berman J, editor. *Cross-Cultural Perspectives. Nebraska Symposium on Motivation.* Lincoln; NE: University Press; 1990: p. 201–34.
17. van de Vijver FJR, Poortinga YH. Towards an integrated analysis of bias in cross-cultural assessment. *Eur J Psychol Assess.* 1997;13(1):29–37.
18. Uzzell BP. Grasping the cross-cultural reality. In: Uzzell PB, Marcel P, Ardila A, editors. *International Handbook of Cross-Cultural Neuropsychology.* London: Lawrence Erlbaum; 2007: pp. 1–21.
19. Ardila A, Bertolucci PH, Braga LW et al. Illiteracy: the neuropsychology of cognition without reading. *Arch Clin Neuropsychol.* 2010;25(8):689–712.
20. Ostrosky-Solis F, Ardila A, Rosselli M, Lopez-Arango G, Uriel-Mendoza V. Neuropsychological test performance in illiterate subjects. *Arch Clin Neuropsychol.* 1998;13(7):645–60.
21. Nielsen TR, Jorgensen K. Visuoconstructional abilities in cognitively healthy illiterate Turkish immigrants: a quantitative and qualitative investigation. *Clin Neuropsychol.* 2013;27(4):681–92.
22. Phelan M, Parkman S. How to work with an interpreter. *BMJ.* 1995;311(7004):555–7.
23. Ertan T, Eker E. Reliability, validity, and factor structure of the geriatric depression scale in Turkish elderly: are there different factor structures for different cultures? *Int Psychogeriatr.* 2000;12(2):163–72.

24. Vindbjerg E, Makransky G, Mortensen EL, Carlsson J. Cross-cultural psychometric properties of the Hamilton depression rating scale. *Can J Psychiatry.* 2019;64(1):39–46.
25. La FJ, Ahuja J, Bradbury NM, Phillips S, Oyebode JR. Understanding dementia amongst people in minority ethnic and cultural groups. *J Adv Nurs.* 2007;60(6):605–14.
26. Purandare N, Luthra V, Swarbrick C, Burns A. Knowledge of dementia among South Asian (Indian) older people in Manchester, UK. *Int J Geriatr Psychiatry.* 2007;22(8):777–81.
27. Lawton MP, Brody EM. Assessment of older people: self-maintaining and instrumental activities of daily living. *Gerontologist.* 1969;9(3):179–86.
28. Ertan FS, Ertan T, Kiziltan G, Uygucgil H. Reliability and validity of the geriatric depression scale in depression in Parkinson's disease. *J Neurol Neurosurg Psychiatry.* 2005;76(10):1445–7.
29. Naqvi RM, Haider S, Tomlinson G, Alibhai S. Cognitive assessments in multicultural populations using the Rowland Universal Dementia Assessment Scale: a systematic review and meta-analysis. *CMAJ* 2015;187(5):E169–E175.
30. Storey JE, Rowland JT, Basic D, Conforti DA, Dickson HG. The Rowland Universal Dementia Assessment Scale (RUDAS): a multicultural cognitive assessment scale. *Int Psychogeriatr.* 2004;16(1): 13–31.

CHAPTER 24

Community participation in primary health care: Meaningful involvement of migrants

Anne MacFarlane and Christos Lionis

LEARNING OBJECTIVES

At the end of this chapter, the reader will be able to:

- Explain the relevance of community participation in primary health care and describe examples of activities
- Critically assess structures and areas of primary health care where community participation projects with migrants could be used in your local setting
- Identify tools and techniques that could be used to meaningfully involve migrants as equals in partnerships

---

INTRODUCTION

In this chapter, an overview of the concept of community participation in primary health care is provided, as well as a description of partnerships with migrants. We offer some practical and innovative examples of structures and areas of work from North America and Europe. Many of these are from family practice settings but could be adapted for care homes, for example. We provide examples of tools and techniques that have been used and reflect on common pitfalls and what guidance is available for best practice. We conclude by discussing what this means in practice and for your interactions with migrants.

CLINICAL VIGNETTE

Yvonne is a GP in a busy inner-city practice in the Netherlands, and over half of her patients are migrants. The practice has just developed a service partnership with a local NGO for refugees and other migrants and they have decided to collaborate on a community needs assessment. Yvonne has seen examples of surveys that can be used quickly for this kind of activity, which looks very appealing. However, one of the NGO community workers, Sara, is encouraging a different approach that sounds interesting but…time consuming. She is suggesting the use of participatory learning and action (PLA) methods to facilitate a dialogue between the practice members and migrants living in the area. This will involve three 3-hour 'PLA sessions'. Yvonne is feeling uncomfortable about this time commitment; GPs are used to working fast and being pragmatic and this seems time consuming. In the spirit of partnership, however, and recognizing that Sara has extensive experience working with refugees and other migrants and getting them involved in health care improvement projects, she decides to give it a go.

From the first PLA session, Yvonne was immediately struck by how different the discussion and interaction felt to other meetings. The atmosphere was welcoming, the ice breaker was fun and relaxed everyone, and the activities were interactive and engaging. Before long, Yvonne was engrossed in conversations and found that she was learning so much from listening to migrants directly about their experiences of the practice, its accessibility, their health care needs, and so on. This created a sense of humility in her. Yvonne realized that she was used to being recognized as the expert about health and health care. Increasingly, as she 'gave in' to the PLA sessions and the dialogue that was taking place, she realized that she was regarding it as an investment in the development of her practice.

After Yvonne participated in the PLA sessions, she was really confident about the needs assessment in terms of the information that it contained, and also the way in which things could be implemented in practice. She observed changes in her consultations because of her new sense of cultural humility and a stronger sense of compassion for migrants. She also observed changes in the wider practice, including at the reception desk. Everyone seemed calmer and more patient in their interactions with migrants. They thought a bit more about what coming into the practice was like from their perspective. The practice was certainly on its way to becoming a more migrant-friendly primary care service.

COMMUNITY PARTICIPATION

Community participation comes from a social justice perspective and emphasizes that the participation of communities and groups who experience poverty and social exclusion is essential to the development of primary health care services in order to shape these services and make them relevant to those with the greatest need (1). This is important if we are to address the inverse care law which has been documented in primary care (2). Thinking about the provision of prevention, treatment, and management of migrants in primary health care often brings our attention to specific health needs and conditions such as reproductive health, managing multimorbidity, or mental health. It often brings our attention to people's needs at different stages of their life course. Of course, there are also many cross-cutting opportunities and tools that encourage us to think beyond a specific condition or patient group. The notion of community-based approaches to primary health care — the process of involving people who use the services in their design, delivery, or development — is one of these.

Community participation in primary health care involves a wide variety of activities, some of which involve clinical primary care services. Community participation in primary health care could include a community needs assessment to inform service design, community representatives working with interdisciplinary teams in primary care to shape the delivery and development of services, or community garden projects to extent the options for social prescribing (3).

A defining feature of community participation in primary health care is that there is a *partnership between diverse stakeholders*. Partnerships may be between clinical and community stakeholders only, or, where there is a research and development focus, the partnership may be between clinical, community, and academic stakeholders. GPs, as community clinicians with a key gatekeeper role, have unrivalled opportunities to collaborate with other community-based services and voluntary groups (4). These community-based services and voluntary groups of users may be natural, informal, and self-help networks within the community (e.g. neighbourhood groups, self-help groups, or religious groups) or more formal ones (e.g. community development organizations or NGOs) (5–6).

From the social justice perspective underpinning community participation, it is important that different stakeholders involved in these partnerships are regarded as equals. They will of course have different backgrounds and areas of expertise, but there needs to be mutual respect. In fact, ideally, ownership for community participation projects would lie with community rather than other stakeholders and they would be involved from the initial stages of design to project governance, analysis, and dissemination (7).

The terminology in the field of migration and health is quite complex (8) and we will follow the terminology as explained in Chapter 1. We would also emphasize that we are aware that there are very diverse individuals and groups within the notion of 'migrant community'. Where appropriate, we will employ the terminology used in specific projects.

WHY COMMUNITY PARTICIPATION IN PRIMARY HEALTH CARE?

The WHO Alma Ata Declaration of 1978 (9) identifies community participation as one of the key components of Primary Health Care:

> The people have the right and duty to participate individually and collectively in the planning and implementation of their health care.

This is in the context of understanding that primary health care reflects, and evolves from, the economic conditions and sociocultural and political characteristics of the country and its communities. This also highlights that communities are a local resource that can shape the development of services and programmes that are appropriate and responsive to their needs (9). The Alma Ata was revisited in 2008 and the emphasis on community participation remained (10). There is also a global growing impetus about participation in health which is reflected in public and patient involvement activity in the United Kingdom (11) and patient engagement in the United States (12) and many other high-income countries. There are multiple terms in use in this field and lot of debate about concepts and terminology (13). Overall, however, we do know that the participation of communities enhances the delivery and uptake of health interventions to address health inequalities and inequities (14,15) and helps increase the acceptance, quality, and efficiency of health care (13).

This broad policy context and research evidence for community participation projects should be extended to migrants. Just like other people, migrants have a right and duty to participate in primary care. Just like other people, they have a right to 'have a voice'. Just like other people, they can be a *resource* for shaping the adaptation of your services so that services are migrant-sensitive and efficient. This fits with sociological perspectives on *experiential knowledge* — knowledge gained through experience, based on the idea that people become experts about health and illness because of their lived experiences of navigating health and illness experiences in their social world (16). Who knows best what it is like to be a refugee in transit across Europe and what the health implications are? There is only one answer: the men, women, and children who are living that experience each day. Furthermore, migrants have what sociologists refer to as *agency* (17), which means that they are thinking, reflective, and reflexive actors who can conform or disrupt existing routines and ways of doing things in their social world. In this way, if migrants are given the opportunity to have a voice in community participation partnerships in primary health care, they can raise our awareness about health and health care issues that we may consider to be fine or good enough (e.g. initiatives to improve health literacy to improve access to health care). They can challenge us to persist in identifying solutions to problems that we consider intractable (e.g. improving the availability and uptake of trained interpreters in all primary health care settings).

This emphasis on service adaptation is very prominent in the WHO Europe Strategy and Action Plan for Refugee and Migrant Health in the WHO European Region (18). This is explicit about the need for health care systems to cope with and respond to migrants' needs. However, the involvement of migrants in health policy, health research, and practice development to inform such health system adaptations is rare. Certainly, there are some specific challenges that may explain this. As mentioned earlier, the migrant community is a heterogeneous community. It is not necessarily a bounded community in a specific geographic or social space. It includes large numbers who are 'on the move' with changing legal status, social identities, and health care entitlements, depending on the progression of their migration journey and/or the legal and governance structures in the countries through which they pass or settle (8). The term *community for migrants* cannot only be defined in one time and space. Migrants have a connection with communities in their country of origin and their new environments at the same time (19). This means that to develop community participation with migrants, a fundamental step is to explore with and learn from migrants how they as individuals understand their identity, the connections they have with other migrants as well as their connections with members of the host community (20).

Regarding research and experimental practices, migrants can be considered 'hard to reach' on the basis of inaccessibility, language discordance, and cultural difference. O'Reilly-de Brun et al. (21), explained that in their endeavours to create academic-community partnerships for health research, they had to consider several issues. University researchers were not familiar with the languages or cultures of the intended migrant research participants and could not engage directly in fieldwork with them. Migrants, particularly undocumented migrants (22), may be reluctant to participate in research that brings them into direct contact with the 'establishment'; therefore standard recruitment strategies were unlikely to generate a participant group.

Notwithstanding these challenges, given the policy context and evidence base, we consider that there is both an ethical imperative and a sense of opportunity about migrant community participation in primary health care development and implementation. They are attending primary care centres, residents in care homes, and visiting emergency departments, so we do need to consider what adaptations are necessary. This moves our attention from *why* community participation in primary health care is important to *what* it involves and *how* to do it.

TOOLS AND METHODOLOGIES FOR INTER-STAKEHOLDER COLLABORATIONS FOR PRACTICE IMPROVEMENT

As mentioned earlier, a defining feature of community participation in primary health care is that there is a partnership between diverse stakeholders. There are different ways to structure these.

In Kansas in the United States for example, the Bethel Neighbourhood Centre (BNC) has an established service relationship with migrants in the city, specifically Bhutanese Chin and Karen refugees and Latin American migrants. The project is composed of community members, health advocates, academic researchers, and health care providers whose goal is to work collaboratively to identify and address gaps in health and health care (23).

Similarly, in Montreal, Canada, the Kahnawake Schools Diabetes Prevention Project is a community-based, participatory research project with the goal of preventing type 2 diabetes (24). This partnership is between family physicians and a Mohawk community, Kahnawake. The Kahnawake community is represented through a community advisory board of 25 volunteers from the health, educational, political, recreational, social, spiritual, economic, and private sectors and the full-time project staff.

In England, from April 2015 all general practices are contractually required to involve patients in service improvement through patient participation groups (PPGs) (25). The current contract states PPGs must be representative of the practice population. However, there are concerns that in reality, the 'usual suspects' (e.g. white, English speaking, middle class) are on patient participant groups rather than a wider representation.

In Ireland, in May 2008, a novel initiative between the Health Service Executive and the Combat Poverty Agency funded 19 demonstration projects to help support disadvantaged communities and local health service interests to work together and plan for the participation of excluded communities and groups in local primary health care services and in the implementation of national primary care strategy. Most of the steps that took place within the project are summarized in Box 24.1 with examples of structures for partnerships, such as the establishment of *community health fora*.

There are three important points to note here. First, whatever partnership structure is being used, it is important to think about the process of developing partnerships. A common pitfall in community participation projects is that partnerships are put together hastily or carelessly or, perhaps, based on a good personal connection between only a small number of people. Typically, these partnerships struggle or do not last very well because important foundation work has not been done to sustain partnerships over time and as they grow.

The Ethics Office of the Canadian Institutes of Health Research (CIHR), in conjunction with its Institute of Aboriginal Peoples' Health, has developed guidelines to assist the development of research partnerships that facilitate and encourage mutually beneficial,

> **BOX 24.1 STEPS FOR COMMUNITY PARTICIPATION IN PRIMARY HEALTH CARE – JOINT INITIATIVE PROJECT, IRELAND**
>
> • Community consultations and mapping of community and Primary Care Team resources in the project area: This was done through public meetings, workshops or focus groups.
> • Joint training for community representatives and Primary Care Team representatives: To develop skills for participatory research and community health needs assessments, or for establishing structures and terms of reference for community representation on Primary Care Team.
> • Training for Primary Care Team members: To raise awareness of community participation processes and methods and the social determinants of health.
> • Training for community representatives: To build the capacity, knowledge, and skills of local volunteers, to raise awareness of Primary Care Team services, and to identify appropriate community participation methods and structures.
> • Development of Community Health Forums: To inform the work of the Primary Care Team.
>
> *Source*: Adapted from Pillinger J. *Formative Evaluation of the Joint Community Participation in Primary Care Initiative.* Dublin: Health Service Executive and Department of Community, Rural and Gaeltacht Affairs; 2010. Available from: http://www.hse.ie/eng/services/yourhealthservice/Documentation/CommunityParticipationPrimaryCare.pdf

culturally competent research. This includes a sample agreement form which covers issues such as who the partners are, what funding is involved, what benefits will be derived from the project for each stakeholder group, what the various responsibilities are, and how the findings will be shared with all involved (26). This form could be adapted to meet the needs of a partnership between a primary health care centre and a local community group working with migrants.

Second, as you can see from the previous examples from different international settings, the area of work in a community participation project may be on identifying health needs and gaps in health care, chronic disease management, or health promotion. This means that there can be diversity in terms of the structures that may be established and the area of work that is undertaken. A common pitfall in community participation in primary health care is that this causes confusion for stakeholders and it can be hard to get everyone 'on the same page' in terms of what they are going to do. This problem can be made more complicated by the fact that the terminology and words used to talk about community participant is very varied (as mentioned earlier). Furthermore, stakeholders are coming from different backgrounds including paid and unpaid personnel involved in community groups, paid or unpaid community representatives, general practitioners, health service planners, and managers and employees working in front-line primary health care services. Stakeholders have different needs and resources in terms of time, money, skill sets for collaborative working, and so on. The upshot of this is that getting 'on the same page' is no mean feat!

Findings from a recent study that analysed factors that promoted or inhibited community participation activities in primary health care, were used to produce a theoretical Framework for Community Participation in Primary Health Care (27,28). In the spirit of community participation, the framework presents guidance on best practice through a series of reflective and interactive activities. Although not specifically designed for migrants, this approach is likely to be useful for migrant communities too. All stakeholders who are interested in coming together for a community participation project in primary health care are invited to work together through the activities to develop a shared view and common approach to progress their work. This is not always possible. If stakeholders cannot physically come together to complete the activities, they could complete them in their own time but should make time to compare their responses together regularly. The essential point is that time taken at the beginning to work through the activities in the framework will lay a solid foundation because it encourages stakeholders to think through:

- What the potential value is of what they are doing
- Whether all the right people are involved
- What resources and capacities there are to do the work
- How will they know if it has made an impact or not

The value of the framework is that it explores these four issues from all stakeholder perspectives and can bring conversations and debates to the surface about issues that have been found to undermine partnerships as they unfold.

Third, all partnerships rely on conversation and debate. A common pitfall in community participation projects is that these are tokenistic rather than meaningful. All too often communities are asked their views, but in fact, their views are not listened to or acted upon because other, usually more powerful stakeholders (the clinicians, for example) have already got a fairly strong idea about what they want to happen. This might be especially relevant with migrants due to language and cultural differences if they are not acknowledged and dealt with. This is really problematic and leads to consultation fatigue for community members. Therefore, it is important to consider how partnership is 'enacted'. This means thinking about how meetings and conversations are set up. Is there a 'safe space' for all stakeholders to come together as equals?

PARTICIPATORY METHODOLOGIES

Participatory research methodologies have their origins in the global south and are committed to knowledge-making and social change (21). While they differ in terms of tools and processes, their overarching connection is the focus on community members as local experts and emphasizing their active participants in projects. Participatory World Cafés were used to facilitate dialogue between all stakeholders involved in the BNC in Kansas (23). This is a simple yet powerful conversational process that works well with stakeholders from different backgrounds and in groups that are larger than most traditional dialogue approaches are designed to accommodate.

Participatory Learning and Action (PLA) is a useful methodology with groups where there are asymmetries of power, such as those that exist between migrants and their health care providers. PLA involves a combination of a mode of engagement and techniques (29). A PLA mode of engagement refers to the kind of environment that is created for dialogues. The aim is for a trusting environment, a 'safe space' where stakeholders are encouraged to respect a diversity of views and experiences, and to learn from each other's perspectives. PLA techniques are based on a shared stock of ideas and experiences from participatory trainers and stakeholders around the globe. They continue to be adapted to specific contexts as required. They are designed to be active, inclusive, user friendly, and democratic. They are visual and tangible, meaning that they are used to generate physical maps, charts, and diagrams. There are useful resources available with examples of how to organize workshops, icebreakers, interactive games, and strategies to facilitate learning between stakeholders and stimulate critical thinking about the issues being analysed, from all perspectives (30,31). Some recent innovative examples of using PLA to involve migrants in research, in the next section, may stimulate ideas for you to use PLA in partnerships with migrants for developing your practice.

The European Refugees–Human Movement and Advisory Network (EUR-HUMAN) project was funded by the EU in 2016 to enhance the capacity of European member states in addressing refugee health needs in the early arrival period (first reception centres) as well as in transit countries and longer-term settlements (longer-stay reception centres in countries of destination). The community participation element of this project was a health care needs assessment with migrants. This novel work, the first to explore health needs of migrants in transit in Europe, focussed on refugees and health care workers in Greece, Italy, Croatia, Slovenia, Hungary, Austria, and the Netherlands. The objective was to establish their health needs, experiences, wishes, and expectations regarding health care and social care throughout the journey through Europe (32,33). The group sessions were conducted through the PLA research methodology. Local staff members from all intervention sites were trained in PLA mode of engagement and PLA techniques. They used PLA flexible brainstorming as a fast, interactive, and visual tool to gather data with migrants (Table 24.1). The fieldwork was conducted in challenging settings – camps at 'hot spot centres', reception centres, and transit centres – with migrants who had varying degrees of literacy and who were under time pressure and, obviously, had many other urgent priorities. However, in most settings, the PLA techniques were employed and yielded data about health needs.

The implications of EUR HUMAN for clinical practice is that a series of educational materials and tools have been developed for practicing primary care professionals to improve health care for migrants (32). There have been exciting implications for community participation in primary care settings as well. In the Greek setting, the government in collaboration with the United Nations Office for Refugees decided to integrate a number of refugees in different parts of Greece, including Crete. The academic unit in Crete that operates jointly with the Municipality of Herakli on health care services is now offering primary health care for more than 70 families of refugees. The PLA techniques mentioned in Table 24.1 have been used further in collaboration between voluntary and non-voluntary community groups and primary care team members to design and offer integrated health care services to refugees.

RESTORE was an EU-funded project which focussed on optimizing the delivery of primary health care to European citizens who are migrants who experience language and cultural barriers in host countries (34). The project took place in Austria, England, Greece, Ireland, Scotland, and the Netherlands. The community participation activity was to involve migrants to work with primary care providers and other key stakeholders to select, adapt, and implement interventions to improve communication in daily practice.

Researchers were trained in PLA and used a PLA mode of engagement and PLA techniques to provide a 'safe space' for migrants to work alongside the other stakeholders. A variety of PLA techniques were used to share ideas about the adaptation process (PLA flexible brainstorming and card sorts) and to plan the steps necessary to actually implement guideline or training initiatives in their setting (PLA seasonal calendar). The adaptation process was extensive in each setting.

TABLE 24.1   Summary of PLA techniques used in EUR-HUMAN and EU-RESTORE

PLA technique	Purpose	Example from EUR-HUMAN	Example from EU-RESTORE
Flexible brainstorming	Fast and creative approach of using materials, such as pictures or objects, to generate information and ideas about the topic.	Generate information about health care needs: • Amputations • Physical disability • No examinations during pregnancy • Depression • Insomnia • Suicidal thoughts	Generate ideas to adapt guidelines and training to: • Include practice nurses • Involve receptionists • Time pressures • Change clinical focus • Develop online learning
Card sort	Interactive method for facilitating and recording brainstorming around topics so that the detail and richness of discussions is captured during the event in a visual way.	Sort the information into categories such as: Disabilities or injuries • Amputations • Physical disability Mental health problems • Depression • Insomnia • Suicidal thoughts Pregnancy-related issues • No examinations during pregnancy	Sort the ideas into overarching topics such as: Adapt target group • Include practice nurses • Involve receptionists Adapt content • Change clinical focus Adapt mode of delivery • Develop online learning
Seasonal calendar	Grid-based diagram used for cooperative planning and democratic decision making. A flexible adaptive tool, it can be used as a 'running record' of stakeholder's planning over time.	n/a	Used to plan out what actions stakeholders needed to take to make the planned adaptations

Source: van Loenen T et al. *Eur J Pub Health.* 2018;28(1):82–7; MacFarlane A et al. *Imp Sci.* 2012;7:111.

In some settings, migrants were included in the training as participants or as trainers. Migrants who were trained community interpreters got involved in delivering training to GPs about working with an interpreter in Ireland. This had an enormous impact on the GPs' knowledge and understanding of the benefits of working with trained interpreters. Therefore, these seemingly small adaptations had a significant impact on the knowledge that was shared between stakeholders during the training. Stakeholders said that the training was transformative and that their knowledge and understanding was broadened as they learned to see things from each other's perspectives.

The RESTORE consortium concluded that PLA was instrumental to the quality and nature of the collaborative work between the migrants, primary care providers, and other key stakeholders involved (35,36).

DISCUSSION: WHAT THIS MEANS IN PRACTICE

Earlier in this chapter, we met GP Yvonne and heard about her interest in improving primary care services for the migrants in her area. Yvonne made a decision to get involved in a service partnership with a local NGO and to listen to their expertise about using participatory methods to progress that partnership. Her concerns about how time-consuming the work was were significant, and certainly the pressures on modern general practice are seriously troubling. However, Yvonne's decision to 'give it a try' meant that she had a transformative experience and she developed an appreciation that it takes time to have meaningful dialogues and to truly listen and learn from migrants. She developed better knowledge about migrants' needs and more confidence about changes needed to service delivery as well as other unanticipated impacts such as enhanced cultural humility and compassion. It is interesting to reflect that these unanticipated impacts can themselves have wider 'ripple effects'. Evidence suggests compassion is crucial in alleviating pain, prompting fast recovery from acute illness, assisting in the management of chronic illness, and relieving anxiety (37).

In this way, we can see that community participation has multiple and intersecting effects on practice. It is less about tools and methodologies to apply in one-to-one encounters and it is not explicitly about the usual focus on managing and treating presenting symptoms. Community participation in primary health care is about 'stepping back', taking time from the hard graft at the coalface to develop partnerships and structures that will facilitate dialogues with migrants and other key stakeholders that can shape professional competencies, practice policies, and health care decision making. The impacts of taking time for community participation may be slower or harder to see when compared with prescribing effective medication, for example. The impacts, however, are worth it given that they lead to new learning, shifts in knowledge, attitudes, and behaviour for more responsive and migrant sensitive care. It is important to think through what this means in practical terms in your day-to-day work. We can refer back to the previously mentioned Framework for Community Participation in Primary Health Care (28) and pose the questions shown in Box 24.2 for consideration by you and your colleagues.

CONCLUSION

In summary, this chapter has focussed on the importance of community participation in primary health care. We have highlighted that taking the time to develop partnerships and structures, and taking time to participate in interactive inter-stakeholder dialogues, is an investment in the development of integrated and compassionate care for migrants. There is plenty of room for implementation and further exploitation of all the innovative tools and methodologies discussed here across different kinds of primary care settings. The questions posed in Box 24.2 are designed stimulate and support you to take steps at the practice level to move toward this way of working. We hope that you will be able to be part of a growing movement in primary care to involve migrants in the adaptation of primary care to meet their wishes, values, and expectations.

BOX 24.2   QUESTIONS FOR CONSIDERATION IN YOUR PRACTICE

What is the potential value of involving migrants in adapting your primary care services?

* Can you convene meetings/add the issue of migrants' involvement to practice meetings?
* Is there agreement among you that this would be valuable?
* Is it a new and different way of working for your practice or are there previous experiences of working in partnership with communities that you can refer to?
* Is there agreement about which structure(s) are desired for developing partnerships with migrants and relevant community organizations?

Are the right people involved?

* Can you clarify if everyone in the practice is on board (clinical, managerial, and administrative staff)?
* Have you talked to some of your individual patients who are migrants to see if they would be interested in adapting your services or if they have information about relevant voluntary and community organizations who have a commitment to health and health care improvement?
* Does your practice already have a patient participation group, and does it reflect the ethnic diversity of your area?
* Are there academic partners and service planners that you can identify to get involved?

What resources and capacities are there to do the work?

* Are there resources in your practice that can be redirected for community participation projects with migrants?
* Is there funding for research and development projects via academic collaborators or service improvement initiatives via health sector agencies?
* What resources can you access to establish a partnership?
* Is there scope for training in participatory methods in your region to develop skills for collaborative working and sharing decision making?

Will involving migrants make an impact on primary care services?

* What knowledge do you have about how migrant sensitive services are already?
* Can your partnerships brainstorm the kind of data that should be gathered to identify changes in practice over time?
* Can your partnerships examine any available data and find ways to maximize levers to change and minimize any identified barriers?

Source: Adapted from MacFarlane A, Tierney E, McEvoy R. A Framework for Implementation of Community Participation in Primary Care: A University of Limerick and Health Service Executive Collaboration. 2014. Available from: https://www.ul.ie/gems/sites/default/files/Framework%20for%20Implementation%20of%20Community%20Participation%20in%20Primary%20Healthcare.pdf

REFERENCES

1. Pillinger J. *Formative Evaluation of the Joint Community Participation in Primary Care Initiative.* Dublin: Health Service Executive and Department of Community, Rural and Gaeltacht Affairs; 2010. Available from: http://www.hse.ie/eng/services/yourhealthservice/Documentation/Community ParticipationPrimaryCare.pdf
2. Watt G. The inverse care law today. *Lancet.* 2002;360:252–4.
3. Brandling J, House W. Social prescribing in general practice: adding meaning to medicine. *BJGP.* 2009;59(563):454–6.
4. Pereira Gray D. Towards research-based learning outcomes for general practice in medical schools: Inaugural Barbara Starfield Memorial Lecture. *BJGP Open.* 2017;BJPG-2016-0507.
5. Sotiropoulos DA, Bourikos D. Economic crisis, social solidarity and the voluntary sector in Greece. *J Power Polit Govern.* 2014;2(2):33–53.
6. Piotrowicz M, Cianciara D. The role of non-governmental organizations in the social and the health system. *Przegl Epidemiol.* 2013;67(1):69–74, 151–5.
7. Jagosh J, Macaulay AC, Pluye P et al. Uncovering the benefits of participatory research: implications of a realist review for health research and practice. *Milbank Q.* 2012;90(2):311–46.
8. Hannigan A, O'Donnell P, O'Keeffe M, MacFarlane A. How do Variations in Definitions of 'Migrant' and their Application influence the Access of Migrants to Health Care services? Health Evidence Network Synthesis Report no. 46. Copenhagen; 2016 WHO Regional Office for Europe.
9. *Declaration of Alma-Ata. International Conference on Primary Health Care.* Alma-Ata; USSR: World Health Organization; 1978.
10. *The World Health Report 2008 – Primary Health Care (Now More Than Ever).* Geneva: WHO; 2008.
11. http://www.invo.org.uk
12. https://www.ahrq.gov/professionals/quality-patient-safety/patient-family-engagement/pfeprimarycare/casestudies.html
13. Sarrami-Foroushani P, Travaglia J, Debono D, Braithwaite J. Key concepts in consumer and community engagement: a scoping meta-review. *BMC HSR.* 2014;14(1):250.
14. Draper AK, Hewitt G, Rifkin S. Chasing the dragon: developing indicators for the assessment of community participation in health programmes. *Soc Sci Med.* 2010;71(6):1102–9.
15. Kenny A, Farmer J, Dickson-Swift V, Hyett N. Community participation for rural health: a review of challenges. *Health Exp.* 2015;18(6):1906–17.
16. Popay J, Williams G. Lay knowledge and the privilege of experience. In: Kelleher DGJ, Williams G, editors. *Challenging Medicine.* London: Routledge; 2006: pp. 122–45.
17. Giddens A. *Central Problems in Social Theory, Action, Structure, and Contradiction in Social Analysis.* London: Macmillan; 1979.
18. World Health Organization Europe. Strategy and Action Plan for Refugee and Migrant Health in the WHO European Region. 2016.
19. Ryan L, Sales R, Tilki M, Siara B. Social networks, social support and social capital: the experiences of recent Polish Migrants in London. *Sociology.* 2008;42(4):672–90.
20. Penninx R. Integration: the role of communities, institutions, and the State Migration Policy Institute (on line journal October 1 2003). Available from: https://www.migrationpolicy.org/article/integration-role-communities-institutions-and-state
21. O'Reilly-de Brun M, de Brun T, Okonkwo E et al. Using Participatory Learning & Action research to access and engage with 'hard to reach' migrants in primary healthcare research. *BMC Health Serv Res.* 2016;16:25.
22. van den Muijsenbergh M, Teunissen E, van Weel-Baumgarten E, van Weel C. Giving voice to the voiceless: how to involve vulnerable migrants in healthcare research. *BJGP.* 2016;66(647):284–5.
23. MacFarlane A, Galvin R, O'Sullivan M et al. Participatory methods for research prioritization in primary care: an analysis of the World Cafe approach in Ireland and the USA. *Fam Prac.* 2017;34(3):278–84.
24. Macaulay AC, Commanda LE, Freeman WL et al. Participatory research maximises community and lay involvement. *BMJ.* 1999;319(7212):774–8.

25. NHS Employers. GMS contract changes 2015/16. Available from: http://www.nhsemployers.org/gms201516

26. Canadian Institutes of Health Research. Guidelines for Health Research involving Aboriginal People, 2008. Available from: http://icwrn.uvic.ca/wpcontent/uploads/2013/10/ethics_aboriginal_guidelines_metis_e.pdf

27. May C, Finch T. Implementing, embedding, and integrating practices: an outline of normalization process theory. *Sociology*. 2009;43:535–54.

28. MacFarlane A, Tierney E, McEvoy R. A Framework for Implementation of Community Participation in Primary Care: A University of Limerick and Health Service Executive Collaboration. 2014. Available from: https://www.ul.ie/gems/sites/default/files/Framework%20for%20Implementation%20of%20Community%20Participation%20in%20Primary%20Healthcare.pdf

29. O'Reilly-de Brun M, de Brun T, O'Donnell CA et al. Material practices for meaningful engagement: an analysis of participatory learning and action research techniques for data generation and analysis in a health research partnership. *Health Exp*. 2018;21(1):159–70.

30. Chambers R. *Participatory Workshops: A Sourcebook of 21 Sets of Ideas and Activities*. New York: Routledge; 2002.

31. Pretty JN, Guijt I, Thompson J, Scoones I. Participatory Learning and Action. A Trainer's Guide. IIED Participatory Methodology Series. Available from: http://pubs.iied.org/pdfs/6021IIED.pdfc

32. Lionis C, Petelos E, Mechili E-A et al. Assessing refugee healthcare needs in Europe and implementing educational interventions in primary care: a focus on methods. *BMC Int Health Hum Rights*. 2018;18(1):11.

33. van Loenen T, van den Muijsenbergh M, Hofmeester M et al. Primary care for refugees and newly arrived migrants in Europe: a qualitative study on health needs, barriers and wishes. *Eur J Pub Health*. 2018;28(1):82–7.

34. MacFarlane A, O'Donnell C, Mair F et al. Research into implementation STrategies to support patients of different ORigins and language background in a variety of European primary care settings (RESTORE): Study protocol. *Imp Sci*. 2012;7:111.

35. Lionis C, Papadakaki M, Saridaki A et al. Engaging migrants and other stakeholders to improve communication in cross-cultural consultation in primary care: a theoretically informed participatory study. *BMJ Open*. 2016;6(7).

36. Teunissen E, Gravenhorst K, Dowrick C et al. Implementing guidelines and training initiatives to improve cross-cultural communication in primary care consultations: a qualitative participatory European study. *Int J Equity in Health*. 2017;16(1):32.

37. Shea S, Lionis C. Introducing the *Journal of Compassionate Health Care*. *J Compassionate Health Care*. 2014;1(1):7.

Index

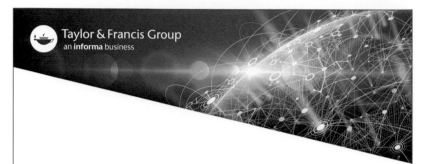